DE-PROFESSIONALISM AND AUSTERITY

Challenges for the Public Sector

Nigel Malin

First published in Great Britain in 2020 by

Policy Press
University of Bristol
1-9 Old Park Hill
Bristol
BS2 8BB
UK
t: +44 (0)117 954 5940
pp-info@bristol.ac.uk
www.policypress.co.uk

North America office:
Policy Press
c/o The University of Chicago Press
1427 East 60th Street
Chicago, IL 60637, USA
t: +1 773 702 7700
f: +1 773-702-9756
sales@press.uchicago.edu
www.press.uchicago.edu

British Library Cataloguing in Publication Data
A catalogue record for this book is available from the British Library

Library of Congress Cataloging-in-Publication Data
A catalog record for this book has been requested

ISBN 978-1-4473-5018-7 paperback
ISBN 978-1-4473-5016-3 hardback
ISBN 978-1-4473-5019-4 ePub
ISBN 978-1-4473-5017-0 ePDF

Cover design by Robin Hawes
Front cover image: iStock; Stock photo ID:1128003503
Printed and bound in Great Britain by CMP, Poole
Policy Press uses environmentally responsible print partners

For Charlotte, Heath, Arlo and Bev
– to reclaim a welfare state, enhanced
by social rights and expectations

Contents

Acknowledgements

To name those who have assisted me over the years, wittingly or unwittingly, to bring this book to fruition and the ideas which it represents would be impossible, but of those whose help, material or otherwise, has been freely and generously given I'd particularly like to thank: Jane Tunstill, Michael Lavalette, David Whiting, Teresa Smith, Gillian Morrow, Jane Lewis, Kevin Morris, Jane Tunmore, David Race, Stephen Wilmot, Bob Hudson, James Donohue, Gerald Larkin, Sheila Emmett and Ursula Sharma. As regards permission to quote from sources I am particularly in debt to *Guardian* writers Dennis Campbell, Sally Weale and Patrick Butler. In different ways such individuals have given me help, insight or inspiration. This book has involved solidifying thoughts and ideas that have been developing for some time from earlier research projects, funded through the public, voluntary sector or research councils and from my university teaching career. Before that I had been employed for example as a nursing auxiliary, as an untrained social worker and as a teacher without a formal training. I've always had a particular interest in 'care' environments – residential and community-based – and what goes on in these settings, how carers apply their expertise and the personal strengths that they bring to bear. It arose that my main research interests over 40 years have centred around the organisation, delivery and evaluation of health and social care along with unravelling changing ideas about professionalism, identity and their cultural boundaries.

I am deeply grateful to all the staff at Policy Press who have been encouraging and supportive from the outset of this project, particularly Laura Vickers-Rendall who successfully saw the book through the labyrinth of anonymous peer review – I'm grateful to her and Christie Smith for undertaking this arduous task, as well as to the three anonymous reviewers whose criticisms of the original proposal have proved useful, also to the reviewer who commented on the original draft. I am also grateful to Elizabeth Stone, Phylicia Ulibarri-Eglite and Amelia Watts-Jones for their advice, help and support throughout this process.

'Acknowledgement' may also refer to an action of showing that one has noticed events that have been set in train over the past decade prescribing a need for an analytical framework to define the concept of 'de-professionalism'. Why have I chosen to write this book and why is the topic important? The original purpose was to write something that would rediscover the notion of professionalism and document the countervailing influence of austerity politics on the 'professional project'. Impacts of this and other neo-liberal leanings concerning the role of the state, outsourcing and privatisation have contributed, it would seem, to a qualitative failure within the UK public sector, stemming partly from reduced funding, but in particular from growing evidence of the sector's inability to recruit, retain, train and reward adequate numbers of professionals to meet society's increased demands. This deficit and fragmentation have, in turn, led to a pattern of 'de-professionalisation'; therefore, an additional aim emerged for this book, to chart these developments and to create a framework for evaluating the effects of the process. The objective was to use research findings, practice experience and other insights to understand how different professionals employed by both large and small organisations learned to work effectively, given the scarce resources, conflicting tensions, risks and compromises pervading the work environment.

The topic is important for three main reasons. First, these cultural changes have prompted a rethink of some of the main theoretical and interdisciplinary perspectives, used as a basis for understanding how different professions have developed their identity. This has involved, sometimes casually, threats to professional knowledge, training and expertise. Secondly, 'de-professionalism' has become a euphemism for intensifying a trend towards public sector retrenchment, which includes outsourcing, underfunding and devolution of tasks. This has caused severe disruptions in respective workforces across the UK and contributed both to a decline in morale and become associated with abuses of power and authority. Thirdly, I believe that public sector workers have become undervalued. This has had implications for the level and quality of care, protection, teaching and other professional interventions. It also diminishes the efficacy of certain areas within public services and reduces productivity, thereby leading to greater social inequalities. Austerity as an accepted norm has become characterised by a political failure to argue against it, even among opposition parties; and this has sent out a message from the UK 'establishment' that in post-crash Britain the capitalist state remains unreformed and is unreformable.

Foreword

Andy Alaszewski

The first part of the 20th century can be called the era of the professions. As governments in high-income countries in the Global North developed different variants of the welfare state so they drew on and incorporated the expertise of the professions. For example, in the United Kingdom when the post-war government decided to set up the National Health Service, the Minister of Health, Nye Bevan, negotiated the structure of the new service with the leaders of the medical profession. The government gave the medical profession carte blanche to run the new service.

As the chapters in this book clearly show, the hegemonic role of the professions and their symbiotic relationship with governments has been undermined in the later part of the 20th century. A number of pressures have contributed to the development of a more hostile environment to professions. These pressures include rising costs, the development of neoliberal ideologies and evidence of professional failures.

The expansion of governments' spending on health, welfare and education in the 1950s and 1960s was facilitated by post-war economic growth in the Global North. This growth ended relatively abruptly in the 1970s with conflict in the Middle East that led to a major increase in the price of oil and associated disruption. In the UK there was a period of stagflation culminating in a financial crisis and run on sterling during which the Chancellor of the Exchequer had to initiate emergency measures including negotiating a standby loan with the International Monetary Fund and controls on public expenditure. Like most economic recessions, this one was time limited and was followed by economic recovery which, in turn, was terminated by the major banking crisis of 2008. As Malin observes in the first chapter, these economic crises created a major challenge to the funding of the welfare state as governments across the Global North sought ways of reducing expenditure. In the UK this search for cost-cutting was formalised by a coalition government elected in 2010 as a programme of austerity in which there was a sustained long-term reduction of public expenditure. Given health, education and social care professions receive the bulk of their income from public funding, this has meant sustained erosion of their incomes and pensions alongside increased pressure of work as demand has continued to rise and staffing levels have fallen.

As Malin argues in Chapter 2, austerity can be linked to neoliberalism, an ideological assault on the welfare state and the professions. The economic crisis of the 1970s fed into and underpinned the emergence of the New Right with a neoliberal agenda to roll back the (welfare) state. Politicians such as Ronald Reagan in the USA and Margaret Thatcher in the UK, sought to slim down the state, by shifting the responsibility for individual health and welfare from the state to the individual. These politicians drew on the work of critics of the welfare state such as the Hungarian economist Friedrich Hayek. In his critique of the Beveridge Report, *Road to Serfdom* (London, Routledge, 1944) Hayek argued that centralised state planning and provision of welfare services would create a culture of dependency in which individuals lost their autonomy and became reliant on the state and its agents, the professions, for the basic necessities of life. Thus, for the New Right, the professions, rather than being agents of progress and human emancipation, act to protect expensive welfare systems that undermine individual autonomy and independence. A key part of the New Right agenda is the reduction of state spending and increased efficiency in the use of resources by reforming the professions that receive and allocate these funds. Paradoxically, in the UK austerity was promoted by Prime Minister David Cameron, who purported to be a One Nation conservative committed to protecting the most vulnerable and marginalised in society. One way he attempted to square the circle was through building a 'Big Society' in which, as the state reduced its expenditure on health and welfare, so voluntary associations or charities would plug the gaps. To some extent this has happened: the roll-out of universal benefits with slower and reduced level of social security benefits has stimulated the growth of food banks run by volunteers to provide short-term relief for those affected.

Alongside the neoliberal ideological critique of the professions, there was more direct evidence of the limitations of the professions. In the UK this took the form of scandals and disasters and associated public inquiries (see Andy Alaszewski and Patrick Brown, *Making Health Policy*, Cambridge, Polity, 2012, pp 114–39). These started in long-stay hospital facilities in the late 1960s, with evidence of harmful practices that professional oversight failed to identify and prevent. In the 1980s and 1990s the failures were evident in the more prestigious sectors of the health care system. In primary care, a general practitioner, Harold Shipman, was killing his elderly patients; in a small general hospital, a nurse, Beverley Allitt, was injecting young children with insulin so that she could revive them; at Alder Hey children's hospital a pathologist was harvesting and storing children's organs without their parents' permission; while at Bristol Royal Infirmary there was a professional club culture in which unacceptably high death rates for young children were concealed and justified.

In Chapter 6, Malin analyses the ways in which governments have responded to these pressures by creating systems to monitor and manage the activities of professions, thereby removing many of their privileges. Governments have used markets forces to undermine the natural monopoly that professions have had over the delivery of services. In the UK the development of an internal market in which hospital funds were dependent on the number of patients treated formed a central element of the 1989 reorganisation of the NHS and has remained a key element of subsequent reforms. In some professional domains marketisation has resulted in total deprofessionalisation. For example, in England the supervision of long-term and recently discharged offenders was undertaken by the probation service, which was staffed by professionally qualified probation officers. In the post-2010 austerity programme, services for low-risk offenders were privatised and provided by staff with no professional qualifications. This was not a great success as the payment by results basis of the new service did not result in the desired reduction of reoffending rates.

Governments have sought to restrict the autonomy of professionals through the imposition of frameworks that structure professionals' work. Thus, in education in England, the government has specified a national curriculum which for teachers in primary or elementary schools specifies both what is taught and how it is taught. The effectiveness of such teaching is then assessed through national examinations, with pupils in English primary school sitting SATS exams when they are 6–7 and again when they are 10–11 years old.

In Chapter 8 Malin outlines the ways in which governments have created additional safeguards to protect the public from professional incompetence, setting up systems of independent inquiry. Thus, in the UK virtually all publicly funded professionally staffed services have independent inspectorates. In England the health and adult social care are inspected by the Care Quality Commission, an independent regulator, and education and children's social care by OFSTED (the Office for Standards in Education, Children's Services and Skills). These inspectorates regularly visit and inspect all services and rate the quality of professional practice. A poor inspection report can have major consequences for an individual professional's career and standing. In addition, these inspectorates have the power to respond to public concerns and other evidence of poor practice by undertaking special investigations.

Since the peak of professional power and autonomy in the 1960s, there has been a steady erosion of professional standing. The reduction of funding and increase in demand have reduced the income and pensions of many professionals while increasing their workload. At the same time, professional autonomy has been substantially curtailed by marketisation, the development and use of guidelines to structure professional practice and external inquiries. It is perhaps not surprising that in many areas of the public service it is proving difficult to train and retain adequate numbers of professional staff.

Note on the author

Nigel Malin holds degrees from the Universities of Manchester, Oxford, Sheffield and the West of Scotland. Previously he has held full-time teaching and research posts at the Universities of Sunderland, Derby, Sheffield and Sheffield Hallam University, including two Professorships and one Readership. He is author/co-author of ten books, including *Professionalism, Boundaries and Workplace* (Routledge, 2000), *Key Concepts and Debates in Health and Social Policy* (Open University Press, 2002), *Evaluating Sure Start* (Whiting and Birch, 2012) and *Community Care For Nurses and the Caring Professions* (Open University Press, 1999). Since 2014 he has been Editor of *Social Work & Social Sciences Review: An International Journal of Applied Research* and since 2015 Associate Editor for the *British Journal of Learning Disabilities*. He currently lives in Sheffield and is undertaking research on the topic of professionalism and identity.

PART I

Policy background and concepts

Austerity as a UK policy context in the early twenty-first century

The election in the United Kingdom (UK) of the Conservative-led Coalition government (2010) followed by subsequent elections in 2015 and 2017 have led to a period that has become characterised as an 'age of austerity', where public spending has been substantially reduced in pursuit of deficit reduction, alongside an ideological commitment to reducing the size of the state. As a defining era of welfare state development, 2010 marked the end of 13 years of New Labour governments. Coming into government in the wake of the economic crash of the mid-2000s and in the middle of a recession, the government introduced stringent austerity measures, including some of the largest cuts in public finance ever seen and some of the most extensive welfare reforms since the introduction of the welfare state (see Taylor-Gooby and Stoker, 2011; Beatty and Fothergill, 2013; Lambie-Mumford, 2015).

The UK government austerity programme has been defined as a fiscal policy and a deficit reduction programme that consists of sustained reductions in public spending and tax rises, intended to reduce the government budget deficit and the role of the welfare state in the UK. It has been presented as both a political and economic project whose effects appear still controversial, and as an inevitable consequence of the 2007–8 financial crisis. During austerity some aspects of the National Health Service (NHS) and education sectors in the UK have been 'ring-fenced' and protected from direct spending cuts – despite expressions of serious problems such as workforce shortages, including recruitment, retention and remuneration of staff. Nevertheless, UK austerity policies have received criticism from the media, and political and academic sources in particular, and have prompted anti-austerity movements among citizens more generally.

At the end of the first full parliament under the austerity programme, the Labour Party and the Conservatives were deadlocked in the polls. At the 2015 general election the Conservative party modified their commitment to austerity with a series of unfunded spending promises, including £8 billion of additional expenditure for the NHS. At the same time, the 2015 Conservative Party general election manifesto proposed making sufficient reductions in public spending and welfare to eliminate the budget deficit entirely by 2018–19 and run a small budget surplus by 2020. The Labour Party's manifesto proposed the less rigorous objective of reducing the budget deficit every year, with the aim of seeing debt as a share of gross domestic product (GDP) falling by 2020 and achieving a budget surplus 'as soon as possible'. This would render the spending reductions proposed by the Conservatives unnecessary, according to some analyses. The Conservative Party won the 2015 general election with an overall majority for the first time in 23 years, which was unexpected as most polls had predicted another hung parliament. An argument made was that one of the reasons for Labour's loss was its lack of clarity on the causes of the budget deficit. Anti-austerity protests followed the election result, but post-election polling for an independent review, conducted by Campaign Company for Labour MP John Cruddas indicated that voters in England and Wales did not support an anti-austerity platform, concluding: 'The Tories did not win despite austerity, but because of it' (Wintour, 2015).

The 2017 general election was held almost three years earlier than scheduled under the Fixed-Term Parliament Act 2011 in an attempt to increase the government's majority to facilitate the Brexit vote process. In this election, the Conservative Party lost their parliamentary majority, but remained in government as the largest single party. Brexit and austerity were blamed for the loss of seats, according to one minister (Gavin Barwell, then Chief Whip). From 2017 the Labour opposition announced a plan to challenge further austerity measures and vote against them in the House of Commons. A Labour spokesperson said: 'We will be using the changed parliamentary arithmetic to drive home the fact that the Tory programme for five more years of austerity (until 2022) will not go on as before' (Stewart, 2017: 14).

It would seem clear, however, that the Conservative government will continue to freeze household benefits until at least 2020, while welfare cap restrictions on certain types of support will remain until at least 2023. Without factoring in the impact of the extra £20 billion increase promised by the Government to the NHS, the Office for Budget Responsibility (OBR), in forecasting government spending as a percentage of GDP, has asserted that state expenditure was expected to fall in every year until 2023. However, a promise was made by the prime minister, Theresa May, in her October 2018 conference speech, to end austerity sooner than originally planned. This might not be fulfilled given the overall economic policy context set by the Chancellor, Philip Hammond, whose aim has been to work within a 2 per cent deficit to GDP target, along with the expectation that an imminent Brexit would make him reluctant to spend earlier than promised. The Conservative government also pledged a budget surplus by the mid-2020s, which will act as a further pressure against raising public spending. The OBR forecasted that, even if spending was allowed to rise to take account of the extra health costs of an ageing population, the deficit would remain roughly flat over the four years to 2025–6, making it likely that some form of austerity will continue as long as the Conservatives remain in power (OBR, 2018; Partington, 2018).

Were austerity policies an inevitable response to the financial crisis? Michael Burton (2016) provides an historical context to austerity, analysing how different governments in various countries have sought to manage public finances during recent recessions. The fiscal crash of 2007–8 turned into the Great Recession and tax revenues tumbled, with public finances across the UK, the United States (USA) and Europe plunging into deficit. Controversial attempts by governments to balance their budgets have focused on the relationship between public spending and public deficit, seemingly with mixed success politically and economically (see, for example, Kushner and Kushner, 2013; Ferguson et al, 2018; Gedalof, 2018).

The fiscal crash started in the USA's 'sub-prime' housing sector. Owing to a lack of investment in, and lack of provision of, social housing, poor families were in effect forced to buy homes they could not afford. Financial institutions provided mortgages and loans to poor families based on the assumption that house prices would inevitably rise, and so if families defaulted on their loans their homes would be repossessed and sold on by banks for a profit. Banks and lending companies found themselves with increasing amounts of bad debt, which they in turn bundled up and sold on through the financial system to hedge funds and various financial interests. The bad debt spread throughout the system until, in 2007, the system fell like a pack of cards. Banks were deemed 'too big to fail', so vast state resources were ploughed in to save them, creating vast pools of state debt (Lavalette, 2017).

The all-encompassing impacts of austerity and state retrenchment have been felt within areas of community participation throughout the UK, particularly as the agency of communities, incorporating a combined approach of risk and 'responsibilisation' (Liebenberg et al, 2015), has become an essential element of central government strategy for local communities. Evidence from several studies (examples being Batty et al, 2010; Hastings and Matthews, 2014; Hastings et al, 2015; Rolfe, 2018) suggests that the agency of communities and the local state may be outweighed by the impacts of austerity. Thus communities, particularly where they have limited capacity in terms of skills, experience and confidence, may struggle to benefit from the opportunities presented by national community participation policy, either because they lack the support to develop organisational capacity or because they are forced into a defensive mode as essential services are cut. The studies noted suggest that austerity and the consequent cuts to local government budgets may be undermining the possibility of tackling inequalities between communities at a local level.

In a 2015 *Guardian* article about benefits, sanctions and food banks, Ken Loach calls for 'public rage' and speaks about 'conscious cruelty'. The word 'austerity' has allowed the UK Conservative government to disguise both intent and outcome. In its original meaning austerity suggests plainness and simplicity, a cosy view of cutting back, perhaps a mythical wartime pulling together (Kynaston, 2008). By comparing the notion of pre- and post-welfare state austerity, it appears evident that the historical period alluded to by Kynaston was defined by rationing, controls and hardship, for instance as regards housing, food, clothing, fuel, bread, beer and tobacco, the black market and the 'brewing up of moral panic' (Kynaston, 2008: 113), whereas the latter has become more defined through a lens of cuts to public services.

> The Government will have to face up to the job of convincing the country that controls and hardships are as necessarily a part of a bankrupt peace as they were of a desperate war. Every inch of useable English soil will still have to be made to grow food. People are suddenly realising that in the enormous economic blitz that has just begun, their problems may be as serious as the blitz they so recently scraped through. (Kynaston, 2008: 103)

'Austerity' has become a weasel word used to promote a government-led rhetoric that there is no alternative, that anaesthetises public anger as we are led to believe that there is no choice (Clough, 2018). Peter Rushton (2018) analyses the various impacts of austerity in order to integrate different forms of inequality that combine in people's lives, for example income/wealth, age and generation, health inequalities, housing, work and insecurity, and the changing role of professionals. He claims that the Blair government reacted well to the dire situation of 2007–8, devising policies aimed at recapitalisation of the banks accompanied by partial nationalisation, a speedy change in monetary policy, involving slashing interest rates, and the injection of funds into the system by quantitative easing, all contributing to staving off the consequences of the 'credit crunch' that shut off finance to the economy. A conclusion, however, is that:

> orthodox economics and neo-liberal ideology cut in, as public debts became an obsession: such debt was redefined as a problem of government spending rather than revenue collapse, and cutting the public sector and all welfare spending came to dominate, making 2010 onwards strongly resemble a return to the policies of the early 1930s. (Rushton, 2018: 24)

Austerity was a choice made by the British government. As Mark Blyth (2013) points out, austerity was not imposed by an outside body, as was the case with the International Monetary Fund in Greece after 2008 or during the notoriously flawed and counterproductive 'structural adjustments' foisted on a number of Latin American countries in the 1980s and 1990s. It was a domestic political decision to 'shrink the state'. When the Coalition government took control, both political parties, Conservative and Liberal Democrat, took pains to convince the British public of the fallacy that, rather than neo-liberal ideology masquerading as 'fixing' the economy, the wholesale dismantling of the welfare state they had in store was essential if the UK was to tackle its budget deficit. The global economic crisis and banking catastrophe of 2008 was unprecedented and therefore warranted an exceptional response, the austerians declared. The argument was that austerity was right, necessary and unavoidable, and that the population ought to be 'all in this together'. However, as Blyth and others may have argued, rampant public spending was not the primary culprit in the UK's difficulties; rather it was the billions of taxpayers' cash pumped into bailing out a failed global banking system:

> We need to remember that the crisis that brought us here was a private sector crisis. Their debts landed on the balance sheet of the public sector through bank bailouts, recapitalisations and unlimited quantitative easing. In other words, taxpayers bailed bankers and the price was a ballooning deficit. That growth and competitiveness would be restored by reducing public spending quickly and drastically has been proven wrong so many times throughout history it's a wonder anyone continues to take it seriously. (Blyth, 2013: 43)

The political economist Robert Skidelsky framed this financial crisis as a puzzle to be solved, posing the question 'Should the British government have opted for austerity after the collapse of 2008 or should it have gone for economic stimulus?' (Skidelsky and Fraccaroli, 2017). The answer suggests that since austerity was the consensus policy in the European Union, the question has a more general relevance:

> [The claim is that] … the idea of austerity gained success mainly because of its political message – austerity's political-economic prescription, in fact, matches the ideology of laissez-faire (or neo-liberalism), a common ground for European and British centre-right parties that dominated the political scene before and during the recession, with the exception of New Labour. The idea that economic growth should come from the private sector and that government's fiscal policy should not interfere with the functioning of the market offered strong political support for policy-makers who wanted to reduce the size and influence of the state. (Skidelsky and Fraccaroli, 2017: 11–56)

Skidelsky asserts that the advocates of stimulus policies may loosely be called Keynesian, reasoning that during a boom, when the economy is at full employment, additional public expenditure would 'crowd out' real resources. This is the view that government spending, whether financed by taxes or borrowing, diverts resources from productive use by the private sector, referencing ideas that go back to classical economists Adam Smith and David Ricardo. A counter position, however, would be that during a slump when the resources of an economy are under-employed, a deficit created through fiscal stimulus is not deferred taxation but a boost to economic activity. As such it creates its own means of repayment by increasing the aggregate income from which the government's revenue is drawn and reducing the government's spending on unemployment; hence no question of 'crowding out' of real resources arises. Skidelsky writes:

> While Keynesianism's original purpose was to 'save' the capitalist system (unable to adjust on its own), its prescriptions have found a favourable response in left-wing parties, e.g. Syriza in Greece, Podemos in Spain, Labour under Corbyn in UK, whose aim is to preserve the state's presence in the economy, and in particular to protect the

social security system, the main target of austerity cuts.
(Skidelsky and Fraccaroli, 2017: 52–4)

Now austerity policies rather than stimulating growth are leading to a dismantling of social systems that operated as a buffer against economic hardship, exposing austerity to be a form of systematic violence, according to Vickie Cooper and David Whyte (2017). Their edited collection provides trenchant examples such as police attacks on the homeless, violent evictions in the rented sector and risks faced by people on workfare schemes who are being driven by reductions in public sector funding. The book references other empirical studies, for example Seabrook (2013), O'Hara (2014) and Mendoza (2015), to demonstrate the human impact of austerity in the UK, resulting in 'a shocking expose of the myriad ways in which austerity policies have to date harmed people in Britain'. Mary O'Hara (2014) specifically documents how whole swathes of the population – the poorest, people with disabilities, women, carers, older people, poorer people from black and minority ethnic backgrounds, children and young people – have been made more financially insecure and increasingly vulnerable as a result of austerity policies. She illustrates how:

> For many, their very dignity has been stripped away as essential state-supported services and benefits have been slashed ... (and that) churches and some mainstream charities were doing much of the anti-austerity heavy lifting through work within communities and charities by campaigning, lobbying, fronting legal challenges and evidence gathering on the spiralling crisis. The main austerity battle was being fought on a small-scale or hyper-local level away from mainstream media. (O'Hara, 2014: 253)

A main feature of Cooper and Whyte (2017) is a challenge to three key 'deceptions' promoted by the British government defending austerity policy: 'We all played a part in the crisis' – a combination of reckless government spending and debt-fuelled personal consumption; 'Austerity is necessary'; and 'We're all in this together'. Various evidence is presented to show that the people most affected by austerity cuts have not only been struggling under the financial strain but are becoming ill, physically and emotionally, and many are dying. An aim of the book is to show how the toll of sickness and death created by the politics of austerity has left none but the most privileged in the UK untouched. Moreover, it is alleged, this scale of death and illness is simply part of the price that has been paid to maintain the basic structure of social inequality.

A conclusion is that the upshot of externalities (the unmeasured impact of financial transactions on bystanders who have nothing to do with the transaction) has been that attacks on the publicly funded services, and social and welfare rights, which are supposed to protect people in almost all spheres of life, have produced 'profoundly violent outcomes'. The research findings focus on:

> the violent capacities of those public and private institutions that have brought turmoil to the lives of those most affected by austerity: JobCentres, The Benefits Agency, Local Authorities, housing authorities, the criminal justice system, third sector programmes, employers in the public and private sectors and debt recovery companies … on the assemblage of bureaucracies and institutions through which austerity policies are made real. These are sites through which highly political strategies, like austerity, are de-politicised and their harmful effect made to appear normal and mundane. (Cooper and Whyte, 2017: 22)

Others writing in the same vein, such as Dorling (2014), Seymour (2014) have addressed a puzzling aspect of the current conjecture: why are the rich still getting away with it? They show how 'austerity' is just one part of a wider elite plan to radically re-engineer society and everyday life in the interests of profit, consumerism and speculative finance. Richard Seymour (2014) focuses on social class, the state and ideology, posing a question about why political and social protest in response is so ephemeral, and why 'the left' appears to be marginal to political life. His polemic focuses on the fact that the 2008 financial crisis led to further benefits to the urban, cosmopolitan class, whereas the excesses of the banks, the risks taken that crystallised following the crisis, have since bred a sense that 'costs' have been concentrated on a group of losers, for example poorer people and those working in and dependent on public services. A conclusion drawn is that it is time to forge new collective resistance and alternatives to the current (capitalist) system.

The United Nations' expert on extreme poverty and human rights, Philip Alston, has spelt out his view that austerity was a political choice, and following a months-long investigation of poverty in Britain branded the UK's benefits sanctions regime as 'cruel and inhuman' (Booth, 2018b). His report highlights the disproportionate impact of austerity on children, disabled people and women, indicates how disabled people are faring under the new universal credit benefits system, and describes the poor as '"easy victims, as they suffer highly disproportionately in terms of their civil and political rights"… the government had inflicted great misery on the British people with punitive, mean-spirited, and often callous austerity policies driven by a political desire to undertake social re-engineering rather than economic necessity' (Chakelian, 2019).

The Secretary of State for Work and Pensions, Amber Rudd, in response dismissed the UN report as 'overtly political and highly inappropriate' (BBC News, 2019). This was in spite of the availability of statistics supplied by the Department for Work and Pensions, which state that 14 million people in the UK are currently living in poverty and local authorities have seen a 49 per cent real-terms reduction in funding from 2011 to 2018 (Booth, 2018a).

Seemingly, there has been no resetting of how economics should work in the future, either by 'experts' or by those working in government. The initial response to the financial crisis had not been austerity, but a bailing out of the banks by the Labour government. Writing with the benefit of hindsight ten years later, the ex-prime minister Gordon Brown has stated that there should have been much heavier costs to bankers and others employed within the financial system and that their actions were rebarbative – 'they should not have been allowed to get away with it and that many more should have been jailed' (Sabbagh, 2018: 22). When governments bailed out their bankers in 2008–9, was it the equivalent of bringing them before a court? And if it was? Danny Dorling (2014) similarly suggests that the growth of the wealthy is making the UK a more dangerous place to live; and that since the great recession of 2008, 1 per cent of the population has grown richer while the rest find life increasingly tough: 'While the rich have found new ways of protecting their wealth, everyone else has sugared the penalties of austerity … Inequality is the greatest threat [society] faces, is more than just economics, it is the culture that divides and makes social mobility impossible' (Dorling, 2014).

Although austerity appears to be failing as an economic idea, the cuts in public funding reduction continue. The banking crisis of 2008 led to a public rescue of private banks, and subsequent austerity measures have been presented as a necessary response to the state of the public finances in a time of national emergency. The aim is to shrink the state and reduce social welfare provision, not just in response to the current crisis but permanently. The Institute for Fiscal Studies (IFS, 2012) has calculated that there would be over 900,000 public sector jobs lost in the period 2011–18. Austerity appears not to be a technocratic exercise in economic management but instead an ideological attack on the foundations of the social contract that formed the basis of the post-war society.

Summary

The UK austerity programme has been defined as a fiscal policy and a deficit reduction programme consisting of sustained reductions in public spending and tax rises. Were austerity policies an inevitable response to the financial crisis? Debt was redefined as a problem of government spending rather than reserve collapse (Rushton, 2018); hence the dismantling of the welfare state became essential to tackle budget deficit (Blyth, 2013). Should the British government have opted for austerity after the financial collapse of 2008 or should it have gone for economic stimulus (Skidelsky and Fraccaroli, 2017)? Austerity policies, rather than stimulating growth, are leading to a dismantling of social systems that operated as a buffer against economic hardship, exposing austerity as a form of systematic violence (Cooper and Whyte, 2017). These authors challenge three 'deceptions': 'We all played a part in the crisis', 'Austerity is necessary' and 'We're all in this together'. Whole swathes of the population, the poorest, people with disabilities, women, carers, older people, children and young people, have been made more financially insecure and increasingly vulnerable as a result of austerity policies (O'Hara, 2014). These groups are singled out as most prominent and are where key professions tend to focus their concern, being where professional support is most highly valued. The question is asked why political and social protest in response is so ephemeral; and the implications of austerity for social class, the state and ideology are considered (Seymour). One per cent of the population has grown richer while the rest find life increasingly tough. Inequality is the greatest threat society faces; it is more than just economics, it is the culture that divides and makes social mobility impossible (Dorling, 2014). The Institute for Fiscal Studies (IFS, 2012) has calculated that there would be over 900,000 public sector jobs lost in the period 2011–18. Austerity appears not to be a technocratic exercise in economic management but instead an ideological attack on the foundations of the social contract that formed the basis of the post-war society.

2

Neo-liberalism as an ideology, an elite project and its impact on austerity

The 2008 financial crisis and the introduction of austerity policies produced a sense that the prevailing economic and policy programme in the United Kingdom (UK), termed neo-liberalism, had suddenly gone off the rails and a new paradigm would have to be grasped. We should begin by defining neo-liberalism. The term gained popularity largely among left-leaning academics in the 1970s 'to describe and decry a late twentieth century effort by policy-makers, think-tank experts, and industrialists to condemn social democratic reforms and unapologetically implement free-market policies' (Shermer, 2014). Neo-liberalism argues that a free-market will allow efficiency, economic growth, income distribution and technological progress to occur. Any state intervention to encourage these phenomena will worsen economic performance. According to some scholars, neo-liberalism is commonly used as a catchphrase and a pejorative term, outpacing similar terms such as monetarism, neo-conservatism and market reform in scholarly writing (Boas and Gans-Morse, 2009).

The 'Washington Consensus', a term associated with the advent of neo-liberalism as an economic paradigm, refers to a set of broadly free market economic ideas supported by prominent economists and international organisations, such as the International Monetary Fund (IMF), the World Bank, the European Union (EU) and the United States (USA). Essentially it advocates free trade, floating exchange rates, free markets and macro-economic stability. The ten principles originally stated by John Williamson in 1989 include policy recommendations covering low government borrowing, thereby avoiding large fiscal deficits relative to gross domestic product (GDP); redirection of public spending from subsidies towards broad-based provision of key pro-growth, pro-essential services such as primary education, primary health care and infrastructure investment; privatisation of state enterprises; deregulation/abolition of regulations that impede market entry or restrict competition; tax reform, including broadening the tax base and adopting moderate marginal tax rates; interest rates that are market-determined and positive (but moderate) in real terms; competitive exchange rates; and a legal security for property rights (Skidelsky and Fraccaroli, 2017).

Springer et al (2016) posit that the term neo-liberalism has become a means of identifying a seemingly ubiquitous set of market-oriented policies as being largely responsible for a wide range of social, political, ecological and economic problems. To view the term as merely a pejorative or radical political slogan, the authors argue, is 'to reduce its capacity as an analytic frame. If neo-liberalism is to serve as a way of understanding the transformation of society over the last few decades then the concept is in need of unpacking' (Springer et al, 2016: 19). Currently neo-liberalism is most commonly used to refer to market-oriented reform policies, such as eliminating price controls, deregulating capital markets, lowering trade barriers and reducing state influence on the economy, especially through privatisation and austerity.

A purpose of this chapter is to consider the relevance of neo-liberalism as an ideology in the framing of austerity policies, particularly as these ideas may have an existential bearing on the present and future direction of public services, including the professional workforce. As a developmental model, neo-liberalism refers to the rejection of structuralist economics; as an ideology, it denotes a conception of freedom as an overarching social value associated with reducing state functions to those of a minimal state (Peters, 1982). In critiquing neo-liberalism in this context, it may be said that greater stress should be placed on factors affecting the quality of life, such as the impact on the environment, social cohesion and personal satisfaction. Neo-liberalism, like many economic philosophies, has tended to place too much stress on measurable variables such as real GDP per capita and ignore the wider and more intangible factors affecting the quality of life.

Evidence suggests that a broadly neo-liberal economic and social policy has seen a widening of inequality of both wealth and income in the Western world (Hay and Beaverstock, 2016). This is down to several factors, such as skilled workers being in a position to command higher wages, but low-skilled workers in flexible labour markets are more likely to see stagnant wages. Firms with monopoly power can increase producer surplus at the expense of consumers. Firms with monopsony power tend to limit wage growth, for example the public sector in employment of civil servants, nurses, police and so on. A monopsony occurs when a firm has market power in employing factors of production, for example labour, and where there is one buyer, such as the National Health Service, and many sellers. An employer with market power in hiring workers has similar market power in setting wages and choosing how many workers to employ.

Social policies in the UK have been devastated under the pretext of rescuing confidence in the financial system. William Davies writes:

> By 2016 there was little sign of economic growth and political events in the form of Brexit and Donald Trump, witnessed popular movements diametrically opposed to the economic common sense that has held sway in the UK and US since the 1970s. These movements are strictly anti-neo-liberal, not in the sense that they rest on a coherent critique of monetarism, or a specific ambition to regulate markets differently. But inasmuch as neo-liberalism embeds particular forms of economic rationality (overseen by economic experts) as the governing principles of nearly all public policy, the very fact that this rationality (and those experts) are being defied or ignored is evidence that something has come unstuck. (Davies, 2017: 13)

Most certainly a main characteristic of neo-liberalisation is a breaking off from 'embedded liberalism' and its adherence to the post-Second World War socio-economic settlement that aimed to achieve full employment and maintain the welfare state, namely the 'neo-Durkheimian' perspective (see Chapter 4). As has been claimed (for example by Wilmot, 2003: 94; Moran, 2004: 31), this 'model' welfare state was a professional state: it depended on professionals both for the expertise needed to formulate policy and to deliver that policy; thereby underscoring the interdependence of professions, the state and the public. Whilst a systematic trend towards liberal paternalism in welfare reforms has been observable in the long term, a sharper shift has occurred since 2010 (Wright, 2016). In light of these developments, the UK welfare system can be understood as entering a 'new phase' of 'fundamental restructuring' (Hastings et al, 2015: 32). The emergence of 'welfare austerity' can be seen as instigating 'a new, more constrained and qualitatively different deal for citizens than that envisaged by the architects of the post-war welfare state' (Dwyer and Wright, 2014: 33).

Another characteristic of neo-liberalisation is a 'remaking of the state', where the state is not 'rolled back' as such but is reshaped and reconfigured to better serve the demands of capital through the installation of 'workfare' regimes, where the unemployed (rebranded as 'job seekers') are corralled into low-waged employment (Garrett, 2018: 8). An example of how the neo-liberal paradigm has come to dominate current economic and political life can be found in the overseas aid sector, where the delivery of aid, both humanitarian and development, has increasingly been privatised (Provost, 2016). There has been a shifting away from delivery by governments to delivery by non-governmental organisations as implementing partners. An implication of this is that, in order to be effective, professionals working within the public sector need to develop a critical approach to their practice and perhaps delve deeper into how power relations operate through the language and culture of neo-liberal capitalism.

Those writing about austerity as a context in which an ideology of neo-liberalism continues to thrive, for example Blyth (2013) and Burton (2016), have argued that this is a creed that directly rolls back the public sphere everywhere in favour of the private sector. Economists Ian Goldin and Chris Kutarna (2016) suggest that granting too much recognition towards neo-liberalism as a pervasive model in the real world has to some extent created a failure in economics teaching and in the economics profession itself by limiting the main discourse to tenets of classical economic theory. In an interview on BBC Radio 4 (16 October 2018), Goldin highlights the poor evidence base of much current economics teaching, over-reliance on theory, the belief that markets are always right and that key assumptions about perfect markets are flawed. He claims that many current students of economics have not been exposed to real life economics, and hence have had a tendency to ignore the self-interest and criminal behaviour of bankers and the fallibility of markets, often shying away from honestly explaining events in the real world: 'Business and science are working giant revolutions upon our societies, but our politics and institutions evolve at a much slower pace. The public therefore have become righteously angry about being left out and stressed about where we're headed' (Goldin and Kutarna, 2016: 10).

Such a system could be seen as anti-democratic – elected politicians have abdicated many of their core powers to the market, and inefficient – the state is locked into generation-long contracts. This political-economic model places profit ahead of people's needs, slashes taxes on big corporations and wealthy people, and tends towards an obsessive deregulation. Neo-liberalism is an historically specific form of capital accumulation endeavouring to engineer a 'counter revolution' against welfare capitalism (Fairclough and Graham, 2002: 221). We are witnessing, feeling and experiencing 'the wholesale extension of a basic feature of capitalist power relations present from the beginning: class domination' (Fleming, 2015: 29). Reflecting neo-liberalism's ascendancy as a financial and cultural force, 'social activity and exchange become judged on their degree of conformity to market culture' with 'business thinking migrating to all social activities' (Holborow, 2015: 34, 35).

This theme has been expanded in Dale-Davidson and Rees-Mogg (2012), in which the authors make an argument that the state will eventually become obsolete as a political entity (as a consequence of neo-liberalism):

> The democratic nation-state basically operates like a criminal cartel, forcing honest citizens to surrender large portions of their wealth to pay for stuff like roads and hospitals and schools. The rise of the internet , and the advent of crypto-currencies, will make it impossible for governments to intervene in private transactions and to tax incomes, thereby liberating individuals from the political protection racket of democracy ... Out of this wreckage will emerge a new global dispensation, in which a 'cognitive elite' will rise to power and influence, as a class of sovereign individuals 'commanding vastly greater resources' who will no longer be subject to the power of nation-states and will redesign governments to suit their ends. (Dale-Davidson and Rees-Mogg, 2012: 32)

Allied to neo-liberalism's pervasive impact on the UK's political, economic and business culture rests a social dimension, that is the notion of a 'cognitive elite' having a right to rise to power, and this view is echoed by David Runciman (2016). He presents a thesis based on respect for experts, namely epistocracy – the rule of the knowers. This paradigm is directly opposed to democracy, because it argues that the right to participate in political decision-making depends on whether or not you know what you are doing. The 19th-century philosopher John Stuart Mill argued for a voting system that granted varying numbers of votes to different classes of people depending on what jobs they did. Professionals and other highly educated individuals would get six or more votes each; farmers and traders would get three or four; skilled labourers would get two; unskilled labourers would get one. Mill, it seems, believed that some points of view carried more weight simply because they had been exposed to more complexity along the way. Jason Brennan (2016) attempts to revive the epistocratic conception of politics, insisting that many political questions are simply too complex for most voters to comprehend. 'Worse, the voters are ignorant about how little they know; they lack the ability to judge complexity because they are so attached to simplistic solutions that feel right to them' (p 10).

In acknowledging the embeddedness of the neo-liberal paradigm, Nicholas Shaxson (2018) defines the present era as driving 'financialisation', characterised as the transformation of business and the rise of finance, with an increasing role of financial motives in all human services, coupled with that of financial actors and financial institutions in the operation of domestic and international economies. Half a century ago, corporations were not only supposed to make profits, but also to serve employees, communities and society. The economist John Maynard Keynes, who helped construct the global financial system known as Bretton Woods, which kept cross-border finance tightly constrained, knew this was necessary if governments were to act in their citizens' interest. He famously said: 'Let goods be homespun whenever it is reasonably and conveniently possible; and above all, let finance be primarily national' (Bullough, 2018: 35). From the late 1970s onwards, finance broke decisively free of these controls, taxes were slashed and swathes of our economies were privatised. As a result our businesses began to undergo a dramatic transformation: their core purposes were whittled down, through ideological shifts and changes in laws and rules, to little more than a single-minded focus on maximising the wealth of shareholders. In contrast to the German manufacturing model, the UK has adopted a financial services industrial model and a smaller public sector.

Evidence of the impact of financialisation on public services has been immediate. For example, a report authored by different economists (Baker et al, 2018) suggests that the total cost of lost growth for the UK caused by 'too much finance' (p 3) between 1995 and 2015 has been in the region of £4,500 billion. This total figure amounts to roughly 2.5 years of the average GDP across the period. The report is said to provide the first ever numerical estimate for the scale of damage caused by the UK's finance sector growing beyond a useful size. Of the £4,500 billion loss in economic output, £2,700 billion is accounted for by the 'misallocation of resources' (p 15), where resources, skills and investments are diverted away from the more productive non-financial activities into finance. The other £1.8 billion arises from the 2008 banking crisis. A main conclusion is that the UK economy may have performed much better in overall growth terms if finance had been more focused on supporting other areas of the economy, rather than trying to act as a source of wealth generation (extraction)in its own right. Shaxson (2018: 15) concurs with the labelling of this form of financial engineering practice as a 'misallocation of resources', and proceeds to use the example of private equity firms to illustrate how a majority of modern companies

– including those helping to finance public sector services – now run their operations:

> through tax havens, fleecing taxpayers, squeezing workers' pay and pension pots, or by buying several companies to dominate a market niche, then milking customers for monopoly profits …Then armed with the enlarged cashflows from these tactics, they borrow more against that company and pay themselves huge 'special dividends' from the proceeds. They retain a 'limited liability if the company goes bust … Private equity investors sometimes do make the companies they buy more efficient, creating wealth but this has become a lesser priority compared to that of financialised wealth extraction. (Shaxson 2018: 92)

Under the Private Finance Initiative (PFI), introduced by John Major's Conservative government in the 1990s but significantly expanded under New Labour, instead of the government building and paying for projects such as schools or hospitals directly, it encouraged private firms to borrow the money to finance their construction, including the full delivery of public services and major infrastructure projects. Under this arrangement the government would agree to pay them back over, say, 25 years, with interest and other bonuses. The 700-odd PFI schemes in Britain today have an estimated capital value of less than £59.1 billion in 2017, yet it has been estimated that taxpayers will end up paying out more than £308 billion for them. Professor Allyson Pollock, a PFI expert, claims this as a gift to the City of London, namely 'one hospital for the price of two' (Pollock, 2018: 67). About £240 billion, a third of the UK government's annual budget, now goes on privately run but taxpayer-funded public services. The chancellor's budget of 2018 announced an abolition of any new PFI contracts, stating that this public–private partnership model was 'inflexible and overly complex' (BBC News, 2018b). Critics of PFI, including the Labour Party and trade unions, state that if existing contracts were allowed to run their course, they would end up damaging the finances of public institutions. The Labour Party has therefore indicated that it would take some contracts back under state control, and paying interest on these projects would cease to be a drain on the public sector. 'But this does nothing to help the many hospitals, councils, police forces and schools. They'll be paying through the nose for many years to come for what are now brand new buildings, but which won't be when the debts are finally paid off' (UNISON representative quote).

The logic of markets and economic evaluation

The phrase 'the neo-liberal era' must be used with care, since it is associated with a bewildering range of meanings (Venugopal, 2015). Gough (2017: 10–11) concurs with this, defining it as a distinct phase of capitalism that began in around 1980. It embraces a dominant set of ideas and of practices and almost certainly continues to have a strong impact on the way our public services are evolving. Its defining ideas include a belief in the superiority of markets and a denigration of much government and collective action. Its defining characteristics include a new international division of labour, the global spread of production networks, trade and financial flows, the dominance of finance, rising profit shares and widening inequalities within countries (Glyn, 2006; Newell and Paterson, 2010; Koch, 2012; Stiglitz, 2013). In this new era the relative power of business corporations and the financial sector has grown, especially relative to trade unions and labour interests, but also vis-à-vis nation states. This stems not only from their lobbying power but also from their structural power, the ability to influence policy without having to apply direct pressure on governments through agents. This stems from several factors, but two have become more important in recent decades: the ability to shift investment and economic activity between jurisdictions and the structural position of finance capital in ensuring national economic survival. The end result is a closer symbiosis or even 'capture' of governments by big business and finance (Hacker and Pierson, 2002; Woll, 2014).

According to Davies (2018), the spirit of competitiveness has entered all spheres of social life; and neo-liberalism represents an attempt to replace political judgement with economic evaluation, including, but not exclusively, the evaluations offered by markets. The central defining characteristic of all neo-liberal critique is its hostility to the ambiguity of political discourse, and a commitment to the explicitness and transparency of quantitative, economic indicators, of which the market price system is the model. 'Neo-liberalism is the pursuit of the disenchantment of politics by economics' (Davies, 2018: 6).

Quantification and measurement have their own affective and aesthetic qualities (Porter, 1995), but the example of market price indicates to an economic sensibility that ambiguity and performativity can be beneficially minimised or constrained. The disenchantment of politics by economics would involve a deconstruction of the language of the 'common good' or the 'public', which is accused of a potentially dangerous mysticism. As manifest in the work of Hayek (1944), this may be an attack on socialism and the types of state expertise that enact it, but it is equally apparent in a critique of the liberal idea of justice (Arblaster, 1985; Posner, 2002). For instance, hospitals and schools may appear to be more valued by the public than fragmented community services; so, in line with consolidating the neo-liberal view, politicians and public service administrators may bolster this so-called normative judgement by resorting to methods of outcome measurement. The targets of neo-liberal critique are institutionally and ontologically various, where substantive claims about political authority and the public are critically dismantled and replaced with technical economic substitutes. However, critics of neo-liberalism have noted that it did not seek or achieve a shrinking of the state, but a reimagining and transformation of it (Peck, 2010; Mirowski, 2013):

> The rise of American and German industrial capitalism had been achieved thanks to new economies of scale and organisational efficiencies associated with large corporations and hierarchical structures, including the birth of management. Science and expertise were now formally channelled into business. Technical advancements in the fields of statistics and national accounts, followed by the birth of macroeconomics in the 1930s, meant that 'the economy' had appeared as a complex object of political management. (Davies, 2017: 7)

The point is that the ongoing growth of a 'social' realm, measured and governed by sociology, social statistics, social policy and professions, meant that the American and European states of the 1930s onwards had far more extensive capacities and responsibilities for audit, intervention and knowledge transfer than previously. The pragmatism of the neo-liberal pioneers committed them to a reinvention of liberalism suitable for a more complex, regulated, Fordist capitalism. Hayek's belief that 'the fundamental principle that in the ordering of our affairs we should make as much use as possible of the spontaneous forces of society, and resort as little as possible to coercion', is capable of an infinite variety of applications (Hayek, 1944: 17). Victorian laissez-faire was only one empirical manifestation of the liberal idea. Restoring economic freedom would not be achieved simply through withdrawing the state from 'the market', but through active policy interventions to remould institutions, state agencies and individuals in ways that were compatible with a market ethos and were amenable to economic measurement. The state is therefore a powerful instrument of neo-liberalism, particularly insofar as it supports deregulated and flexible labour markets. The state is also a major provider and designer of public services, and it appears clearly that some increase in de-professionalisation lies at the heart of the UK austerity agenda, symbolised by profound cuts to services in the form of efficiencies, pay cuts, rationing, reducing staff training and development, along with negative effects on overall economic productivity.

Liberalism is associated primarily with the uncertainty of outcomes: 'to be neutral is to have no answer to certain questions' (Hayek, 1944: 80). By contrast, political activity is interpreted as an instrument of planning, as a project of determining outcomes and reducing uncertainty. Most analyses of neo-liberalism have focused on its commitment to 'free' markets, deregulation and trade, but what is the nature of neo-liberal authority? On what basis does the neo-liberal state demand the right to be obeyed if not on substantive political grounds? To a large extent, it is on the basis of particular economic claims and rationalities, constructed by economic 'experts'. The state does not necessarily cede power to markets, but comes to justify its decisions, policies and rules in terms that are commensurable with the logic of markets. The authority of the neo-liberal state is heavily dependent on the authority of economics to dictate a legitimate course of action, understanding that authority – and its present crisis – requires us to look at economics, economic policy experts and advisors as critical components of state institutions. It is such 'experts' whose views might seem to matter more than those of professionals who have experience of working for these organisations. As such, it is the market-based principles and techniques of evaluation that therefore determine how much state organisations can afford to spend and by how much they may choose to reward their employees.

Globalisation and audit culture

A neo-liberalist ideology characterised by four interrelated characteristics, rationalism, capitalism, technology and regulation, is thought to have caused the expansion of globalisation (Scholte, 2005). Those writing within the Marxian tradition (for example, Giddens, 1971; Bauman, 1998; Edgell, 2012) highlight the decisive role of capitalism, whereas Weber and neo-Weberians emphasise the influence of rationalism (Weber, 1976; Beder, 2000). By illustration, capitalism refers to a distinctive way of organising economic activity oriented to making a profit, and this aspect of capitalism is regarded as a key force behind globalisation. 'The unceasing concern to accumulate a surplus or fail constrains capital to seek out cheaper production sites and new markets for their products, which in practical terms means the world' (Edgell, 2012: 222).

Rationalism refers to a type of knowledge that is thought to have assisted the growth of global thinking, and hence globalisation. Rationalist knowledge does not recognise boundaries based on nationhood, religion, ethnicity and so on, and in this sense is thought to have encouraged globalisation.

Globalisation was initially seen as threat to the welfare state. It was believed that the economic pressures generated by neo-liberal globalisation would inexorably lead to welfare state retrenchment or its dissolution and replacement by a lean 'competition' state (Cerny, 1997). Yet the global rediscovery of poverty (Noel, 2006), the challenges to territorially based conceptions of social rights posed by the increasing flow of migrants, not to mention the enhanced transactional spread of policy ideas and definitions of 'best practice', or the reverse, a loss of autonomy in professional practice, unalloyed de-professionalisation (Demailly and De La Broise, 2009; Frostenson, 2015), have put social policy issues on the global agenda. While neo-liberal ideas came to the fore in the UK during the 1980s, they have not been uncontested. For Deacon (2007) the battle over global social policy has come to centre on the contest between a neo-liberal emphasis on safety nets for the very poor versus universal policies that include the middle class. He went so far as to suggest that:

> powerful states (notably the USA), powerful organisations (such as the IMF) and even powerful disciplines (such as economics) contend with other powerful states (notably the EU, China and Brazil), other powerful organisations (such as the ILO) and other disciplines (such as social and political science) to engage in a war of position regarding the content of global policy. (Deacon, 2007: 16).

As such, globalisation has become associated with the idea of de-professionalisation, defined as low productivity resulting from deskilling and where a rise in low-skilled jobs becomes blamed for static wages. Freedom of movement of labour is currently synonymous with freedom for employers to degrade pay and conditions at one end of the labour market and freedom to asset-strip poorer economies at the other end. It does not have to be so, but foreign workers would not be so attractive to employers if they could not be exploited and had to join a trade union. The position of using reserve armies of overseas labour objectively sustains exploitation and the neo-liberal enterprise.

Changes in the patterning of paid work – for instance, the combination of telephone, computer, and information and communication technologies in call centres – has significantly augmented managerial power, and this phenomenon can only be understood properly through the prism of globalisation. Faced with the imperative of globalisation, management constantly seeks greater wage flexibility, functional and numerical flexibility. Thus the competitive pressures associated with economic globalisation induce shifts in workforce composition and labour demand, which naturally have additional impact throughout the care and education sector in the UK.

It is not just routine work that is being deskilled and outsourced; the trend is for knowledge work to be Taylorised – transferring all discretion from workers to management along with the fragmentation and simplification of tasks. Contemporary globalisation has certainly put additional competitive pressure on capitalist enterprises to lower costs and be flexible in every sense, although there are major social costs and hence limitations to this neo-liberal economic project. A multilayered perspective evaluating the role of individual professionals within a specific sector will consider the changes in their authority and autonomy from removing an area of activity from professional control and influence, and the resultant destabilisation of a workforce (Demailly and De La Broise, 2009). Any measures taken by an employer to lessen the need within an organisation for specialist 'professional' knowledge and expertise may become experienced as a weakening of individual and collective status and may even lead to discrediting of the organisation at a national level. Take for example the use of untrained workers in private G4S prisons or the much-reported abuse of elderly and disabled residents living in care homes.

De-professionalisation may be symptomatic of an audit culture (Power, 1999), directly linked to models of community sector funding and organisational sustainability; and particularly the commissioning process driving public services. If austerity finished tomorrow, it is likely that de-professionalisation would continue, driven by the neo-liberal model of service provision as described. Critiques of this model acknowledge the privileging of economic growth, competition and market forces, whereby this ideology has been combined with managerial technologies, currently expressed in the quality systems regime that requires organisations be continuously audited and assessed for conformance and monitored and reviewed for effectiveness. The audit culture, manifested for example through performance league tables, box-ticking and collecting data on service inputs/outputs, refers to the way in which techniques and values of accountancy have been transposed to fields beyond accounting, and have become a central ongoing principle in the governance and management of human conduct (Shore, 2008: 279). Shore argues that this creates new kinds of relationships, habits and practices. It follows therefore that issues of ethics and the moral behaviour of workers are not private or even organisational business, but become public through the adoption of numerous audit traces (Power, 2014), including codes of conduct, risk management registers, critical incident logs, timesheets, continuous improvement records, training files and so forth. Anthropologists Shore and Wright explain how

> Central to this process has been the re-invention of professionals themselves as units of resource whose performance and productivity must constantly be audited so that it can be enhanced. The discourse of audit has become a vehicle for changing the way people relate to the workplace, to authority, to each other, and most importantly to themselves. (Shore and Wright, 1999: 559)

Summary

Neo-liberalism embeds particular forms of economic rationality as the governing principles of nearly all public policy (Davies, 2017). Its relevance, as both an ideology and as a pragmatic approach, is that it has been defined as a remaking of the state, where the state is not rolled back as such but is reshaped, reconfigured to better serve the demands of capital -where, for example, the unemployed are corralled into low-waged employment (Garrett, 2018). Professionals need to develop a critical approach to their practice and possibly delve deeper into how power relations operate through the language and culture of neo-liberalism. In the current era the relative power of business corporations and the financial sector has grown, especially relative to trade unions and labour interests, but also vis-à-vis nation states. This stems from two main factors: their ability to influence policy without having to apply direct pressure on governments through agents – the ability to shift investment and economic activity between jurisdictions, and the structural position of finance capital in ensuring national economic survival (Gough, 2017). Neo-liberalism represents an attempt to replace political judgement with economic evaluation, including, but not exclusively, the evaluations offered by markets. Quantification and measurement have their own affective and aesthetic qualities (Peck, 2010; Mirowski, 2013). The point is that the ongoing growth of a 'social' realm, measured and governed by sociology, social statistics, social policy and professions, meant that nation states from the 1930s onwards had far more extensive capacities and responsibilities for audit, intervention and knowledge transfer than previously. The pragmatism of the neo-liberal pioneers committed them to a reinvention of liberalism suitable for a more complex, regulated, Fordist capitalism.

Globalisation was seen initially as a threat to the welfare state. It was believed that the economic pressures generated by neo-liberal globalisation would inexorably lead to welfare state entrenchment or its dissolution and replacement by a lean 'competition' state. Yet the global rediscovery of poverty, the challenges to territorially based conceptions of social rights posed by the increasing flow of migrants, not to mention the enhanced transactional spread of policy ideas and definitions of 'best practice' – or the reverse, a loss of autonomy in professional practice, unalloyed de-professionalisation (Demailly and De La Broise, 2009; Frostenson, 2015) – have put social policy issues on the global agenda. De-professionalisation may be symptomatic of an audit culture, directly linked to models of community sector funding and organisational sustainability; and particularly, the commissioning process driving public services. If austerity finished tomorrow, it is likely that de-professionalisation would continue, driven by the neo-liberal approach to service provision. Critiques of this approach acknowledge the privileging of economic growth, competition and market forces, whereby this ideology has been combined with managerial technologies, currently expressed in the quality systems regime that requires organisations be continuously audited and assessed for conformance and monitored and reviewed for effectiveness.

3

Public services, the UK economy and the Brexit debate

Moderate interpretations of neo-liberalism are grounded on the assumption that the state should fight deprivation but not income inequality because the latter is understood as a precondition of economic prosperity (Béland, 2007; Jenson, 2012). Social investment has become a social policy concept that can be seen as a way to find a new economic legitimacy to social programmes (Esping-Andersen, 2002; Morel et al, 2012; Mahon, 2013; Midgley et al, 2017). Seen as part of the Keynesian policy paradigm as a means of increasing economic productivity, social investment was understood to play a positive role in economic regulation, especially during downturns when social benefits helped to maintain consumption. Rather than depicting social programmes as a pure cost for the economy, as traditional neo-liberal thinkers do, social investment suggests that in a so-called knowledge society investment in human capital (training and education) and social programmes such as universal access to child care and early childhood education are good for the economy.

Max Weber argued that modernity had a disenchanting impact in the way that much had been promised through positivist social science, characterised by primacy of observation in its epistemology, the role of theory, causality, laws and value freedom, and by bureaucratisation. This approach subsumes the particular within the universal and reduces qualities to quantities. In Weber's analysis, modern science and bureaucracy lack any 'outward' or public sense of their own intrinsic value to humanity, making them cold, impersonal and anonymous forces – those same characteristics of markets that Hayek deemed valuable (Weber, 1991). The disenchantment of politics by economic ideology depends for its progress, however, on unspoken ethical commitments on the part of its advocates (Davies, 2017: 11). For example, this becomes self-evident when the question of scientific and social scientific methodology arises. In order for objective representations to be generated, certain presuppositions and practical procedures must be adjudged to have a normatively binding force.

The stronger the claim to value neutrality, the more rigidly these procedures must bind, leaving value neutrality to become an ethos in its own right (Du Gay, 2000).

Although neo-liberalism as a creed may be preoccupied by a desire to maximise the potential of management in pursuing policy interventions, those in the Weberian tradition (Freidson,1970; 2001) emphasise that the professions – who are charged with carrying out public policies – develop strategies to advance their own social status. This may involve persuading clients and potential clients about the need for the service they offer, cornering the market in that service and excluding competitors. Professionals are distinguished by their concern to provide effective services to people rather than producing inanimate goods (Rogers and Pilgrim, 2014: 108). What is distinctive about neo-liberalism as a mode of thought and government, however, is its desire to invert the relationship between technical rationality and substantial ethos. Where Weber saw modern rationalisation and capitalism as dependent on certain ethical precepts, Hayek and his followers believed that various technical forms of quantitative evaluation could provide the conditions for and guarantee of liberal values. This technocratic turn diverts the attention of the liberal away from moral or political philosophy – from credentialism and valuing of specialist knowledge and skills – and towards more mundane technical and pragmatic concerns. Prosaic market institutions and calculative devices become the harbinger of unspoken liberal commitments manifested through the employment of knowledge workers and entrepreneurial professions (Davies, 2017; Friedman, 2000).

> Power has shifted too far towards big business and managerial unitarism since 1979. Politicians seduced by neo-liberal economics have enabled the dominance of a financial model of corporate governance serving short-term profitability and shareholder value, detrimental to even minimalist industrial democracy. It is now evident to parts of 'the establishment', not just to left-wing observers, that inequalities under British capitalism have contributed to exclusion and disadvantage. This disconnection influenced Brexit, though externalities of the EU and immigration were blamed. The main culprit is a failed 30-year domestic experiment with neo-liberalism and deregulated flexible labour markets. (Dobbins and Dundon, 2016: 24)

Towards dismantling the public sector

Outsourcing a local authority in its entirety became a long-held Conservative Party municipal fantasy begun in the era of Nicholas Ridley, local government minister under Prime Minister Margaret Thatcher. Large Tory-run authorities such as Cornwall, Suffolk and Barnet embarked on their own high-profile versions of this model, claiming that impoverishment gave them no choice but to pursue large-scale privatisation. Jumping forward to the present era, the recent (March 2018) fate following the budget crisis in Northamptonshire has demonstrated wider problems of local government finance caused by the legacy of years of poor practice, outsourcing, mismanagement and a failure of governance. The social policy writer Melanie Henwood (2018), in describing health and social care provision in the area, reported that eligibility for local government services has become tightened and also that a failure to meet statutory duties leaves the most frail and vulnerable citizens without basic support. This has become part of a wider national picture.

In a similar vein, a report in the national press asserted that 'British entrepreneurs have quietly but determinedly turned to the public sector to make money – albeit small amounts at the moment' (Osborne, 2018). Here it was claimed that changes to the commissioning of National Health Service (NHS) services had forced local service providers to consider private companies. The 2013 Health and Social Care Act had succeeded in fragmenting the service as a whole, opening up everything by law to private as well as NHS bidders. Transactions such as mergers, acquisitions, joint ventures and commissioning have been subject to a range of changing regulatory bodies, such as Monitor, the Competition Commission and the Office of Fair Trading (Sanderson et al, 2017). The Competition and Markets Authority (CMA) oversees enforcing competition to ensure that would-be suppliers can sue the NHS if any service is not put out to tender. These events collided with the harshest NHS funding cuts in its 70-plus year history. Significant problems associated with private NHS providers have sometimes appeared understated, such as the large 'credit card bills' for paying the debt to private companies, some based outside the United Kingdom (UK) and not paying UK taxation, through the Private Finance Initiative (Powell, 2019). Different variants of the 'internal market' have become deeply ingrained in the NHS over the last 30 years or so and have been increasingly entrenched within both general European Union (EU) and UK competition law and sector-specific competition regulation. A process of 'juridification' has emerged whereby laws, such as contract law and EU public procurement and competition laws, have increasingly come to regulate the NHS (Powell, 2019). At national level contracts have included the following 'services': a nine-year contract to provide sexual health services for local councils in the north-east of England; a £700 million deal to run district nursing, dementia care and support for vulnerable children in Bath and North-East Somerset; a contract to run GPs' surgeries in Essex; a partnership to deliver start-up loans for the government; healthcare, including dentistry, in a number of low-category prisons; and a contract with NHS England to give flu jabs at schools in Devon. It might be worth noting that since 2010 Virgin Care Services Ltd has bid for and won at least 400 NHS contracts worth almost £2 billion, between 2013 and 2018 becoming one of the UK's leading healthcare providers. According to a leading UNISON spokesperson, although there was nothing untoward about the arrangements, the growth of the company and the lack of transparency over the contracts must raise concerns among campaigners:

> the company has even been prepared to go to court to win contracts– moves that have cost the NHS dearly, concluding that (the company) appears to be paid more for doing less. While the NHS remains dangerously short of funds, taxpayers' money should not be wasted on these dangerous experiments in privatisation. (UNISON, 2018a)

A further example of a lack of transparency concerns the case of the company Carillion, the 'big four' UK accounting firms acting as a cosy club and failing to identify or simply ignoring catastrophic internal problems. This firm was forced to continue bidding for government contracts so that it could survive (or not); it eventually entered compulsory liquidation in January 2018. This became a story of an inquiry where openness and honesty seemed early casualties and of a system that appeared to have favoured profit, dividends and shareholders' interests over the common good. The claim was that the whole system for delivering essential public services through companies driven, by definition, for profit guarantees that such a pattern of events would continue. 'The Conservative Party's neo-liberal dogma appears to be at war with common sense' wrote Owen Jones (2018: 6), referencing franchises such as the UK privately run rail system, as an inefficient fragmented mess: when it fails it will eventually be sold off to another group of profiteers.

This characterisation of neo-liberalism as organisational breakdown coupled with government bail-out has seemed endemic through similar scandals that have occurred in local government, the NHS and the care sector. For example, in 2011 the financial collapse of the care home chain Southern Cross – owned by private equity group Blackstone – furnished evidence of the sheer recklessness of privatisation (Coward, 2011; Scourfield, 2012). The care sector has become an opportunistic site for greater and more extensive capital accumulation (see also Gallagher, 2014). Given this development, it is vital to recognise that for the private sector the determining motivation is to drive down labour costs and increase profitability (Boffey, 2014). This factor has become increasingly important with regard to the delivery of care for older people in the UK since the introduction of the NHS and Community Care Act relating to the adult and learning disability sector, where large corporate providers now prominently nestle (Harris, 2003; Humber, 2016). For example, it seems that Four Seasons Health Care, the nation's second biggest provider of care homes for older people, is hundreds of millions in debt and has closed or sold many homes (Davies, 2018: 23).

Residential care has perhaps become perceived as a commodity to be traded and exploited for its surplus value like any other commodity, and as a consequence 'the quest for profitability means that business values, reductions in costs and income generation have been prioritised above the quality of care' (Scourfield, 2013). One of capitalism's failures is not to properly value non-monetary work such as care – an answer must be to address the fundamental power imbalances that allow employers to shift risk onto their employees by forcing them to become self-employed contractors or refusing to pay them for breaks. There may be a need to replace punitive benefit sanctions and replace them with a welfare-to-work system that puts much more emphasis on training and support for people to find a job that is right for them, so that individuals may become promoters of their own skills. The UK has had too many low-skill, low-paid jobs offering poor prospects of progression. According to the professional human resources organisation CIPD (2018a), 'The government's rhetoric of an immigration system that only works to attract the brightest and the best doesn't tally with what employers want or need.'

The structural carelessness integral to the evolution of neo-liberal social policy was highlighted in 2011 by the abuses committed against residents at Winterbourne View Hospital in Bristol, owned by the Irish investors Castlebeck (O'Toole, 2012). A Serious Case Review (SCR), undertaken for the South Gloucestershire Safeguarding Adults board, was scathing in its assessment that whilst the 24-bed hospital charged the NHS on average £3,500 a week to treat each patient, this was 'no guarantee of patient safety or service quality' for 'uniquely disadvantaged' individuals (Flynn, 2012: 145). Castlebeck cynically, but entirely in tune with neo-liberal rationality, prioritised 'decisions about profitability, including shareholder returns, over and above decisions about the effective and humane delivery of assessment, treatment and rehabilitation' (Flynn, 2012: 144). Following this SCR a Government White Paper, 'Transforming Care for People with Learning Disabilities – Next Steps' (DH, 2015), was released. Its recommendations placed a strong emphasis on delivering personalised care and support planning along with personal budgets, with personal health budgets for people in receipt of NHS Continuing Health Care, introduced in 2014 following the Care Act of the same year.

A strong emphasis on demonstrating in the future a more professionalised form of care for adults with a learning disability was evidenced in this White Paper, intended to give teeth to 'quality standards' via the service model proposed. This would use performance indicators as a form of 'social investment' to assist commissioners. These cultural changes, as applied to community learning disability services, emphasised workforce development, based on providing 'personalised support and treatment approaches through holistic assessments and non-aversive treatment strategies using positive approaches' (DH, 2015). The success of this strategy has become partially dependent on the efficacy of an Integrated Personal Commissioning Programme that was introduced in April 2015, aiming to blend health and social care funding for those many individuals with the highest care needs. However more recent evidence shows that some care home practices still remain invisible to any form of rigorous external scrutiny or accountability, that too many assessments are over-lengthy, that many people are placed in residences too far away from home and, importantly, there is an even higher use of restrictive interventions in patient services. The last includes face-down/prone restraint, use of seclusion methods and an increase in the number of patient-on-patient assaults recorded nationwide, for example 9,000 in 2017, suggesting that safeguarding may not have improved to the extent promised (ADASS, 2016; HCPC, 2016; BBC Radio 4, 2018; S. Ryan, 2018).

The care sector and UK immigration policies

How has neo-liberal managerialism along with austerity adversely impacted on the jobs of those employed in the care sector? Interrogating cuts to services as socially and politically contentious places the notion of de-professionalisation at the heart of assessing the impact of the commercial model within the NHS and social care. How have these cuts helped to downsize professional service-inputs in the form of efficiencies, pay cuts, rationing, reducing training and staff development, all of which potentially affect overall economic productivity? Pointing to examples of reported incapacity to deliver, along with variations in overall standards nationwide, has become a media-driven way of highlighting ineffectiveness (Kitzinger, 2000; Butler and Drakeford, 2005). For example, we rely on migrant medical staff in our NHS because we have not trained sufficient numbers of our own young people. People have perhaps been manipulated by EU policy, where the winners have been big business (a ready supply of cheap labour) and government (lower costs in terms of training doctors and nurses).

The Conservative government's attitude towards immigration control appears under scrutiny as doctors, teachers and even landlords have been press-ganged into delivery, according to one author, 'In hospitals, schools, lecture theatres, letting agencies and other parts of the public sector, the government's current immigration policy [which] has erected a border within, along which people delivering vital services are coming to terms with unwanted new powers' (Usborne, 2018: 13). This suggests that professionals on the frontline, sometimes unwillingly, have become effectively embedded in measures of deterrence. The 2016 Immigration Act has outsourced immigration control to the general population, leading to discriminatory mistakes as a result of imposing strict document checks in GP surgeries, hospitals and care homes. In essence this undermines the core principles of the NHS, erodes trust in doctors and puts patients at risk, posing unnecessary demands on professional services to check immigration status and becoming a distraction from carrying out main responsibilities.

Social care practices operate within a framework that emphasises political economy and provide possibly the best example in the UK of how de-professionalisation as a growing trend enters and is sustained within a large public sector workforce. A key feature of this policy dynamic is to illuminate that the labour process, associated with a multiplicity of care roles and tasks, has become more fragmented, more surveilled and riper for even greater exploitation. It is entirely within the neo-liberal frame of reference to employ more immigrant, low-waged employees to service the paid care sector, but in theory this cuts across deep strands within government immigration policy to offer jobs only to the brightest and the best – those with professional qualifications.

In the UK social care sector, a natural priority is to care for older people and those living with long-term conditions. While we are most familiar with industrial and factory automation, service robots, which include systems for use in domestic, personal and healthcare settings, have become a fast-growing sector (Prescott and Caleb-Solly, 2017). Despite its potentially beneficial impact, introducing further technology into the care sector is apt to render the work arid when its deployment is driven by the imperative to extract more surplus value from the hard-pressed caring workforce (Taylor, 2014). The UK is now faced with a shortage of carers, and care professions are recognised as being poorly paid. The development of robotics and autonomous systems (RAS) is having an increasing impact in many sectors that are developing assistive and companion robot technologies and should prioritise applications that will relieve the burden on care workers of dull, repetitive and strenuous work. Technology to support caring and more flexible working is both a means of supporting the well-being and employment prospects of carers, and in itself is an area of economic growth that should be fostered and incentivised (Carers UK, 2017). In theory this scenario creates opportunities for a more professional role, with a focus on the human-to-human aspects of care, and as a consequence it may become necessary to reassess training needs for some care roles that will in the future require technical knowledge related to customising and deploying RAS technologies.

Social rights and collectivist values

In a general sense, the neo-liberal model eclipses social rights as an ambiguous domain, despite a prominent observation that the EU may tendentiously strengthen the power of the political elite; and by implication social rights have been enhanced by the UK being a member of the EU. One ambiguity perhaps arises over a clarification of what has actually been achieved in the enshrinement of social rights that are numerous and highly various and come to expression in different ways. They may be described briefly as rights that are intimately connected with human dignity and the right to lead a dignified life. Examples of social rights include the right to work, to health, to housing, to social care (Mikkola, 2007; Lind, 2018). The realisation of these rights is dependent on many factors: how social programmes are organised; how solidarity is expressed in law; how well individuals are able to support themselves; what people consider the appropriate role of collective measures to be; and what they believe economic justice and equal treatment require. European integration has been a fact for decades, and its organs have had to handle tough economic challenges, but constitutionally guaranteed social rights have never been amongst its primary goals. The EU's competence in these fields has always been extremely limited. It seems clear that the role and position of social rights in European law has certainly strengthened one professional group in particular, the legal profession. Whereas the EU has been facing a major financial crisis, social rights have never been so strongly expressed in its fundamental documents. These documents are the Treaty on European Union and the Charter of Fundamental Rights of the European Union (the EU Charter). These fundamental documents represent binding law, both for the member states and for the European institutions. The foremost organ for their interpretation is the Court of Justice of the European Union, but social rights are also expressed in the Community Charter of the Fundamental Social Rights of Workers (hereafter the Community Charter), which the European Economic Community enacted in 1989. This charter has influenced the development of social policy in the EU, and the Court of Justice uses it as an interpretative tool.

The UK's welfare state has become part of a progressive consensus to protect the social and economic rights of individuals, and the diminution of role of the state in securing this objective manifests itself through the reduced contribution of professional services. Taking a broadly Marxist optic highlights 'the prevailing social order's systematic tendency to create unsatisfying work … This perspective is at odds with the implicitly reformist logic of the feminist ethic of care (used in the context of the 2010 Equality Act) which implies that a change in values might bring about a transformative impact *within* the social and economic fabric of capitalism' (Garrett, 2018: 158–9; see also Chapter 2). In contrast, Edmiston (2017) claims that the current period of austerity has instigated a shift in the pace, direction and character of welfare reform, and that such developments have had a noticeable impact on the 'depth of social citizenship in the UK' (Edmiston, 2017: 265). Here the argument is that an undermining of the effectiveness, inalienability and universality of social citizenship has become manifested through cuts in welfare. The term 'welfare' is used here to refer to the social rights of citizenship, and includes the provision of services, goods and transfers, such as housing, healthcare, social security, education and personal social services. The ability to fully exercise other social, civil and political rights is greatly dependent on a minimum level of income (Marshall, 1950); and professional interventions to uphold these rights present as a necessity.

Government spending on health, education and well-being is required for the meaningful exercise of citizenship. This includes a legal right to social justice, for instance in cases involving family break-up, divorce or domestic abuse, where government reforms of legal aid fees have resulted in hampering the defence of people who lack the necessary financial resources to seek protection. Recently this has led to an increase in unrepresented defendants and therefore a higher risk of the miscarriage of justice. Cuts in legal aid entitlement mean that criminal barristers are refusing to take on new publicly funded cases despite the fact that government reforms are meant to shift more money down to junior barristers, and there is some evidence that the criminal justice system is creaking at the seams (Fouzder, 2018).

A further characterisation of neo-liberalism is its pragmatism and its tendency to inject precariousness into the lives of working people – it deploys the rhetoric of 'flexibility' and 'innovation' whilst injecting uncertainty into lives in and beyond the workplace (Mahmud, 2012). The prevailing ideology of the last 40 years has been of privatisation, deregulation and most recently austerity. Professor Diane Reay blames the centre ground in UK politics for a lack of countervailing policy, including the Labour Party, which 'depicts a fabricated reality' (Reay, 2018: 453). Although social justice may be part of their rhetoric,

> Their actions are essentially about protecting the status quo, and a privileged establishment. We have an elite, homogeneous, political and media bubble, based disproportionately on the reproduction of elite families. Outside it, children are going hungry, homelessness is increasing, and inadequate welfare payments are inexplicably delayed. The suffering of poor people seems to be endless, with 30% of children growing up in poverty. It is hard to see any irony in their circumstances. (Lightfoot, 2018: 28)

The age of globalisation has seen the pay of lower- and middle-income groups in North America and Europe stagnate. Most of us have seen not a recovery but a ripping up of our social contract – so that over 7 million Britons are now in precarious employment. But the highest earners are way ahead of where they were in 2008 (Chakrabortty, 2017). Feeding more wealth to the already rich attacks our social structure and causes greater inequality, whereas what is needed is improved access to universal and free high-quality education and public services, strengthened worker protection and government initiatives to stimulate the infrastructure required for a sustainable, high productivity economy.

Such measures are all within the potential remit of a government committed to restoring a firmer foundation to collectivist values.

However, by 2019 a picture emerges of a Conservative government continually missing its targets of reducing national debt in gross domestic product, resulting in a prediction of austerity possibly lasting until 2025, and public sector services not only run for profit but the 'rich and super-rich accumulating by dis-possessing an increasingly indebted working class and unemployed poor' (Garrett, 2018: 95). This impacts directly on the role of professional workers employed for example in health care, education, social care and legal services, where the framework of managerialism, a manifestation of the neo-liberal model, continues to demand greater efficiencies, including questioning the need for a highly trained and educated workforce (see Chapter 2).

In 2018 an International Workers Day/Labour Day conference declared that UK citizens have a basic human right to engage in productive employment (Griffiths, 2018), yet the claim is that record UK employment levels disguise the reality that many new jobs, especially in deindustrialised regions, are low paid, insecure and low skill. This is a legacy of a deregulated flexible labour market policy since 1979, exacerbated by the 2008 financial crisis.

> The human capital ideology that labour market supply of trained workers automatically creates its own demand from employers is a hoax, evidenced by rising underemployment. A new political economy of work is urgently needed that places job quality centre stage. For example, the state, nationally and locally, should intervene in depressed regions to guarantee better jobs grounded in necessities such as health and social care, housing, transport and green projects. (Dobbins and Plows, 2017: 571)

These authors make the argument that a government could create new human-centred social contracts to stop extreme cases of profit/shareholder maximisation and labour exploitation. Neo-liberalisation has both affective and material dimensions and impacts differently in separate national and local settings depending on what suits market forces. For example, public-funded services run by the private sector may choose to buy into professional skills in a niche way by modifying or expanding a worker's traditional role, or sometimes making unreasonable workload demands.

Taking the example of probation and criminal justice reform, one commentator has recently declared that through the erosion of an ethical commitment, 'the culture of public service has been sacrificed on the altar of privatisation' (McCulloch, 2018). Since the New Labour government's ending of the social work qualification for probation, and through the endorsement of the introduction of 'independent providers' and a 'tough on crime' mantra, the result has done little other than fill prisons. Despite a fairly obvious belief that crime can never be tackled through technical controls and contracts alone, and despite a professional recognition that challenging relationships are perhaps the key to rehabilitation, the successor Conservative government initially promised 'transformative rehabilitation' and to consider 'fresh alternatives to prison reform' (House of Commons Justice Committee, 2018). However, all of the evidence suggests that this has involved little more than a strengthened ideological commitment to the outsourcing of probation – 'an untested and deeply unpopular privatisation process' (HM Inspectorate of Probation, 2017), according to the probation officers' trade union. This outsourcing and privatisation by different Ministers of Justice has been despite the fact that prior to privatisation each of the 35 probation areas was rated as 'good' or 'outstanding' by the government's own monitoring (HM Inspectorate of Probation, 2017; Webster, 2017).

As part of a more encompassing polity stressing the centrality of paid employment within societies structured to service the needs of capital, it has been argued however that neo-liberalism as an economic approach has become characterised by low growth, less equitably distributed (Dorling, 2014; Midgley et al, 2017; Greener, 2018; Rushton, 2018; Van Oorschot et al, 2017). The approach has found key supporters within the universities, increasingly modelled on corporate businesses. Affirming the values of the market, academic institutions are apt to amplify and mimic private sector practices underpinned by notions of performance, customer, enterprise and entrepreneurship; and characterised by upbeat words: creative, participation and empowerment (Holborow, 2015). In the decade since the 2008 crash workers have suffered the worst squeeze in wages in modern times – a process that links privatisation, deregulation and the shifting of power from workers to bosses. According to one commentator, the same decade has seen the biggest financial crisis in a century, the biggest slump since the Great Depression and the slowest recovery since the Second World War. Living standards have flatlined and public spending has been cut, creating perfect conditions for an age of insecurity. People who express concerns about the hollowing out of industrial communities by globalisation have been lectured about free trade. Those worried about migration have been called racists (Elliott, 2018a). An 'identitarian' doctrine has claimed that globalisation had created a homogeneous culture with no distinct national or cultural identities (Jones, 2012).

Ideology, the UK economy and Brexit

The neo-liberal model helped to shine a light on the outcome of the UK EU referendum in June 2016, given that Prime Minister Theresa May continued to show concern that people voted 'leave' because they wanted respite from globalisation. However, it also appeared that several Conservative MPs voted leave because they thought that Britain wasn't globalised enough. This difference expressed a profound dilemma for English conservatism. It illustrates an argument about the relationship between economic liberalism and social cohesion that has been brewing since the Tories were expelled from power in 1997. It contains a dispute over Margaret Thatcher's legacy, made more acute by the financial crisis and its ongoing social repercussions. It leads to questions of whether public discontent today is better explained by excessive exposure to market forces (individual greed driving rampant inequality) or misapplication of market forces (prosperity obstructed by a meddling state). 'The EU is a transnational juggernaut geared to neo-liberalism; whereas the European Left sees the EU as promoting democracy, egalitarianism and social liberalism, but the reality maybe somewhat different' (Elliott, 2018a: 39). The four pillars of the EU single market – free movement of goods, services, people and money – would appear to be the axioms of market fundamentalism. For some on the left, however, Brexit was welcomed because the EU's bias in favour of multinational capital, its hard-wired monetarism and its obsession with balanced budgets meant that it is more Thatcherite than social democratic (Elliott, 2018c).

Theresa May pledged to 'end austerity' in her speech to the Conservative party conference in 2018, but implied that the government would need to secure a 'good Brexit deal' before it could outline its approach to tax and spending over the following years. Nevertheless, in the October 2018 budget Chancellor Philip Hammond declared that austerity was 'coming to an end' and peppered his speech with spending pledges and a surprise income tax cut. He opted to spend almost all of a £68 billion windfall handed to him over the next five years by the independent Office for Budget Responsibility. In the case of the NHS and social care, this created a £2 billion boost for mental health funding; with a rise of £20.5 billion a year to the NHS budget in real terms by 2023–4. An extra £650 million in social care funding for local authorities in

England was provided for the following year 2019–20. A big picture scenario was presented by the chancellor for stable but unspectacular growth of 1.5 per cent up to 2023, based on the assumption of a smooth Brexit. If this were not to be the case, his assertion was that the economy and public services would suffer. For instance, despite the fact that the Conservative government had promised a long-term plan for the NHS and social care, a credible workforce analysis estimated that there were around 100,000 staff vacancies within the NHS alone, along with a prediction that this number would rise significantly if the UK cannot attract relevant skills from abroad (Campbell, 2017g; Matthews-King, 2018; NHS England,2018a). The opposition leader, Jeremy Corbyn, described the 2018 budget as offering 'half measures and quick fixes, ideological tax cuts to the richest in our society while austerity grinds on' (Kentish, 2018); whilst the Resolution Foundation thinktank noted: '(the government) has significantly eased – but not ended – austerity for public services. However, tough times are far from over.' The TUC General Secretary, Frances O'Grady, took a sharper tone: 'Working people cannot be fobbed off again with promises of a better tomorrow that never comes … [this budget] does not undo the austerity that has devastated public services.'

The likely impact of Brexit on the 2018 budget was spelled out by the National Institute of Economic and Social Research (NIESR), indicating that the Chancellor of the Exchequer could raise spending on public services above and beyond the £20 billion promised for the NHS -but only if Britain retained the closest possible post-Brexit relationship with the EU (NIESR, 2018). This economic forecaster body warned that a 'no-deal Brexit' would erode almost all this extra spending power and cause public borrowing to rise, while also warning that the pound would fall in value, inflation would rise and the economy would barely grow for several years. NIESR said that a 'soft' Brexit deal would constitute the UK retaining access to the EU economic area and customs union. Compared with a soft Brexit scenario, a no deal would cause annual output to be about 5.3 per cent smaller over ten years. Economic growth would only be 0.3 per cent in both 2019 and 2020, compared with 1.9 per cent and 1.6 per cent in a soft Brexit scenario.

Yet a soft Brexit deal would similarly be financially costly to the UK, in terms of a so-called 'divorce settlement'; therefore, this was opposed strongly by several – mainly Conservative Party – politicians. To leave would be to surrender influence because the best deals were done on the inside, according to Angela Merkel, who claimed that the UK would not find it comfortable negotiating from 'outside the room' (Behr, 2018: 6; Connolly and Boffey, 2018; Martin, 2018). The EU would naturally tend to believe that privileges of membership are unavailable to non-members; that Britain must decide what it likes about its current arrangements and then negotiate a price for retaining them. Conservative Party cabinet ministers Boris Johnson and David Davis left the government during the summer of 2018, possibly feeling the shame at admitting the cost up close, involving owning the weakness of one national government trying to negotiate with a continental bloc. A feature of a multinational union is that common positions, once established, are not readily changed, and the act of leaving means automatically having your own national needs downgraded. Axiomatically, each EU leader values their seat at the table more than they may value any aspect of their bilateral relationship with the UK. This will pose real challenges for politicians and opens up a very live possibility that many highly and medium-paid professionals may choose to move to the EU to work, as it is viewed as offering better prospects.

It may also seem evident that any 'model of Brexit', as conceived at the time, would not overturn a socio-economic approach, based on a blend of austerity and neo-liberalism, thus failing to offer any special advantages to professionally trained individuals who may choose to work in the UK in terms of their valued recognition. One exception to this rule was in the case of medical practitioners expressed through the medical training initiative (MTI). This bespoke policy has acted as an exchange scheme for non-EU medical practitioners as its objectives are 'training-focused', to share knowledge, experience and best practice. It is 'a national scheme designed to allow a small number of doctors to enter the UK from overseas for a maximum of 24 months, so that they can benefit from training and development in NHS services before returning to their home countries' (Academy of Medical Royal Colleges, 2019: 14). Leading evidence suggests that a failure of successive UK governments to invest in education and training, encouraging employers to recruit from overseas, while failing to tax businesses fairly, has meant that the social and economic costs this recruitment model imposes on communities has not been mitigated (UNESCO/OECD, 2014; Shaw, 2015; Berlyne, 2016). One commentator has remarked, somewhat cynically, that 'In the medium to long-term, all the low-skilled jobs will be done by the British-born, all the high-skilled jobs will be done by foreigners who don't have to speak English and who will have been trained and educated abroad' (Tom Swallow, independent blogger).

A question arises: why support a leave campaign dominated by those who want less regulation in the workplace and more of the economic policies that have caused so much damage? For example, the Institute of Economic Affairs, one of the largest supporters of Brexit, has frequently promoted through its website the benefits of more immigration as a way of achieving economic growth. Even in the final stages prior to leaving the EU, the Conservative government seemed anxious to establish a lenient immigration policy sympathetic to all EU business interests (BBC News, 2018a). Will Brexit impact on the role and status of different professions who already work in the UK or who may choose to work here as a result of this policy? Understandably, this will depend on the perspectives of employers along with the differing levels of skill that individuals bring with them. The neo-liberal position is that it is primarily markets alone that determine the pay and conditions of workers. A result has been to extend privatisation and diminish the public realm. Most government departments face drops in their real-terms spending per person up to 2024 under the Conservative government's plans, concluding that austerity is not over but has been reshaped by the 2018 budget to meet the politics of the age.

Post-Brexit entry standards for professional workers

The EU in its development reflects the position of professional groups, iteratively offering an inbuilt communitarian-styled solidarity as envisaged in a conventional trade union. It would seem clear that the decline in bargaining power in an overly casualised UK labour market has held down wages, and that both stronger trade unions and regulation are needed to raise low-income earnings and productivity. For example, Elliott (2018b, c) highlights that there has been a noticeable demise of trade union collective bargaining from a 1970s high of 70 per cent to 26 per cent in 2018, coupled with a failure to recognise union power and rights. Failings of the global and UK economies have included cuts to public services, wage stagnation and a fall in living standards, suggesting that strategies are needed to ensure that technological advances increase productivity not unemployment, along with appropriate training and education to reduce the skills gap.

Highly skilled may not mean highly paid – for instance, is it simply a case of the state choosing to allow markets to flourish and as a result of this process thereby undervaluing particular professional jobs, for example that of a teacher, a health or social care worker? Is there a systemic reluctance to address properly the professionalism engendered within these roles and to remunerate them accordingly? Several UK Home Office reports have produced a system intended to be non-discriminatory between EU and non-EU citizens, based on skills not nationality (MAC, 2018). The objective has been an end to freedom of movement and no preferential access, notwithstanding a few possible exceptions such as workers employed in food management, health and social care, if accompanied by a bespoke trade deal. Estimates from sectors such as social care, where there have been reports of around 80,000 UK vacancies at any given time, may be interpreted as employers needing many more workers, whether high, medium or low skilled. The conclusion, however, has failed to unravel necessary workforce requirements in terms of quantifying this distinction, and does not accommodate the need for a professionalised workforce. Evidence from the private sector is that the majority of care services have come to rely rightly or wrongly on a low-skilled, low-paid workforce, denying recognition that this role may demand a higher level of skill, knowledge, experience and indeed status.

In October 2018 the prime minister, Theresa May, stressed that in January 2021 there would be a stop placed on the number of low-skilled EU citizens entering the UK to work; and a preference would be given to workers with high-level skills earning a specified minimum salary, for example £30,000. Another reported pledge by the prime minister has been to reduce migration by giving priority to migrants, including those from the EU, earning more than £50,000 (Fazackerley, 2018). A further intention would be to bring down the overall annual immigration target to below 100,000. On consideration, some sectors may receive an exemption to this rule, for example social care and agricultural services, if a bespoke trade measure could be agreed between the UK and the EU country involved. At the same time Helen Dickinson, Chief Executive of the British Retail Consortium, speaking on the BBC Radio 4 *Today* programme, expressed caution about a policy that curbs the amount of low-skilled labour, opting instead for a more robust policy that is 'demand-led', and questioning also whether the Government's chosen policy would actually reduce the overall numbers involved – as it may lead instead to an increase in the number of non-EU citizens with high-skill levels entering the country (see also German Retail Blog, 2017).

This conclusion was soon confirmed in a policy initiative that emerged towards the end of 2018, when the Ministry of Health and Social Care stated that it intended to relax immigration rules to let more foreign doctors come to Britain to fill widespread NHS gaps. The Conservative government agreed to significantly expand from 1,500 the number of doctors allowed to come to Britain each year under the MTI, predictably resulting in the maximum number of non-EU medical practitioners able to come rising to around 3,000. Through the MTI, more trainee doctors from countries outside the EU would be offered the opportunity to learn from experienced consultants within the UK national health system. This policy was presented as an inevitable consequence of the NHS's inability to recruit and retain enough doctors and the impact on patient care, this forcing some A&E units to close temporarily or permanently, for example (Campbell, 2018c). While Brexit may allow the NHS to escape from any Transatlantic Trade and Investment Partnership deal, there are concerns that post-Brexit trade deals might include health care (Powell, 2019). By the end of 2018 it was still unclear as to what the Conservative government's post-Brexit immigration system should be. The prime minister and colleagues, leading the debate, expressed a desire to halt the numbers of low-paid workers entering the country, whereas leading business representatives opposed the move. 'The (post-Brexit) system will be based on skills ... and income is an indicator of skills', Sajid Javid, as Home Secretary responsible for immigration, told the Radio 4 *Today* programme in December 2018. Nonetheless, it would be a choice to pay incoming social care workers a low wage, despite the fact that they may, as individuals, be highly skilled.

Why aren't we training our own doctors, nurses, teachers and social care staff? Evidence from the Office of National Statistics demonstrates that the number of EU citizens coming to the UK for work had by 2018 fallen to a six-year low, and suggested for example that many EU nurses have since 2016 left the UK because they were unclear about the nature of their work and pension rights (O'Carroll, 2018). A dominant argument has been that anything that places a restriction on immigration would inhibit the UK's ability to solve its public service recruitment problems. A tougher language test has affected EU recruitment; and the Recruitment and Employment Confederation, the professional body for the recruitment of industry, stated that the public sector, including the NHS and schools, would face up to seven more years of skills shortages based on current demand. By the end of 2018 the Conservative government agreed that there would be no numerical cap on the number of highly skilled individuals entering the UK. 'We must remember that highly-skilled does not mean highly paid', affirmed the Deputy Chief Executive of NHS Providers in an interview on the BBC Radio 4 *Today* programme on 19 December 2018 – 'junior doctors start pay can be 27k, nurses 23k, and a health care assistant (HCA) 17k'. As a representative of mainly private sector providers, she may have not concealed an interest in reducing pressure to raise wages, as a large proportion of the human services sector continues to survive driven by a policy reliant on market-based principles.

By the end of 2018 the government appeared to be interpreting this advice flexibly, by considering that a straightforward cap would be harmful to business interests and other parties, and therefore agreed to resolve this dilemma by putting it out for formal review. The Home Secretary emphasised a policy focus on skills, abandoned any previous immigration target (as not being achievable) and insisted that 'bringing net migration down' was a realistic objective. For highly skilled but lower paid staff protected by existing visa rules, which for example offered permission for one year entry with no extra right of entry for accompanying family members, there may still be a strong disincentive to apply to work in the UK.

An outcome of the Brexit process may be to introduce the equivalent of tariffs to be imposed on employers choosing to import labour from either EU or non-EU countries, thus not necessarily making some foreign workers less expensive to employ. One impact may be to incentivise UK employers to up-skill the indigenous workforce, with an advantage of creating greater stability consistent with any future UK industrial strategy. The UK has a poor record of training and up-skilling, with a low percentage of employees rising above entry-level work. A prevailing argument has been that for too long taxpayers have been subsidising businesses by allowing employers to bring in low-skilled workers – this is because the UK tax system has to provide top-up social security allowances such as housing benefit and universal credit for some workers. A change making it harder for employers to import cheap labour may incentivise them to recognise the qualifications of such workers and help to lead a campaign for a broader recognition of professional skills and expertise within the UK workforce. This action may also empower trade union leaders, including those professions where significant staff shortages appear widespread, such as nursing, midwifery, general practice and hospital medicine, along with professions working in mental health and social care. There is a further argument that, had union representation been an established feature of the high finance arena, individuals would have felt protected in voicing their concerns. Whistleblowing mechanisms are stronger today, but this doesn't prevent the lone voice who seeks to expose looming catastrophe from the constraining solitude that only a trade union can overcome, empower and protect.

The Brexit debate offers a convenient backdrop in that in the UK a rather polite liberal view observes, for example, that 'foreigners' have now become essential to staff care homes and hospitals (Hinsliff,

2018a). This acknowledges a blithe acceptance of how free-market economics along with the extensive use of zero-hours contracts impacts on employment conditions in so many sectors, and perhaps shows contempt to taxpaying 'foreigners' who fund the training of our doctors and nurses. The government's cuts in medical and nursing training can be seen as fundamentally reactionary in a scenario where there may be a preference for investment in the economy and health service, and stronger regulation of employment conditions. A by-product of this model is that some of the world's poorest countries have transferred billions to the UK in the form of trained medical staff. Neo-liberal austerity states look to cut the costs of welfare, and by a clever transfer of words those in favour use words such as 'resilience' (positive) to address and talk up the attitudes of those enduring the consequences of cuts in areas such as 'schools, businesses, police and fire departments, hospitals, community mental health centres and the like'. (Garrett, 2018: 144–7).

The way combined globalisation, technology, demographics and financial imbalances are developing could aggravate regional divisions and wealth inequality, claims an Organisation for Economic Co-operation and Development (OECD) report on social mobility, examining how populism has affected economics and demonstrating discontent with the status quo (see Dumas, 2018; OECD, 2018). The OECD report studies the disposable income of the richest 10 per cent of the population across its 34 member countries, which is now nine times as high – compared with seven times 25 years ago. The top 10 per cent own well over 90 per cent of that wealth and the bottom 40 per cent just 3 per cent, which helps explain why populist politicians have been gaining ground. In the 20th century institutions developed to share the fruits of growth – compulsory schooling, higher education, central banks, credit unions and friendly societies, trade unions, the welfare state. Whereas the 'ethic' of a welfare state has become seriously undermined along with its vision based on collectivist principles, a coming technological change could create further upheaval because artificial intelligence (AI) means humans will no longer have the cognitive playing field for themselves. This so-called 'fourth industrial revolution' will expand the range of ideas, perhaps more than its predecessors and possibly lead to more wage inequality and social unrest. More left-leaning thinkers offer the same solutions: progressive taxation, investment in education, cradle to grave welfare states and collective bargaining.

A bigger picture scenario suggests that some professions may have lost authority because the state has lost authority. Nation states everywhere are in an advanced state of political and moral decay from which they cannot individually extricate themselves, asserts the political scientist Rana Dasgupta (2018). Why is this happening? He claims that 20th-century political structures are drowning in a 21st-century ocean of deregulated finance, autonomous technology, religious militancy and great-power rivalry. The argument is made that nation states have also lost their moral aura, which is one of the reasons tax evasion has become an accepted fundament of 21st-century commerce. The destruction of state authority over capital – a further feature of neo-liberalism – has become the objective of the financial revolution that defines the present era. As a result, states have been forced to shed social commitments in order to reinvent themselves as custodians of the market. There are, however, limits to self-organising markets, and it is axiomatic that democratic institutions play a crucial role in compensating for capitalism's failings through regulation and institution-building. One commentator has claimed that a main threat to capitalism has appeared following a decline of the Enlightenment spirit, and the accompanying public realm is under assault from ultra-libertarian values (Hutton, 2018).

This has drastically diminished national political authority in both real and symbolic ways. In 2013 Barack Obama called inequality 'the defining challenge of our time' (Newell, 2013), but US inequality has risen continually since 1980. Capitalism has been sustained by inherited moral values that are now all but exhausted. Neo-liberal economics – in which market forces are allowed to operate freely – represented a new belief in individualism, and a long tradition of property rights traditionally ensured that self-interested action also produced public benefit. However, such rights, including the laws underwriting economic and financial innovation and parliamentary democracy, have been gradually captured and shaped by those who could benefit most from them. The outcome is a reduced ability to generate real wealth combined with exceptional economic and social inequality, as well as a worldwide breach of the vital trust between voters and their representatives (Kingston, 2017).

The picture is the same all over the West: the wealth of the richest continues to skyrocket, while austerity cripples the social democratic welfare state. The reason the nation state was able to deliver what achievements it did was that there was, for much of the 20th century, an authentic fit between politics, economy and information, all of which were organised on a national scale. National governments possessed actual powers to manage modern economic and ideological energies, and to turn them towards human ends. But that era is over. After decades of globalisation, economics and information have grown beyond the authority of national governments. Western governments possess nothing like their previous command over national economic life, and if they continue to promise fundamental change it is now at the level of public relations and wish fulfilment. Without political innovation, global capital and technology will rule us without any democratic consultation, and therefore become the natural leader. The assault on political authority appears as an epochal upheaval.

Summary

Social investment has become a social policy concept that can be seen as a way to find a new economic legitimacy for social programmes (Midgley et al, 2017). This has been viewed as a means of increasing economic productivity; it plays a positive role in economic regulation and investment in human capital (training and education) and social programmes such as universal access to childcare and early childhood education, viewed as good for the economy. Those writing in the Weberian tradition, such as Freidson (1970, 2001), emphasise that the professions – which are charged with carrying out public policies – develop strategies to advance their own status. Professionals are distinguished by their concern to provide effective services to people rather than producing inanimate goods (Rogers and Pilgrim, 2014). What is distinctive about neo-liberalism as a mode of thought and government, however, is its desire to invert the relationship between technical rationality and substantial ethos (Davies, 2017). Neo-liberalism has been characterised as organisational breakdown coupled with government bail-out thanks to a range of scandals that have occurred in local government, the NHS and the care sector. Residential care, for example, has been perceived as a commodity to be traded and exploited for its surplus value like any other commodity, and as a consequence the quest for profitability means that business values, reductions in costs and income generation have been prioritised above the quality of care (Scourfield, 2012, 2013). One of capitalism's failures is to not properly value non-monetary work such as care – an answer must be to address the fundamental power imbalances that allow employers to shift risk onto their employees by forcing them to become self-employed contractors. The argument is that there needs to be a greater emphasis on training and support for people to find a job that is right for them and which will ensure that individuals may become promoters of their own skills.

Interrogating cuts to services as socially and politically contentious places the notion of de-professionalisation at the heart of assessing the impact of the commercial model within the NHS and social care. How have these cuts helped to downsize professional service-inputs in the form of efficiencies, pay cuts, rationing, reducing training and staff development, all of which potentially affect overall economic productivity? It is entirely within the neo-liberal framework to employ more immigrant, low-waged employees to service the paid care sector, although in future UK government policy is expected to offer preference to those with higher-level skills. At one level, the development of AI/RAS within the care sector could, in theory at least, create opportunities for a more professional role, with a focus on the human-to-human aspects of care. Austerity has instigated a shift in the pace, direction and character of welfare reform, with these developments having a noticeable impact on the 'depth of social citizenship in the UK' (Edmiston, 2017: 265). This has affected legal rights to social justice, divorce or domestic abuse, where government reforms of legal aid fees have resulted in hampering the defence of people who lack the necessary financial resources. A further characterisation of the neo-liberalist approach is its pragmatism and its tendency to inject precariousness into the lives of working people. The argument is made that a firmer foundation should be restored to collectivist values, as austerity leaves a legacy of deregulated flexible labour market policy. A new political economy of work is needed urgently that places job quality centre stage, and for government to create new human-centred social contracts to stop extreme cases of profit/shareholder maximisation and labour exploitation (Dobbins and Plows, 2017).

Most public services have seen evidence of a strengthened ideological commitment to outsourcing, privatisation and deregulation. Of equal concern, the public services sector has become characterised by low growth, less equitably distributed. The neo-liberal model helps to shine a light on outcomes of the UK EU referendum in June 2016, given that both main political parties continue to show concern that people voted 'leave' because they wanted respite from globalisation. Will Brexit impact on the role and status of professionals in the UK? It would appear that a 'successful' Brexit will not overturn or even damage the neo-liberal economic model and may offer advantages to highly skilled professional people who choose to work in the UK, as future immigration policy is likely to give preference to such individuals. Strategies are needed to ensure that technological advances increase productivity not unemployment, and effort is required to reverse the demise of trade union collective bargaining (Elliott, 2017, 2018a). Technological change such as AI, along with global capital – a 'fourth industrial revolution' – may lead to more wage inequality and social unrest. Left-leaning thinkers continue to offer the same solutions: progressive taxation, investment in education, cradle to grave welfare states, collective bargaining. A bigger picture scenario suggests that some professions may have lost authority because the state has lost authority (Dasgupta, 2018).

PART II

Theoretical frameworks and ideology: professionalism and de-professionalism

4

Perspectives used in studying professions: sociology, social philosophy

Introduction

What are our criteria for judging teachers, health care staff, social workers and those employed in the criminal justice system as 'professional' and what are the impacts of current changes and challenges on the nature of the 'professional project', where professionals need to become accountable to the interests of a changing public amid a growing background of tighter resources and demands for citizenship rights? There are several rich theoretical perspectives shaping professionalism as a concept, demonstrating that there is more than one valid view of a social action or a social phenomenon. However, most social scientists agree on some basic characteristics of professionals (see, for example, Rogers and Pilgrim, 2014: 108):

- Professions are interest groups and engaged in competition with each other and other groups in society, up to and including the state.
- Professionals are concerned with providing services to people rather than producing inanimate goods.
- The social status of professionals tends to increase as a function of length of training required to practice.
- Professions have a distinctive place in the class system, because their opportunities for income derive from their knowledge and qualifications and they claim a specialist knowledge about the service they provide.

At the heart of the 'professional project' is a belief that professionals need to strive both economically and socially. The services that professionals provide are characteristically different from the goods that are sold by a manufacturer or a retailer, in that they are intangible and the purchaser has to take them on trust (Macdonald, 1995). The growing number of people working in professional, managerial and administrative occupations has been related to the importance of large-scale public, private, voluntary and third sector organisations both in the United Kingdom (UK) and elsewhere. It has also been connected with the expanding numbers of people working in sectors of the economy where the state plays a major role – for example, in government, health and social welfare, education and criminal justice.

Main theoretical perspectives

The following represent examples of the main theoretical perspectives used as a basis for developing an analytical framework for understanding both the policy and practice dimensions relating to how professionals develop their identity. In this chapter and Chapter 5 different disciplinary-based perspectives are outlined briefly, for example from sociology, social policy, economics and management. The intention is not to impose an artificial ordering but to capture aspects of the manner in which the notion of professionalism has become defined in contemporary practice. It begins with reference to some leading sociological thinkers.

Neo-Durkheimian

Structural, functionalist accounts, which see professions as a static/stable social stratum that offer a socially cohesive role, a disinterested integrative social function.

Taking the neo-Durkheimian perspective asks of the professional questions such as 'in performing your role how far do you prioritise being disinterested, dispassionate and bringing cohesion, unity or integration to your work?' The background UK historical context is located within the welfare state, whose focus and direction became structured by a commitment to two modes of coordination: bureaucratic administration and professionalism. This welfare state was a professional state: it depended on professionals both for the expertise needed to formulate policy and to deliver that policy, thereby underscoring the interdependence of professions, the state and the public (Moran, 2004: 31).

Durkheim thought of the increasing struggle for existence, which accompanied the growth of material and moral density and of social volume, as necessitating a greater division of labour. Improved productive capacity was seen as a consequence of specialisation in response to generated social needs. He was particularly clear about the tendencies of modern industry: 'it advances steadily towards powerful machines, towards greater concentrations of forces and capital, and consequently to the extreme division of labour. Occupations are infinitely separated and specialised' (Durkheim, 1966: 39). For Durkheim the nearest approach to accommodating an increasing specialisation of economic activities was through 'syndicates', composed of either employers or workmen, though he is careful to observe that this was only a rather formless and rudimentary beginning of occupational organisation (Turner and Hodge, 1970: 20). He was concerned to emphasise that the division of labour provided a basis for cooperation and interdependence and has been subjected to serious criticism for an overemphasis on social integration generally. Nevertheless, he neither ignored the analysis of conflict and competition, and recognised a distinction between a minimum necessary cooperation and total cooperation (Durkheim, 1966).

Professions continue to play a pivotal role in the concepts of welfare states and their transformation to service-driven societies, which are characterised on the whole by an expansion of expert knowledge and professionalism. From an historical perspective the rise of professionalism and the emergence of 'professional projects' are characteristic of civic societies (Bertilsson, 1990). Strong state intervention is needed to ensure at least health, housing, education, training and social security for all workers, research and power for industry and infrastructure for transport, local government and other forms of spatial and social democratic integration to allow all aspects to work together. The ideological difference is not the intervention, which is functionally indispensable, but the underlying values: in the conservative model the social integration is hierarchical, while the social democratic model is egalitarian.

The developing welfare states had a vital interest in the expansion of professional projects. For instance, as they promised access to social services for the citizens, they had to provide and expand the markets for professionalised work. From the public's perspective these services offered by the professions became a gauge for the success of the attempts of welfare states to translate the concept of social citizenship into the practice of social services. The mindset around social services represents a generational perception contrasting earlier and later post-Second World War expectations and was deeply ingrained with the creation of local authority social services departments (Seebohm Report 1968), when personal social services grew to be more embedded in British culture (Sainsbury, 1977). Both the economic and social order then became less about production and more about consumption, and the emergent professional classes responded actively to new opportunities to serve varied and wide-ranging public interests.

A depiction of the positive qualities of professions was labelled, in sociological terms, the 'trait' approach, where individual professions were categorised and their work described fairly uncritically. One of the principal reasons why the trait theorists (such as Etzioni, 1969; Toren, 1972) identified nursing, social work, teaching and the remedial professions as 'semi-professions' was that they did not appear to have developed dominance in discrete areas of knowledge. Despite the considerable growth of the caring professions, substantially based on claims to knowledge and skills, they would not satisfy this criterion (Hugman, 1991). An alternative view is that 'professional attributes are the symptom and not the cause of an occupation's standing' (Howe, 1986: 96). For instance, the term 'professional' implies competence, efficiency, altruism and integrity. An equally uncritical account of professions was that of 'structural functionalists' (for example, Parsons, 1939; Goode, 1957; Marshall, 1939), who tended to view the professions as a stratum of society providing a socially cohesive role. Notions of public service as a set of values, a code of behaviours and forms of practice became institutionalised, granting a position of considerable privilege that historically has had to be earned. According to Goode (1969), many of the characteristics that have been proposed are derivative, the two core characteristics in his view being a lengthy period of training in a body of abstract knowledge and a strong service orientation. Elsewhere (Goode, 1957) he described the characteristics of a professional community as a sense of identity associated with shared values, an agreed role definition, a common technical language and a recognition that the professional group has power over its members.

Barber (1963: 670–2) looked for characteristics of professionalism that might be regarded as having greater functional relevance for the relationship of professional to client or for society generally. He identified four such characteristics: a high degree of systematic knowledge, orientation to community interest, control through a code of ethics emanating from a voluntary association, and a system of rewards that is primarily a set of symbols of work achievement. Interactionist perspectives are similarly relevant to such integrative accounts, seeing professionalism as a function of a dialogic process between a person's self-identification and their interactions with others. For example, the interface between the social work profession and nursing is characterised by status, unclear boundaries and public perceptions of the social work task (Wilmot 2003: 94).

Neo-Weberian

Frameworks that emphasise professions developing strategies to advance their own social status, persuade clients/potential clients about the need for the service they offer, and corner the market in that service and exclude competitors. This concept acknowledges two main directions: social closure and professional dominance (Rogers and Pilgrim 2014: 108–9).

Max Weber acknowledged that 'members of positively privileged acquisition classes are typically entrepreneurs', and that these included 'members of the "liberal" professions with a privileged position by virtue of their abilities or training, and workers with special skills commanding a monopolistic position, regardless of how far they are hereditary or the result of training' (Eldridge, 1971: 89, quoting from Weber, *Social Stratification and Class Structure* (1949)). Examples of social classes included 'the intelligentsia without independent property and the persons whose social position is primarily dependent on technical training such as engineers, commercial and other officials, and civil servants, (and that) these groups may differ greatly among themselves, in particular according to costs of training' (Eldridge, 1971: 90). Notably relevant to understanding Weber's stance on the cultural development of professions was his concept of 'social status' (*Standische Lage*). This applied:

> to a typically effective claim to positive or negative privilege with respect to social prestige so far as it rests on one or more of the following bases: (a) mode of living, (b) a formal process of education which may consist in empirical or rational training and the acquisition of the corresponding modes of life, or (c) on the prestige of birth, or of an occupation....A social 'stratum' stand is a plurality of individuals who, within a larger group, enjoy a particular kind and level of prestige by virtue of their position and possibly also claim certain special monopolies. (Eldridge, 1971: 91)

Social closure

A neo-Weberian framework argues for the predominance of material interests, introducing technical qualifications as characteristic and a basis for professional promotion. Professions were seen as under pressure to systematise their knowledge and thereby make it potentially accessible to lay members of society. A revived version of Weber's ideas centre on the importance of qualifications and expertise as well as property as opportunities for income in a market society. At the heart is a need to understand the meanings and motives of actors who operate in this way – by cornering the market, professionals offer a service that is closed off from others. It follows that it is important to study the motives and meanings of individuals and their embodiment in a professional project. Society is to be seen as individuals pursuing their interests, and this activity generates more or less collectively conscious groups, seen as the representatives or practitioners of ideas that legitimate the pursuit of their interests. Social groups engage in social closure in the course of furthering their interests, and they attempt both to exclude others from their group and to usurp the privileges of other groups.

According to Weber, their knowledge and qualifications give professions a significance on a par with those whose class position derives from either their capital or their labour power. The collective actions of groups can usefully be conceptualised as a strategy of social closure. In the economic order, the professional project is pursued in two main areas: the legal closure and monopolisation of the market and the occupation; and the exclusive acquisition of the knowledge and education on which the profession is based. The professional project is an 'ideal type' (Weber, 1978: 342), and the phrase acknowledges that the ideal type contains elements that are more or less present and occasionally absent. Weber uses the concept of professionalisation as an analytical tool, which includes examining attributes of professional behaviour – how formal training is established, how political activity leads to legally controlled licensing and certification, and how a formal code of ethical practice is developed.

Social closure cannot exist unless it is believed that the particular tasks that a profession performs are so different from those of most workers that self-control is essential. For instance, professionals internalise their work, their modus operandi, and continually make judgements about when, where and how to intervene. This has led to an inherent moral and ethical creed defining their behaviour. Integrity is demonstrated by how tasks become learned, based on standards that individuals internalise to perform a set task effectively, embedded most cogently in ways of mentoring and offering higher-level work supervision.

Features relating to social closure include monopoly, self-regulation, indispensability, self-importance, along with possessing high value and having high rank/status. Monopoly is essential to professionalism, as is freedom of judgement or discretion in performing work, both being intrinsic qualities; this constituting an antithesis to a 'managerialist' model, opposed to freedom of judgement, and asserting that organisational efficiency improves through minimising discretion (see, for example, Clarke and Newman, 1997; McKimm and Phillips, 2009; Alvesson, 2013).

In order for professionals to maintain their social status, they must convince those outside their boundaries that they are offering a unique service, and so they develop various rhetorical devices to persuade the world at large of their special qualities (high quality of care based on individual qualification; mystique of expert knowledge and self-importance; manipulation of the media). To do this they must justify a peculiar knowledge base that has a technical or scientific rationality on the one hand, but on the other is not so easy to understand that anybody can use it. Medicine as a whole can be seen to provide such accounts to the world. However, this persuasion is precarious, taking the example of alternative medicine and psychiatry, with regard to their coherence and credibility of scientific knowledge.

Exclusionary patterns of professionalism are characterised by hierarchical, bureaucratic patterns of self-regulation and self-administration: 'tribalism' and occupational closure; claims for 'autonomy' and self-determined decision-making; identity construction based on 'belonging' to a professional community; an expert–lay divide; and, specifically within the context of delivering health and social care, a gendered division of the workforce. For example, although within the UK there may have been evidence of a breakdown of tight gender divisions in the NHS, in social care a pervasive pattern of de-professionalisation as a result of poor working conditions has become particularly noticeable owing to its associated gender pay gap along with the feminisation of care work (Gray and Birrell, 2013; Manthorpe, 2002).

Professional dominance

It is often the case that a profession is controlled by its elite membership, which attempts to establish an order that limits competition through formal monopolies (Weber, 1978). Weber constructs 'a continuum of recurrent social action, on which such phenomena as "usage", "custom", "convention" and "law" can be placed. A "law" presupposes that there is a "staff of people", whose members will use "physical or psychological coercion" if some sanction deviates from the prescribed course' (Swedberg, 1998: 84). Exclusionary closure is the exercise of power in a downwards direction and is primarily concerned with the definition of the membership in such a way as to exclude those whom the professional body and its elite regard as 'ineligibles' (Parkin, 1979). The occupational quest is for a monopoly in the market for services based on their expertise, and for status in the social order as Weber terms it. Weber traced the development of hierarchy as a diffuse social form to its influence on industrial society as a model for the organisation of large social groups. Hierarchy is frequently portrayed as a technical solution to the separation of design and execution of work tasks. Expertise, normally subsumed as a criterion of professionalism, is interpreted to mean the technical competence that Weber concluded was the basis of bureaucratic efficiency (Weber, 1966).

Professionals have power over their clients; the latter, convinced of the need for the service they are offered or seek, are dependent on professionals. An imbalance of specialised knowledge keeps the client in a state of ignorance, insecurity and vulnerability. This power balance is reinforced if the professional operates on their own territory rather than that of their client, for example by treating people in hospital rather than their own home (Rogers and Pilgrim, 2014: 109). The development of professional specialisms, associated with the middle rather than the working class, led to the coming of the expert and the technician. The new occupational professions emerged, some evolving from the old status professions, for example bone-setters into orthopaedists, domestic workers into trained nurses, almoners into social workers, lawyers into advocates (Dingwall and Lewis, 1983; Freidson, 2001: 18–35). The few intellectual occupations trained in the medieval universities, the original status professions (Elliott, 1972) of law, medicine, the ministry and university teaching, expanded in size and were either transformed or split up into separate disciplines. This development towards so-called esoteric knowledge, typifying specialisation, ingrained the separation of professionals from their client base.

Taking accountancy as an example of a 'professional project' (Macdonald, 1995: 187–204), as the economic world became increasingly complex and the legislation required to regulate it followed suit, professional practice came to entail an esoteric collection of areas of knowledge. Accountancy includes a basic skill of bookkeeping, auditing and legal provisions, and provides services in the fields of taxation, insolvency and bankruptcy. To become a knowledge-based occupation, it was necessary to assemble, define and isolate a particular cognitive domain to which it could restrict access, and in the journey towards professionalisation the difficulty in defining the occupation, its jurisdiction and its knowledge base was one of the stumbling blocks that halted progress.

Professionals exercise power over their new recruits – thus a dominance hierarchy is common in professions, with senior practitioners and trainers exercising control and discipline over their juniors. Power enjoyed in the upper ranks of a profession can only be secured by submission and deference in early junior days, as trainees are dependent on their superiors for career progression (Rogers and Pilgrim, 2014: 109). This may not apply as much today in both public sector and private organisations where a culture of managerialism is predominant. Here career progression may become more dependent on the whims and persuasions of general managers rather than senior professionals acknowledged for their expertise and experience of working within a specific discipline. Cultural work to establish the legitimacy of their practice must set about 'producing the producers' (Larson, 1977: 71); that is, ensuring that all future entrants have passed through an appropriate system of selection, training and socialisation, and been turned out in a standardised professional mould. This will involve the attempt, at least, to control the educational input and is closely connected to the development, definition and monopolisation of professional knowledge.

Professionals seek to establish a dominant relationship over other occupational groups working with the same clients. They may seek to exclude existing equal competitors or they may seek to usurp the role of existing superiors. In medicine, in addition to excluding competitors, they also subordinate them (obstetricians directing the work of midwives) or limit their therapeutic powers to one part of the body, for example dentistry or optometry (Rogers and Pilgrim, 2014: 109). The profession pursues its 'professional project' where there are other actors in the field. Relations with them may have both market and status consequences and none is more fateful than those with the state, with whom a regulative bargain must be struck (Abbott, 1988; Cooper and Law, 1995). The occupation must also have dealings, sometimes cooperative, sometimes competitive, with other occupations in and around their potential jurisdiction and with educational institutions. Both may have impact on the course of the professional project. The new occupational professions grew, some evolving from the old status professions, some from the informal economy or major developments in social policy, for example educational psychology, health visiting and youth work. In social work, a professional hierarchy of training as applied to different contexts arose with therapeutic case-work as the gold standard compared with residential work, day care and domiciliary work.

The pursuit of professional dominance may be achieved through discretionary specialisation, involving tasks where direction or fresh judgement must often be exercised if they are to be performed successfully. Different occupational groups may offer different solutions to problems. A dominance over other occupational groups is created by recognising an overarching expertise to the task at hand, which, no matter how narrow, minute or detailed, requires a broad knowledge of the current evidence to discover what type of intervention will likely produce the best outcome. The tasks and their outcome are believed to be so indeterminate as to require attention to the variation to be found in individual cases. Inevitably, such tasks will almost certainly engage in some routines that can be quite mechanical. It follows that there needs to be an added sensitivity to the necessity of altering routine for individual circumstances that require discretionary judgement and action. Such work has the potential for innovation and creativity, thus distinguishing it from mechanical work (Freidson, 2001: 19). The two most general ideas underlying professionalism are the belief that certain work is so specialised as to be inaccessible to those lacking the required training and experience, and the belief that it cannot be standardised, rationalised or, as Abbott (1991: 22) puts it, 'commodified'. These distinctions are the foundation of the social processes that establish the social and economic status of professional work.

With regard to reflecting on personal identity, an individual will likely choose to focus on specialist knowledge and expertise, as this relates to belonging to a group possessing a kind of monopoly of resources in the paid-work environment. Such a mindset touches on how far one sees oneself as belonging to an interest group or professional community, and therefore in competition with other occupations for business, contract work and the like. Moreover, the perspective is characterised by its consideration of how far individuals believe that their identity has become shaped experientially and incrementally through performing different roles.

Neo-Marxist

Frameworks with a focus on power relations where professionals fit into a social structure characterised by two main groups: those who work to produce wealth in society and those who own the means of production and exploit these workers, expropriating surplus value as profits.

The Marxian sociology of the professions is chiefly concerned with two problems: professions in relation to the state and the proletarianisation of professional occupations. For example, social workers would be seen in a contradictory position, as being both agents of social control acting on behalf of the capitalist state and employees of that state – and so vulnerable to the same problems of any group of workers. Upholding a Marxian tradition of analysis, Oppenheimer (1975) claims that the knowledge-based professions have had control over their work eroded by the state bureaucracies that employ them since they have been subjected to 'bureaucratic subordination' (p 115). As a result, their control over their specialised skills has diminished (de-skilling), and consequently they have become part of the working class (proletarianisation). Gough (1979) highlights the contradictory position of professionals in capitalist society – they are not capitalists but they serve the interests of the latter. There is little controversy over the role of professions as mediators between the state and its citizens. Their employment is in the gift of state-funded services, now all too often privately outsourced. With private companies having taken over large chunks of public services in the UK, many professionals have been co-opted to swell the entrepreneurial ranks and have complemented their professional practice for example by engagement in lucrative roles at private health care firms (Jones 2014). The Report Inquiry on the Mid-Staffordshire NHS Trust (Francis, 2013), which focused on 'doing the system's business – not that of patients', offers evidence to illustrate that power lies in a cult of managerial ideology.

Saks's account of the neo-Marxist perspective upholds the notion that our understanding of professions should be based on the relations of production, rather than the relations of the market, as he regards the activities of professional occupations as being either partially or wholly tied to the interests of the bourgeoisie (Saks, 1995: 11–34). As the work of Braverman (1974), Carchedi (1975) and Poulantzas (1975) demonstrates, the precise nature of the linkage here depends on where the line of class cleavage is drawn between the bourgeoisie and the proletariat. The adherents of this more critical Marxist approach agree that professional groups in one way or another play a significant role as agents of capitalist control in contemporary Western society. Somewhat cynically, Marxist authors may view the public services ethos of professions 'as a convenient myth which conceals not simply occupational self-interests, but also the supervisory and disciplinary tasks that professional workers perform for the dominant capitalist class ' (Saks, 1995: 27). It seems fairly clear that the role of professions in Western industrial societies such as the UK and the United States

(USA) is largely compromised, assuming that the state, which has increasingly acted as a formal employer of professionals and effectively underwritten the privileges of professions, is relatively autonomous of any particular faction of capital but represents the long-term interests of the capitalist class as a whole. For structural Marxists, for example Saunders (1983), the prospect of professions ultimately functioning in anything but the long-term interests of the bourgeoisie is theoretically precluded. However, authors such as Abbott and Sapsford (1990), who accept the social control dimension of the operation of professions and deny professional altruism, do not see this as irrevocably linked to dominant class interests. Instead they view certain professions as acting more neutrally, as a moral agent, serving society's wider needs. Ultimately these assumptions need to be based on carefully formulated and empirically grounded argument.

This neo-Marxist framework emphasises power relations insofar as, for example, the origins of the notion of de-professionalisation are seen as based on ideas taken from Taylorism (or scientific management), which came to dominate managerial ideas about how best to control alienated labour (Edgell, 2012: 57–71). Braverman's 'de-skilling' thesis, focusing on the USA in the 20th century as the most advanced capitalist economy, draws upon Marx's theory of work on industrial capitalism in that he starts from the proposition that in such a society workers are constrained economically, by the absence of alternatives, to sell their labour to employers who are similarly constrained to seek a profit or go out of business. This is the capitalist mode of production, and at its core is the unequal relationship between employer and employee. Braverman's aim was to examine 'the manner in which the labour force is dominated and shaped by the accumulation of capital' (Braverman, 1974: 53). For example, schools and the teaching profession may thrive or fail dependent on the extent to which they are able to attract external support from local businesses and local finance to fulfil their educational ambitions. Power is just one of a number of topics that have been pursued in the sociology of the professions (Macdonald and Ritzer, 1988), and probably the most prominent of related theoretical approaches derive from Marx and from Foucault.

As Marxian sociology is primarily structuralist in nature, the explanation of what happens to the professions in these contexts is seen as the outcome of the workings of a society based on capitalist relations of production. For the working professional, questioning seeks to discover how far individuals see themselves as agents of social control and whether the outcomes or results of one's work might be seen through this lens. The state is a dominating partner in the narrative of professional development, and professionals may feel vulnerable because of perceiving themselves as state-dependent or state-constructed. In his discussion of professions, Johnson (1982: 188) emphasises the plurality of processes at work in modern society and the lack of coherence of the objectives of dominant groups and the state. He focuses on the 'processes of professionalisation' that are integral to state formation. Marx's materialist theory of human society, based on analysis of structure and system, demonstrates that the basis of stratification – and every other aspect of society – is to be found in the means of production and the relations of production that are based on them. It follows that state formation, polarisation of social classes and monopolisation of the means of production constitute processes in which the professions are bound up.

Relevant to this perspective is the idea that professionalism – as a mediator within the power nexus – can be regarded as a set of boundary-defining practices. For example, the practitioner may adopt a persona in which his or her emotions or prejudices are backgrounded and subordinated to the client's task in hand (Deverell and Sharma, 2000). This merging of identity becomes evident in the following framework, which centralises the notion that the mapping out of discourses occurs within an historical time-frame, and this impacts on the way in which certain professions, for example the medical profession and the social work profession, have become viewed by the state or by the public.

Summary

This chapter has set out some of the main frameworks used to study the work of professions from a classical sociology perspective. It is possible to compare and contrast individual disciplinary perspectives and apply them to a specific field of activity, for example teaching and education, delivering health and social care or criminal justice work. The perspectives can be used to understand and validate the work of professionals, and each framework may reflect a separate emphasis and contextual prism. As Rogers and Pilgrim (2014: 107) have concluded: 'When sociologists first began to investigate professionals they provided a set of rather flattering descriptions. This was because, by and large, they were prepared to accept definitions provided by professionals themselves.' These tended to emphasise that practitioners have unique skills, which are put altruistically at the service of the public, namely the trait definitional approach.

For many 'ordinary people' the word 'professional' still tends to imply both special skills and ethical propriety. It may imply competence, efficiency, altruism and integrity. Hence, the converse of this is the everyday notion of what it means to be 'unprofessional' – to behave incompetently, inefficiently or unethically. One academic writing on the subject of 'snobbery', describing it as becoming part of political discourse and responsible for building social divisions, refers to the 'professional and managerial elite of PME' as characteristically socially and culturally remote from the white working class (Morgan, 2019: 117). He poses the question 'why does the working class resent professionals but admire the rich?'. An answer given is that members of the working class are more relaxed about wealth, especially where it is seen as the outcome of hard work. This type of ideology states that the rich are wealth creators: it is sometimes difficult to appreciate what some professionals do or what they contribute to the national economy (Morgan, 2019: 117).

The neo-Durkheimian framework stresses disinterestedness, bringing cohesion and implies commitment to welfare state values or similar and particular codes of behaviour, whereas the neo-Weberian framework emphasises social closure, where professionals develop strategies to advance their own status, place a premium on specialist expertise and show a concomitant desire to corner the market for that service. Another feature of this model, professional dominance, focuses on how professionals exercise power over others, for example over clients, new recruits and other occupational groups where there is competition for serving a particular client group. The neo-Marxist model tends to focus on the web of power relations that underpins professional relationships, including that which a profession holds with the state, which traditionally may have been a main employer or commissioner of professional activity. This account stresses the proletarianisation of professional occupations where there is manifestly a clear dependency on the contract with the state. The professional project, however, remains rather loosely circumscribed within this power nexus:

> The debate for example between Marxian and Weberian sociologists on the nature of social class, hinges to an important extent on the former's insistence that Marx was correct to give social production a unique position in sociological explanation, and that capitalism has an inherent tendency to monopoly, which enables the owners of the means of production to dominate all markets and therefore

society. Weber's definition of capitalism, on the other hand, emphasises a number of features – rationality, the capitalist spirit (or enterprise) and formally 'free' markets in capital, labour, goods, services and raw materials; and it does not suggest that the owners of the means of production necessarily 'exploit' or achieve monopolistic positions in any of these. (Macdonald, 1995: 36)

5

Perspectives used in studying professions: social policy and public administration

Introduction

The sociology of professions makes an important contribution to the study of stratification – more important than is often realised (Macdonald and Ritzer, 1988). A reason for this is that the professions started to appear in their present form contemporaneously with modern capitalist industrial society. As modern society is knowledge-based, professions as knowledge-based occupations, are an integral part of, for example, how the modern class system developed. A further reason is that the professional project has the market as one of its main themes, and it has become an aphorism that modern, industrial, capitalist society is a *market* society.

Structuralist accounts of disciplinarity define the discipline or perspective as a framework for understanding and interpreting information and experience, for judging the validity and adequacy of solutions to problems by defining what is acceptable, appropriate and useful. Structural views tend to focus not least on how human agency is constrained by influences external to the individual. In the structuralist scenario, disciplinary change is resisted unless it is in approved directions and influence appears unidirectional: the community is shaped by the discipline (Lattuca, 2001: 24).

In contrast a post-structuralist perspective directs attention to the community, portraying the discipline as a heterogeneous social system composed of individuals with varying commitments to ideas, beliefs and methodologies, and to interaction among those individuals. By focusing on the communal construction of meaning, the existence of multiple perspectives and the linkage of individual perspectives to social processes, post-structuralism replaces the idea of a structure with the more fluid concept of a space in which persons and ideas exist in relation to one another. Because meanings are seen as socially constructed, disciplines are sites of ontological, epistemological, methodological tensions, and these tensions animate structures such as subject matter and methods (Lattuca, 2001: 25). The structural perspective abstracts underlying frameworks that are believed to define a phenomenon, for example how a profession has evolved; or to define a belief system, for example how individuals construct their identity. A post-structural approach eschews abstraction and attends to the local and the particular, which are time and context bound.

Post-structuralist/social constructionism

> This perspective demonstrates power as dispersed and not simply located in any elite group, involving mapping out discourses associated with particular social periods and places. Social constructionism involves meaning and interpretation, and what we claim when labelling something as mental illness or child abuse – socially constructed or naming of pre-existing phenomena?

Drawing on more than one theoretical tradition since it can be defined as a school of thought selecting doctrines from various schools, this perspective is eclectic. Post-structuralism goes beyond eclecticism in framing the significance of professionalism as a core concept; seeing the notion of professions or a professional project as a social construction created through human interaction with other people and the natural world. It embraces a form of social constructionism that involves naming, even inventing 'kinds'; but once constructed or invented has real consequences, in the enabling and constraining of behaviour, for those so named (Williams, 2016: 208). For example, this framework poses the question 'Is your power/authority in the work-place defined more by your professional expertise than by the organisation or by both?'

Similarly, the 'mapping out of discourses associated with a specific time period' (Derrida, 1978) becomes pertinent to understanding the changing role and attitude of the state towards different professions. One of the main intellectual leaders of this tradition is Foucault (for example, 1965, 1973 and 1980), who considered that social analysis entailed examining a 'heterogenous ensemble consisting of discourses, institutions, architectural forms, regulatory decisions, laws, administrative measures, scientific statements, philosophical, moral and philanthropic propositions – in short the said and the unsaid' (1980: 44).

Let's take two examples of this notion of mapping out discourses: the role of politics towards the medical establishment at the inauguration of the National Health Service (NHS) in 1948 (collectivism) and the framing of the United Kingdom (UK) Health and Social Care Act 2013 (neo-liberalism). For the first it was clear that doctors became recognised as a professional elite on the inauguration of the NHS, with the state choosing to act as their protector. The profession gained significantly during this period: 'the medical technocrats seeking to maximise the opportunities to deploy the tools of medical science played a leading role' as '[Minister of Health] Bevan paid a heavy price in terms of concessions made to buy off opposition, both from consultants and local government' (Klein, 2010: 19–20). This enmeshes with a contemporary state of affairs during the period we call 'austerity' where, owing to a perceptible imminent collapse of the NHS along with social care, particular professional groups such as nurses and midwives take on a centre-ground media and political focus as the Conservative government moves to win them over (Elgot et al, 2018). The government decides to intervene in a 'protector' role by introducing measures to increase recruitment and retention, offering higher pay to these professions so that services are not mothballed – 'beds unused due to insufficient staff' (Campbell, 2018h).

The second example chosen in which mapping out discourses becomes a useful device for understanding how professions are viewed in the policy-making process is apparent through documenting how knowledge becomes manufactured and therefore real for civil servants in a study of their behaviour in the framing of the Health and Social Care Act 2013. In a detailed empirical analysis of the policy-making process, the argument is made that the received view of professionals applying formal knowledge acquired in professional criteria was both misguided and misleading (Maybin, 2016). Instead a contrasting view of the work of professionals, and in particular civil servants, who are arguably more important in policy-making, presents a scenario containing a different mode of information and knowledge gathering.

This entails an ongoing flow of knowing, practical, situated, interactive and embodied, that emerges out of organisational practices – structures of meanings, rules, routines, competences, materials, spatial arrangements and affects – that make government organisations tick. In this example policy-making becomes the result of a process of building connections between a policy in development and powerful ideas, people and instruments, revealing the 'policy know-how' required by civil servants to be effective in their jobs. 'Civil servants worked to interpret what might make sense, given what they knew about current political agendas and existing policy commitments, the guiding principle was one of coherence with known agendas and commitments' (Maybin, 2016: 118).

The Whig narrative – as applied to the development of the welfare state

Mapping out discourses in order to identify the position and 'lived in' experience of a professional group is in some ways consistent with a conventional Whig interpretation of history approach (Butterfield, 1931), which centres on the notion that historians are moulded by the environment of the time and place. In the 19th and early 20th century, the course of history was viewed as a demonstration of the principle of progress, expressing the ideology of a society in a condition of remarkably rapid progress. After the First World War, historians such as Toynbee (1948), Berlin (1954) and Carr (1964) made a desperate attempt to replace a linear view of history with a cyclical theory – the characteristic ideology of a society in decline – claiming that there is no general pattern in history at all. Sociology as the science of society was a response to this growing complexity to understand events. In a similar fashion it is said that Butterfield denounced the Whig interpretation 'in a sparkling invective although lacking precision and detail' (Carr, 1964: 19–20) stating that it studies the past without reference to the present. For example, an analysis that examines empirical evidence of the inauguration of the NHS and the respective roles of different actors along with claims that they are working towards progressive ends may refute any assessment of contemporary events that appears to undermine this claim. Butterfield asserted that this kind of interpretation was therefore 'unhistorical' (Butterfield, 1944: 2–5).

In the context of the development of welfare states, in Britain and elsewhere, the general character of social services has been described recently as witnessing a consistent theme of marked 'disruption' (Martinelli et al, 2017). It is claimed that 'disruption' has been caused by public sector disengagement and the recent tendency to adopt market elements and commercial logics in the design and distribution of social services. Applying the Whig narrative lens, Matzke (Martinelli et al: 376–90) states that the normative core of a 'social citizenship-based, progressive agenda' identifies undesirable traits in recent developments of social service fields. To recall, this social citizenship perspective, led originally by Marshall (1950), stipulates entitlement to a minimum standard of social care, if needed, as a privilege that comes with citizenship; as a membership right. Such a conception of social rights insists on the importance of the public sector in supplying and financing social services rights as complementary features, not alternatives, to a notion of social rights that would focus on redistribution and income transfers.

Most evidence suggests that there is a lot of trust in the professionalism and expertise of public sector employees (Hood, 1995) and an overall positive appraisal of the long-term historical trajectory of publicly provided service infrastructures and social benefits. Steinmetz (1993) labels this perception of social policy improvement a Whig narrative of the welfare state. In historical perspective, the 'darker' side of early social policy intervention has not gone unnoticed, and many historiographic accounts have pointed out the repressive nature of local poor relief and institutional regimes (Townsend, 1962; Morris, 1969; Rose, 1971; Jones, 1972; Fraser, 1973; Barham, 1992; Scull 1979). Emancipation and professional development, along with broadened access and dropping many of the old poor-relief lineages have been the building blocks of a story of social service modernisation often told. This scenario occasionally appears to form the backdrop against which the late 20th-century transformation – from public service to public management – is eyed with reservation. Some observers have been worried about a decline of professional norms and public service ethos (Noordegraaf, 2014 ; Hupe et al, 2015), others have been critical of possible repercussions of market logics for quality and availability of social services, and still others fear new forms of exclusion or a new 'welfare paternalism' (Clarke and Newman, 1997; Garrett, 2018) to result from marketisation and managerialism.

This summary gives an insight into an historical narrative that aims to demonstrate the evolution and direction of how a particular profession becomes symbolised through an enactment of the principle of progress – sometimes expressed as the unfolding of an ideology as, for instance, in increasing our understanding of the notion of 'collectivism' (Heywood, 2000: 121). The Whig interpretation had a close affinity with the more well-known economic doctrine of laissez-faire, also 'the product of a serene and self-confident outlook on the world, that the facts of history were themselves a demonstration of the supreme fact of a beneficent and apparently infinite progress towards higher things' (Carr, 1964: 21). The reconstitution of the past in the historian's mind is dependent on empirical evidence, and the process of reconstitution governs the selection and interpretation of the facts, in other words what makes them historical facts. Replacing a linear view of history with a cyclical theory is evident in the work of a more contemporary writer, Snyder (2018: 1–94), who has eyed the current American and European socio-economic scene by contrasting the 'politics of inevitability' with the 'politics of eternity'. He writes: 'those swayed by inevitability see every fact as a blip that does not alter the overall story of progress; those who shift to eternity classify every new event as just one more instance of a timeless threat' (p 44).

This is relevant to the present argument as it questions whether 'mapping out discourses' according to time and place is consistent with a positive transformational approach, by highlighting the changing outcomes of a profession's continuous dialogue with the state as seeking recognition of embedment and progress. The inevitability perspective prioritises the contextualisation of time and place in understanding how a profession advances its course. Snyder describes a dysfunctional state as a provider – education, pensions, healthcare, transport and other forms of social assistance – as a logical outcome of the neo-liberalist economy following the financial crisis of 2008, where deregulation of campaign contributions in the United States in 2010 magnified the influence of the wealthy and reduced that of voters. The politics of eternity takes over: 'As economic inequality grew, time horizons shrank, and fewer (Americans) believed that the future held a better version of the present. Lacking a functional state that assured basic social goods, citizens lose a sense of the future, with a stabilisation of massive inequality' (Snyder, 2018: 38).

Following the analogy, just as inevitability promises a better future for everyone, the politics of eternity places one nation at the centre of a cyclical story of victimhood. 'Time is no longer a line into the future, but a circle that endlessly returns the same threats from the past' (Snyder, 2018: 46). In the politics of eternity, no one is responsible because we all know that the enemy is coming no matter what we do. Eternity politicians spread the conviction that the state/government cannot aid society as a whole, but can only guard against threats. In contrast to the inevitability paradigm, Snyder concludes that no one is responsible because we all know that the details will sort themselves out for the better. The eclectic/post-structural framework recognises that power is dispersed, is not concentrated in any elite group and is not tempered by the actions of the state in the way the latter perceives the practices and functions of any given professional group. Hegemony equals the struggle for influence and is no guarantee that progress is inevitable, although perhaps we may become more optimistic owing to rationalism, humanism and technology (see for instance Gramsci, 1971; Fukuyama, 1989).

Mapping out discourses – as applied to directions in community care policy

The notion of discursive practices characterises an account without endorsement of any self-conscious collective activity of professionals, who are advancing their own interests or acting for example on behalf of the state (Rogers and Pilgrim, 2014: 111). Professions may emerge, advance or retract dependent on a range of technological, financial and cultural considerations and on the existence of certain policy conditions that augur a need for urgent reform. Taking the example of the development of the community care policy in the UK, which began during the latter half of the 20th century, it has become clear how financial cuts to services may have reversed, possibly permanently, any progressive trend to provide social justice for those vulnerable individuals targeted as beneficiaries of that policy. The reforms that were introduced at the end of the 1980s, leading to the NHS and Community Care Act 1990, expanded the idea of needs-led or community-led planning. The crisis in funding and the curtailment of local government financial autonomy, as well as how policy created opportunities to shift the burden of responsibility for care from the state to the individual, gradually illustrated how professional practitioners and their employing organisations would become faced with a number of dilemmas (Malin, 1997).

Whereas it seems now to be the case that most providers, for example NHS commissioning groups, say that their priority is to provide 'high quality care packages that are safe, clinically appropriate and meet people's needs' (Ryan, F., 2018: 24) an expanding body of evidence shows that this has not been possible, and a resulting decline in standards marks a return to a past era of institutionalisation (Flynn, 2012; CQC, 2016b; Leonard Cheshire Disability Organisation, 2016). Over the past 40 years campaigners have fought for the basic right of vulnerable citizens to independent living and care in the community, against a long-standing prejudice that treats disabled people as children to be cared for or dehumanises them as objects to be put away. The independent living movement in the UK has fought for disabled people to be seen as ordinary adults, with the same rights to fundamental freedoms as anyone else (Evans, 2003). But as austerity measures have kicked in, such progress has been increasingly under threat, and the question is then asked whether the clock is turning back (F. Ryan, 2018). Losing the right to live independently, and with care packages slashed, entering a nursing home or being 'interned' in a care home sometimes appears to be the only option.

The policy, and indeed practices, associated with the provision of community care to vulnerable citizens might hence be labelled as a kind of discursive practice where power does not lie within the boundaries of any elite or professional group. To some extent the forces behind the policy have gone out of control, as it has become shaped by the financial politics of the time. It is a reaction, not a pro-action, to outside events, and lacking of any self-conscious collective activity of any professional group to advance its own interests. Although at one level we may be currently witnessing a crisis in social care, this interplay of events may have created an opportunity for the evolution of a more professionalised social care workforce as a protector of the rights of vulnerable people.

What has been indicated as a post-structuralist perspective was embodied at a theoretical level in the work of Foucault (1973, 1980), for example. A key characteristic has been to deny the possibility of universal explanation – 'incredulity towards meta-narratives' (Mambrol, 2016) – which includes both philosophical positions, for example, the 'isms' previously alluded to in this chapter, along with economic theories such as Keynesianism. Foucault uses the term 'discourse', not just of language but of thought and action; and his ideas have appeal for the sociologist of the professions because his central concern was with the relationship between knowledge, power and authority.

Foucault's exposure of the power structures intended to control us and how power is used to control knowledge demonstrates that what authorities claim as scientific knowledge is really just a means of social control (controlling the mind is a more effective means of social control than punishing the body). Foucault (1980) considers that social analysis entails examining 'a heterogenous ensemble consisting of discourses, institutions, architectural forms, regulatory decisions, laws, administrative measures, scientific statements, philosophical, moral and philanthropic propositions – in short the said and the unsaid' (Rogers and Pilgrim, 2014: 110).

This perspective might ask of individual professionals whether they feel subjected to bureaucratic subordination; and as part of an eclectic/ post-structuralist critique, it then would go on to demonstrate power as dispersed and not simply located in any elite or otherwise non-elite group. Foucault's view is that the emergence of modern society was accompanied by an epistemic shift from a classic to a modern form of knowledge, which is organised into (scientific) disciplines. Power in modern societies does not depend on the prowess and prestige of individuals but is exercised through an impersonal administrative machinery operating in accordance with abstract rules. Individuals are constituted by power relations, power being the ultimate principle of social reality. Power should not be conceptualised as the property of an individual or class, not a commodity that may be acquired or seized, but rather it has the character of a network. The threads (of power) extend everywhere and equate to the processes by which subjects are constituted as effects of power. 'Power produces, it produces reality; it produces domains of objects and rituals of truths' (Foucault, 1977b: 27).

Foucault's reflections on psychiatry and medical knowledge (Foucault, 1965) deal with structured inequality and ideology, where he conceptualises the relationship between forms of applied knowledge and their external environment, and later between the constitution of professional expertise and the organisation of professions as social entities. In creating the myth of *true* community-based services, it is possible that the institution becomes dispersed rather than dismantled (Foucault, 1973; Scull, 1979). Much of Foucault's work, however, was concerned with the body and doctors' relation to it via what he calls 'the gaze' (*le regard medical*), so that it would be of more interest to sociologists of medicine and of health and illness (Bowling, 1995; Gomm and Davies, 2000; Barry and Yuill, 2016). Health care professions have had a central role in this regard with their interests in diagnosis, testing, assessment and observation, and the treatment, management and surveillance of sick and healthy bodies in society. As noted earlier, in the post-structuralist account there is a failure to endorse the notion of self-conscious collective activity of professionals to advance their own interests; instead the level of abstraction at which Foucault operates may be gauged from the terms he uses: 'Power derives its bases, justifications and rules to define subjection of man as an object of knowledge for a discourse with a scientific status' (Foucault, 1977b: 23).

Managerialism

A contemporary perspective relates to managerialism and the changing patterns of professional governance that are embedded in professional practices, and which are associated with demands for increased efficiency in the provision and delivery of services and greater responsiveness to user demands.

A social policy dimension is a feature of modern times, as governance is becoming increasingly embedded throughout professional practices to weigh up demands for efficiency, accountability and achieving more responsiveness to stakeholder and client groups. Social policy analysts reflect a broadening concern with both the theory as well as the practice of welfare and adopt a range of different theoretical perspectives (such as neo-liberalism, conservatism, feminism and social democracy), leading to different conclusions about the viability and desirability of different policy measures. A social policy framework therefore focuses on the organisation, delivery and evaluation of 'services' – health care, criminal justice, housing and the like. This framework also includes the need to understand the impact of partnership-working and inter-professionalism as a pragmatic response to progress policy initiatives and the role of methodology in measuring varying social needs, along with other dimensions of organisational culture, for example modes of leadership, how to manage change and how to maintain employee morale.

Scientific management was seen as a way for managers and owners of industrial production to control labour in order to increase the productivity of profit-based organisations (Taylor, 2003). This theoretical school therefore developed a narrow focus on the needs and concerns of management in industry. Taylorism emerged from this manufacturing production context, embodying principles of work organisation, notably the transfer of all discretion from workers to management and the fragmentation and simplification of tasks, including managerial control over the pace of work. It involves a mechanistic view of organisations: through time and motion studies and careful observation, specialised tasks could be set for workers to maximise productivity. Managers could better govern the organisation by using their secretive knowledge of goals and processes. Managers' first priority was productivity and setting goals, followed by other aspects of work culture, such as the well-being of workers. The theory of managerialism assumes that the interest of managers and workers are the same and that unions are unnecessary.

Those areas of employment that have remained relatively highly unionised have been the professions and public sector occupations (lawyers, doctors, teachers, civil servants), as opposed to what remains of the manufacturing sector. While those in certain professions – law, financial services, medicine, and the higher echelons of business – have seen their incomes rise markedly, even in the period of economic recession associated with the banking crisis of 2008, others in the lower reaches of the service sector, where employment patterns tend to be more casual, have fared less well (Ellison, 2009: 19–20). Managerialism, as part of an enormous architecture of performance management visible for example in hospitals, schools, community care, probation and legal services, is a trait shared across areas of public policy and is illustrative of a progressive shift away from a simple concern with policy outputs and a move towards policy outcomes (Newburn, 2012). This perspective is based on efforts to measure and compare governance arrangements and governance performance. Its key objective is to consider how governance frameworks can be translated into operational indicators, and how these might be used in decision-making processes (Savedoff and Smith, 2016: 85–104). There are significant challenges in measuring governance in all dimensions of the public sector, and typically the UK offers a fairly rudimentary framework for developing relevant metrics, based on the concepts of the structure, processes and outcomes of governance. Decentralisation, contractualisation and the competition of providers are key elements of framing social policies, nationally and locally, along with incentive structures (see, for example, DoH, 2010; DHSC, 2012; Health and Social Care Act, 2013; Care Act, 2014).

It has been claimed that power has shifted too far towards big business and managerial unitarism since 1979: 'politicians seduced by neoliberal economics have enabled the dominance of a financialised model of corporate governance serving short-term profitability and shareholder value, detrimental to even minimalist industrial democracy' (Dobbins and Dundon, 2017: 522). Public sector managerialism is perhaps not sympathetic to the demands and expectations of a workforce of trained, independent, self-actualising professionals. Increases in managerial control and the participation of service users mean that the classic exclusionary tactics of professions are no longer appropriate, resulting in a transformation towards more integrated and collaborative forms of service provision.

One impact of managerialism has been the creation of new agendas for accountability in organisations as a response to wider social policy trends and economic and political developments in service delivery, specifically within the realm of professional accountability. This issue looms large in services that are contracted out, and in many cases where accountability criteria are set by governments. For service providers, these are sometimes difficult to comprehend and unwieldy, and have therefore resulted in tragic consequences for clients and families in the delivery of services, such as in the areas of ageing, disability, homelessness and mental health, to mention only a few (Hughes and Wearing, 2017: 141–64).

From a critical point of view, key actors in service delivery such as politicians, the media and senior public servants are involved on a regular basis in attempts to gloss over and revamp the standard setting and performance accountability of social services. Politicians, for example, are clever at image-managing the perceptions of their policies, even to the point of lying and not seemingly being held to account for these deceptions. Media and official attention on social problems, such as child abuse, can manufacture incorrect and untruthful claims about the role of social work and its responsibilities... (Hughes and Wearing, 2017: 153).

The managerialism perspective seeks to understand whether changes taking place in individual professional practice have led to greater collaborative working among professional groups, also furthering an understanding of main barriers to inter-professional working. Introducing the notion of partnership-working as a management tool has created a methodology whereby different professionals have been increasingly asked to work together across traditional agency boundaries in order to solve social problems (Glasby and Dickinson, 2014). In the current mixed economy approach to delivering public services, individuals often become valued by the depth or range of their partnership, networking and teamwork activity across different sectors involved in public services. Similarly, at a political level, there has been merit in crafting partnerships with other organisations, such as citizen groups and non-governmental organisations. A common reason to care about the structure and strengthening of governance is policy failure. And for the managerialist framework, this may form the subject of a repeated pattern in which specific policy areas are proposed, and then fail owing to bad design, implementation, corruption, ineptitude or unforeseen consequences (Greer et al, 2016: 27).

A principal theme taken from a social policy/economics narrative lies in relation to evaluating the effectiveness of professional interventions within partnership-working. A number of research studies – for example, Sako (1992); Kramer (2006); Murphy (2006); Welter (2012) – have reviewed theories of transaction-cost economics, relational contract theory, alongside networks and management strategy, noting that there has been much theorising about intermediate (or network) modes of coordinating production in recent decades. Whether partnership-working means losing professional identity has become an important factor in analysing effects of managerialism; and building trust has been seen as crucial in achieving collaboration (Gambetta, 1988; Huxham and Vangen, 2005). Gambetta and colleagues review the idea of trust from the standpoint of different disciplines, considering how trust is variously regarded. A conclusion is that there is a fragility of trust in the context of social and political life. Dasgupta (1990) explores the role of trust in economic transactions and shows how rational agents may be expected to search actively for it. He demonstrates that trust is a peculiar resource that is increased, rather than depleted, through use.

Partnership-working usually occurs because there is a need to go beyond involving known individuals or professionals to invite wider representation and expertise. This may be because of government guidelines or because there is a realisation within the organisation that previous policies have been unsuccessful owing to limited resources or expertise (Charlesworth and Thorlby, 2012). Thinking about partnership-working raises difficult questions about the challenges of operating and managing collaboratively. For example, how does one lead a complex team made up of different professions and organisations and create shared aims and vision, when a particular financial model restricts control of the process?

Democratic or collaborative professionalism

This forms a perspective that seeks to demystify professional work and to forge alliances between professionals and excluded constituencies of patients, users, students, parents, voluntary and third-sector organisations and members of the wider community with a view to building a more democratic education, health care or criminal justice system and ultimately a more open society.

This framework involves being sensitive to a wide range of stakeholders, some of whose voices have traditionally been silent in decision-making (Whitty, 2008). Within lies a critique of managerialism as reactive, demanded or prescribed and insufficiently proactive or enacted (Leaton Gray, 2006). The framework requires individual professionals to conceive themselves as agents of change rather than victims of change; although some have argued that democratisation of the professions has diminished the intellectual leadership that professionals once provided (for example, Furedi, 2004a, b; Hammersley-Fletcher et al, 2018). Ironically, the managerialist attack on traditional modes of teacher professionalism has opened up new possibilities, for example the increasing recognition of the importance of the student voice in school decision-making (Fielding, 2004; Leren, 2006; Quaglia and Corso, 2014; Quinn and Owen, 2016).

This perspective extends the notion of accountability specifically insofar as it translates into a dilemma of how to maximise democratic surveillance or control. Corbett's (1991) framework for public sector accountability identifies four broad dimensions to organisational accountability in the human services. Such a framework raises questions about the conduct of professional practice, either directly or indirectly, in terms of upwards, downwards, inwards and outwards accountability processes and techniques (Hughes and Wearing, 2017: 154–6). This model acknowledges four dimensions: accountability to the government executive and parliament (upwards); accountability to the user, client and consumer, as in traditional community development and the managerial model (downwards); accountability to the organisation, which includes processes of internally-driven evaluations and internal audits (inwards); and accountability to the public, for instance by leaking certain information to media outlets, or 'whistle-blowing' (outwards). This framework raises certain tensions and dilemmas, such as how democratic and user-focused accountability mechanisms conflict with each other.

In professional practice, responsibility is a more all-embracing concept than accountability; as for example one can be accountable without taking responsibility, as in 'just doing our job'. We cannot, however, be responsible without demonstrating accountability; and this framework augurs a more robust foundation for pursuing a course of action based on democratic values underpinned by a broader constituency. Managerialist and consumerist approaches to public services stress individual values and downplay collective values such as social justice, fairness, proportionality, reducing discrimination and structural inequalities, and employee solidarity. Outsourcing and transforming methods of delivering public services may have removed some elements of direct democratic control. Each time that the UK central government has attempted to bring in a legal framework to shift public services out of direct control, there has been a parallel move to increase regulation. This tension between direct control of services and arms-length rule-making is an intrinsic feature of accountability (Gulland, 2012: 271–7).

Drawing on a political science paradigm, the concept of *social democracy* represents an ideological strand which endorses a reformed or 'humanised' capitalist system. This strand has roots in a previously outlined framework, namely neo-Durkheimian, which views professions as a stable force in society. Social democracy stands for a balance between the market and the state, a balance between the individual and the community. Its chief characteristic is a belief in reform within capitalism, underpinned by a general concern for the underdog in society, the weak and vulnerable (Heywood, 2000: 75).

The three traditional pillars of social democracy have been the mixed economy, economic management and 'the welfare state serving as a redistributive mechanism' (Heywood, 2000: 76). The Whig narrative perspective, as outlined earlier, encompassed the forward march of social democracy hand in hand with the long boom of the post–Second World War period , and when this came to an end, with the recession of the 1970s and 1980s, the underlying contradiction of social democracy (between maintaining capitalism and promoting equality) came to the surface. The prevailing view was that this tension resulted in a widespread abandonment of traditional social democratic positions and the adoption of more market-orientated values and policies (neo-liberalism).

Hierarchies, markets and networks are well-established 'models of coordination' or 'governing structures' with different co-ordinating mechanisms (Powell and Exworthy, 2002: 15). A political narrative for evaluating the course of professions at the turn of the 20th century became embedded through partnerships and quasi-markets as a key feature of New Labour's main operating code. This was seen to reject both state hierarchies, or the 'command and control' of Old Labour, and the market mechanisms of the previous Conservative government, favouring instead a Third Way of intermediate or network forms of organisation (see, for example, Giddens, 1998; Powell, 1999; White, 2001; Lewis and Surender, 2004). During this period many so-called partnership initiatives were marked by uncertainty of purpose: whether the aim was outcome-orientated (doing something that makes a difference, for example New Deal for Communities) or process -orientated (working in new ways to make a difference, for example Sure Start, Health Action Zones). This posed major practical problems for many professionals whose interventions were judged by a range of stakeholders in different ways.

To take the example of Sure Start Local Programmes, most were founded on the twin concepts of inter-professionalism and parental involvement. As regards the first, inter-professionalism recognised an imperative for different workers and expertise to collaborate to achieve a greater understanding of each other's roles, although often professionals simply had been exhorted to initiate multi-agency working with little training or guidance (Anning and Edwards, 1999). There emerged actual/potential conflicts for individuals working in multi-agency teams about models of understanding, about roles, identities, status and power, about information-sharing, and around links with other agencies (Campling and Payne, 2000; Freeman et al, 2000; Roaf, 2002; Nicholas et al, 2003; Robinson and Cottrell, 2005; Salmon and Rapport, 2005; Barr and Ross, 2006). Furthermore, it became clear that inter-professionalism itself had potentially confusing related concepts, since some research studies failed to differentiate between multi-, inter- and transdisciplinary ideas with regard to emphasis on sharing, collaboration, mentoring and transferring information and skills, seeing only the last of these as referring to true collaboration (Orelove and Sobsey, 1991; Leathard, 1994; Lacey, 2001; Edgley and Avis, 2006; Malin and Morrow, 2007, 2009).

The democratic or collaborative professionalism framework draws upon a social policy, managerialist approach in that it tends to rely on effective leadership to forge alliances between professionals and other constituents, groups and colleagues within the workplace. This has aimed to be a more evidence-based framework built on good practice, strong relationships, a rooted affirmation of the values of professionalism coupled with a critical understanding of the wider social context around which different workers operate. This can mean different priorities, different values and different aspirations across these groups. A leadership vision has become central to most professional practice, where effective leaders require the skills and confidence to shape culture in a positive direction, for instance by communicating a vision and avoiding tokenism. Interestingly, the notion of existential authenticity in leadership serving the people professions has been communicated by one author as a singularly important form of leadership in terms of promoting continuous professional development (Thompson, 2016).

A popular approach to leadership that has been the focus of much research since the early 1980s is the transformational approach. Transformational leadership has been described as part of a paradigm that gives more attention to the charismatic and affective elements of leadership, using emotional intelligence and other qualities such as modelling, inspiring a shared vision, building trust with others, offering rewards and promoting collaboration. Teamwork and cooperation are highly valued by these leaders; in short, they create environments where people can feel good about their work and how it contributes to the greater community. 'Managers are people who do things right and leaders are people who do the right thing' (Northouse, 2010: 2–12). Because of such factors as growing global influences and generational differences, leadership as it is exercised in a professional context will continue to have different meanings for different people (see also Bryman, 1992; Grint, 2005; Carpenter and Dickinson, 2008; Ladkin, 2010; Antonakis, 2011; Gill, 2011; Mackian and Simons, 2013; Schedlitzki and Edwards, 2014; Rickards, 2015;).

Professionals such as doctors, nurses, teachers and social workers have traditionally relied on self-regulation and professional standards to provide accountability to their fellow professionals. The role of self-regulatory bodies is to use peer or elite knowledge to ensure that the standards of the profession are maintained. However, pure self-regulation by the professions has come under increased pressure in recent years as trust in professionals has declined (Smith, 2004; Donaldson, 2006; Jay, 2014; Jones, 2014; Rogowski, 2016). This has led to an increase in independent or semi-independent regulatory bodies, covering professional practice and including more lay members as individual professionals increasingly become guardians of the public conscience. The effective realisation of inter- and multi-agency working has significant implications for future professional training and continuing professional development needs, and this represents one outcome from developing a model of democratic or collaborative professionalism. As such, a model has been initiated by managerial reforms that potentially offers individuals new professional opportunities. The result might be gained through achieving a balance between defining an individual's proper role and staking out the territory too rigidly alongside recognising the contribution of individual expertise as deployed differently in collaborative contexts.

Summary

The post-structuralist account demonstrates power as dispersed and not simply located in any elite group, but lying in administrative machinery, and focuses on key discourses or events associated with particular social periods and places as having a formative impact. Managerialism as a model is presented as a pervasive feature of modern times: its characteristic patterns of professional governance have become embedded ubiquitously in professional practices to weigh up demands for increased efficiency, accountability and achieving greater responsiveness to clients and users. This framing of professional development in the context of broader societal trends has become the harbinger of an increased flexibility, mobility and individualisation within any given workforce.

A contrasting framework, democratic or collaborative professionalism, extends the ambit of professionalism so the directions and ideals of different actors achieve greater sensitivity to the interests of a wide range of external stakeholders, for example service users, patients, students and community representatives. Across the UK education sector, collaborative professionalism has become a watchword for how teachers and other educators transform teaching and learning together to work with all students to develop fulfilling lives of meaning, purpose and success. It is evidence-informed, with educators actively caring for and having solidarity with each other. Of relevance to both democratic and collaborative professionalism is ingrained the notion of finding new ways of deepening accountability towards more collectivist values – social justice, human rights, gender equality and employee solidarity.

6

De-professionalism: an analytical framework

Introduction

A central concern of this chapter is to consider some of the evidence for an evolving process of de-professionalisation, and to pose the question as to whether the direction and substantive nature of this process may have been emboldened by austerity. In Chapters 1–3 it has been suggested that de-professionalisation lies at the heart of the United Kingdom (UK) austerity agenda, symbolised by profound cuts to public services in the form of efficiencies, pay cuts, rationing, and reducing staff training and development, along with negative effects on overall economic productivity. The suggestion is that globalisation has become associated with this process, along with its resultant destabilisation of the public sector workforce. The notion of a democratic or collaborative framework, described in Chapter 5 as a device for studying professions, articulates a version of professional development in the context of broader societal trends involving increasing flexibility, mobility and individualisation, arguably leading to a changed socio-economic climate, namely that of de-professionalisation.

It goes without saying that there is a need to ensure that individuals are properly trained and able to undertake particular tasks to work in the public sector and that any differences in rewards are both fair and proportionate. Previous reforms to public services have entailed outsourcing coupled with a dogmatic adherence of the public sector to the purchaser/provider split. This has meant that local authorities, the National Health Service (NHS) and others no longer directly provide in-house services, but commission them from external private sector providers through forced competition, where costs are minimised to win a contract. If all austerity has done is to reinforce a trend going back to the New Right of the 1980s, encouraged by New Labour in their turn (with their academies, Private Finance Initiative-supported schemes, extended partnerships and so on), then this should in effect be regarded as continuity rather than radical change.

An aim is to develop an analytic framework for understanding the context in which a process of de-professionalisation exists within an employment culture dominated by capitalism, globalisation and inequality. The argument is that this is a feature of a deepened marketisation of public welfare systems, extending the logic of competition in everyday life, where the notion of meritocracy appears to contradict the principle of equality. Over the past few decades, neo-liberal meritocracy has been characterised by the sheer scale of its attempt to extend entrepreneurial competition into all aspects of everyday life and by the power it has gathered by drawing on 20th-century movements for equality (the creation of the British welfare state being an exemplar). Meritocracy, rather like social mobility, is presented as a means of breaking down established hierarchies of privilege.

A starting point is to highlight the social and political roots of de-professionalisation, which seem to reject a socially cohesive role characteristic of a neo-Durkheimian perspective on professions, along with the value of specialist knowledge, skills and acquired status offered by a neo-Weberian perspective. Drawing on an alternative neo-Marxist framework that emphasises power relations, the origins of de-professionalisation are seen as based on ideas taken from Taylorism (or scientific management), which came to dominate managerial ideas about how best to control alienated labour (Edgell, 2012: 57–61). Ideological reference points where the notion of de-professionalisation takes shape therefore include:

- *Neo-liberalism* as a blend of market individualism and social or state authoritarianism is an ideology with the central pillars of the market and the individual. The principal neo-liberal goal is to roll back the frontiers of the state, in the belief that unregulated market capitalism will deliver efficiency, growth and widespread prosperity. This is reflected in a preference for privatisation, economic deregulation, low taxes and anti-welfarism. Individualism as a normative concept, in the form of ethical individualism, argues for the right to make choices rather than being forced to accept what is available.
- *Taylorism–Post-Fordism* ideas emerged from within an industrial and manufacturing production context that notably endorses the transfer of all discretion from workers to management. Unlike traditional Fordist production, Post-Fordism has proclaimed the empowerment of workers while demanding flexible application of many skills to different tasks, under conditions of computerised surveillance and control (Burrows and Loader, 1994). Both approaches – Taylorism

and Fordism – represent distinct branches of managerialism: the primary goal of Taylorism was to improve efficiency using the existing technology, whilst Fordism tended to focus more on replacing labour by machinery and recruiting unskilled workers to attend to the machines.

- *Lifelong -learning* has become an ideology focusing on the economic imperatives of developing a more productive and efficient workforce: it makes the flexible reskilling of individuals a compulsory life project, rather than offering the time-limited period of traditional study to acquire fixed qualifications. Since 2010 governments have planned to increase the demand for skilled workers by focusing on skills rather than qualifications. The connection with de-professionalisation is the way that more of the cost has been shifted onto learners and employers (Callender, 2012).

- *Equality* as a formal rule may be described as unjust where it treats unequals equally and therefore fails to reward people in line with their talents and capacities. De-professionalisation in the workplace fails to acknowledge any difference between those possessing and those not possessing relevant qualifications and acquired skills.

Theoretical definitions of de-professionalisation

De-professionalisation might be described as the antithesis of professionalisation, which is an attempt to translate one order of scarce resources – special knowledge and skills – into another – social and economic rewards (Larson, 1977: xvii). This definition of professionalisation tends to be the result of the particular emphasis given to different key aspects of professionalism: status and pay, expertise and standards, values and ethics (Edmond and Price, 2012: 30). A more nuanced way of examining the concept of professionalisation, and implicitly that of de-professionalisation, is through the lens of 'street-level bureaucracy', an expression coined by Michael Lipsky in an article (Lipsky, 1980) developed since the 1970s (Hupe and Hill, 2007; Lipsky, 2010; Hupe et al, 2015). Lipsky equates the term 'street-level bureaucrat' with 'the public services with which citizens typically interact. In this sense, all teachers, police officers and social workers in public agencies are street-level bureaucrats without further qualification'. He adds that street-level bureaucracy stands for 'public service employment of a certain sort, performed under certain conditions … Street-level bureaucrats interact with citizens in the course of the job and have discretion in exercising authority' (Lipsky, 2010: xvii). The concept embeds both bureaucratic and professional characteristics and encompasses the development of professional roles in public policy delivery. Lipsky acknowledges that there may be differences between street-level bureaucrats arising from professional status. He emphasises the common characteristics of street-level bureaucrats despite the diverse nature of the public services workforce to which this term refers – receptionists, benefits clerks, judges, doctors, police officers, social workers, teachers and so on (Lipsky, 2010).

Tony Evans (2015: 283), a professor of social work, claims that this would perhaps make sense if one were to assume the de-professionalisation of staff in street-level bureaucracies. However, while professional workers, across a range of different settings, have seen changes that have constrained their work, they have also seen changes that have increased their power and status. In England, for instance, the professional status of social workers has been embedded in law for over a decade (Care Standards Act, 2000). Social workers are now registered, and only social workers registered by the professional body can operate as social workers. Furthermore, the number of social workers employed within social services in England increased by 24 per cent in the decade 2000–10, though it has fallen severely since (HSCIC, 2016). Evans's studies of social work activity have examined the continuing role of professionalism as a factor influencing front-line discretion, concluding that the professional status of social workers has been an important factor in the levels of discretion expected and afforded in their practice. Kate Morris, another social work professor, has researched this area of professionalism in relation to scrutinising both professionals' decision-making and outcomes for children in a variety of comparable neighbourhoods in terms of referral rates and the probability of children ending up being assessed or looked after. A stated aim of this research was to establish how poverty and deprivation are understood and responded to by social workers in the frontline of child protection (Featherstone et al, 2018).

Many street-level bureaucrats, as organisational professionals (Evetts, 2009), working in public agencies responsible for delivering public policies, have to deal with standards in doing their work that have various sources: public policy, their organisation and their occupation. Whether the process of professionalisation can be fulfilled is likely to depend on the nature of these standards and the way in which they support or maybe oppose each other (Van der Aa and van Berkel, 2015). Many of these standards have been changing profoundly over the last decades in ways that potentially affect the promise of professionalism. Expectations regarding public services have been changing, and new standards are being set by public policies and managers. The role of occupational standards may change in various ways and may be reduced, resulting in de-professionalisation, which may thwart the promise of professionalism. A general assessment of recent social policy changes is difficult, given differences between welfare states and policy fields. However, scholars on welfare state development (Taylor-Gooby, 2008; Bonoli and Natali, 2012; Davies, 2017; Martinelli et al, 2017; Greener 2018) agree on a number of general changes occurring in social policy fields across countries:

- the alignment of social policy and social protection with economic policies;
- a greater emphasis on the conditionality of welfare state arrangements; and
- especially since the economic crisis of 2008, the reduction of spending on social policies and services and a greater emphasis on the value of financial efficiency.

Such policy changes influence the standards that social policies set for service delivery, put existing occupational standards to the test or give rise to new occupational standards. For example, workers are expected to have a greater focus on the labour market attachment of their clients, to focus more on the financial efficiency of their services or to implement disciplinary instruments, such as financial sanctioning. These new policy standards do not necessarily fit well with existing occupational standards, as the literature on social workers made responsible for implementing these policies has shown (Jordan, 2001; Evans, 2013, 2015). Various authors have produced evidence indicating a growing discrepancy between the self-identity of social workers as critical agents in structural social change and policy development, and the actual role that they have come to play in the technical delivery of neo-liberal social policies (see, for example, Clarke and Newman, 1997; Kirkpatrick et al, 2005; Garrett, 2009, 2014; Lavalette, 2011; Rogowski, 2011, 2016; Marston and McDonald, 2012).

De-professionalisation offers an alternative standards narrative, revealed in the processes of performance management in the workplace. On the one hand, output targets, as well as the external definition of these targets by policy-makers or managers, may conflict with occupational standards and professional ethics and may be experienced as an attack on professional discretion. On the other hand, performance management may go hand in hand with deregulation and less bureaucratic control, thus actually increasing room for occupational standards (Kirkpatrick et al, 2005; Newman, 2005; Hill and Hupe, 2014). Rather than being seen as an attack on 'pure professionalism' (Noordegraaf, 2011) at the cost of occupational standards and professional autonomy, the exact impact of these changes needs to be conceptualised, depending on the nature of the changes themselves, as well as on the existing working and occupational contexts in which they are introduced, resulting in many professionals adapting creatively to new expectations.

Changes in the governance and management of social policy implementation potentially affect the organisational standards for service provision: organisational goals and professional goals sometimes may not directly coincide. Standards might include the redistribution of responsibilities for policy-making and implementation, for example between professionals and professional managers, along with the introduction of quasi-markets for service delivery (see, for example, Øvretveit, 1995; Buse et al, 2005; Malerba et al, 2017). Additionally they cover the stimulation of inter-agency cooperation among health, social care, education, housing, criminal justice and financial sectors (see, for example, Glendinning et al, 2002; Needham and Glasby, 2014; Blomberg et al, 2016; Frost and Robinson, 2016; Webb, 2017) and overall the introduction of new management methods within agencies.

The emergence of the professions as distinctive occupational groups proclaiming the exclusive competence over a particular field has often been identified as the product of specialisation, the division of labour characteristic of modern forms of production and knowledge (Weber, 1987). Thus the emergence of the professions was seen as an integral part of the process of rationalisation: the increasing complexity and extensiveness of knowledge and information led to specialisation and the division of labour. De-professionalisation can then be seen as the rejection of the 'labour of division'(Fournier, 2000: 73) along with the incommensurability characteristic of Weber's definition of professions. Incommensurability proposes that the social position and status of a profession may be such that it is not able to be judged by the same standard as anything else, or indeed has no common standard of measurement: boundaries are thrown up between the sphere of competence of the professions and other spheres of activity. In terms of the attempt through various defensive strategies to place professional activity apart from, outside, the sphere of ordinary relationships and activity, and in particular, outside the market, incommensurability supports the view that professions may thus be better seen in terms of the labour of division than as an outcome of the division of labour. In other words, they are not the technical outcomes of the intellectual division of labour but are constituted and maintained through processes of isolation and boundary construction.

As more boundary layers are created to establish professionalisation, so there would appear to be a skilled effort on the part of outsiders (members of the public, private service providers, government) to question and re-evaluate professional knowledge. More broadly, there has been a wide repudiation of the 'experts', most notably in the 2016 American election and UK Brexit referendum vote to leave the European Union. The Conservative government minister Michael Gove is alleged to have made a statement that 'people in this country have had enough of experts. I'm on the side of the people. We should be less tolerant of those who get it wrong' (Mance, 2016). Said in June 2016 amidst the EU leave debate, this was viewed as a more fine-grained attack on the conventional rhetoric of the establishment. Although his speech may have sounded like an attack on expertise as such, it could also be interpreted more as a critique of modern technocratic government, a claim that the public are sick and tired of we-know-best lectures from economists and professional politicians. The difficulty that ordinary people have in making sense of the language of elite policy-makers is a real issue and language can be seen as within the purview of experts and sometimes used to control us (Thompson, 2016). What researchers in an Ipsos MORI survey identified as 'a presumption of complexity' meant that many respondents thought that it was hopeless to even try to understand an issue in question, often leaving politicians and 'experts' vulnerable to provocation and their position being challenged (Ipsos MORI, 2016: 35) Professionals working in different sectors are frequently challenged over some of their decisions, the quality of service they or their organisation provides, and the organisational structures in which they operate. This critique can even take on a rather sinister existential overtone as, for example, one ex-Minister for Health posited that 'the most important factor to tackle inequalities in education is teacher quality' (Milburn, 2016: 40; see also Asthana, 2016).

Whereas a professionalisation process of separation and boundary creation continues to consolidate an unravelling, the rather less sophisticated de-professionalisation narrative moves in an opposing direction. Parents may disapprove of their child's lack of progress in a particular school or what they may perceive as bullying by a peer group, and hence threaten legal action against the school. Social workers may be criticised following the action of taking a child into care or for failing to obtain a favoured adult placement. Here de-professionalisation can be used as a term to represent a process of disaggregation, dismantling or chipping away at an established position of authority, even when such disapproval might apply only within a specific context to any one or group of individuals representing a profession. In summary, the concept of de-professionalisation can be defined in the following multidimensional way as being made up of the following elements:

- Removal of professional control, influence, manipulation; destabilisation of their mode of professionalisation and of their professional ties (Demailly and De La Broise, 2009). In practice, unalloyed de-professionalisation produces a sharp diminution of autonomy at work and a collective powerlessness to conceive of any positive reconstitution of a lost professionalism. This is the transfer of power dimension.
- To discredit or deprive of professional status, also privately experienced as a weakening of status, respect or tendency away from a position of strength or equal status. It is associated with measures for lessening the need for specialist knowledge and expertise (Rogers and Pilgrim, 2014: 107–11). This is the status and market strength dimension.
- The obverse of professionalisation, in which it is assumed that there is a plurality of professionalisation processes (Demailly, 2003; Kuhlmann and Saks, 2008); otherwise regarded as a function or a by-product of a normally hierarchical process where certain jobs become vulnerable and subordinate, and professional identity is scapegoated, replaced by insecurity and a lack of belonging. It is also depicted in the form of an emerging social class: 'the precariat is faced by systematic insecurity' (Standing, 2014: 270). This is the transformative-contextual dimension.
- An inversion of a specific mode of professionalisation, producing a loss of autonomy in the practice of a profession and subordination to external supervision (Adcroft and Willis, 2006; Frostenson, 2015). The conditions of the 'new capitalism' have created a conflict between character and experience, the experience of disjointed time threatening the ability of people to form their characters into sustained narratives, resulting in a loosening of bonds of trust and commitment, and divorcing a person's will from his behaviour. This is characterised as a loss of anchorage and self-understanding of the employee as a consequence of this ceaseless change (Sennett, 1998: 30–1). This is the managerialism dimension.

- An urge, as a creative practitioner, or indeed a practitioner of any kind, not to be identified with one genre or activity and to be in general a critic of specialisation and a champion of 'dabbling' (UEA Centre for the Creative and the Critical, 2018). The idea and act of de-professionalisation is really a critique of the construction of the professional or trained practitioner by conventional means, by outsiders including the media or by other members of the profession. It also accommodates the notion of value: for instance, the idea that someone may not be good at or trained in the skills of a particular project or genre or form they have embarked upon. This is the divergence from the genre dimension.
- Actions taking place within the historical trajectory followed by and in the space occupied by a group's particular mode of professionalisation. The spatio-temporal framework that forms the context of this process can be considered at various sociological levels (macro-, meso- or micro-) depending on whether one is referring to public policies, organisational change or daily work routines. This is the reconstituting professionalities dimension (Delamotte, 2016).

The last dimension points to what has been denoted as 'de-professionalisation of society' (Demailly and De La Broise, 2009: 15–17), a process that is changing the mode of bureaucratic professional regulation characteristic of European societies. This mode of producing and regulating public policies did, after all, grant an important role to professional groups, represented by their associations and trade unions. It has been argued that the state on the one hand and the market on the other seem to be sharply reducing the role of occupational groups in the regulation of public policies and to be depriving that role of its legitimacy.

Somewhat distinct from the above is a definition of de-professionalisation based on the notion of de-skilling'(Braverman, 1974; Edgell, 2012: 56–73). This focuses on the impacts of breaking down a professional task (or work process) into elements, creating a more atomised position in the workplace (Heywood, 2000: 133). A recent example of breaking down a work process into a linear narrative-form can be given by the partnerships that have characterised the implementation of some of the UK's policies and professional practices towards disadvantaged children and families, examples being Whole Family Approaches (WFA) and Sure Start. The argument here is that the importance and outputs of work processes trumps the perceived contribution of individual professionals. An overall effect of reliance on these partnership or multidisciplinary structures may be to weaken or diminish the role of specific professionals. For instance, in delivering WFA there may be a statutory or policy requirement for partnership in specific areas of practice. The chosen model includes a series of activities collectively defined as participation, engagement and multidisciplinary focus, which may include to enable a process of engagement with the family; to assess and review; to develop multi-agency involvement as regards decision-making; and to strengthen coordination of services. Similarly, there are audits of work processes, introduced to establish and measure impact and outcomes, and these provide an evaluation framework for managers and professionals to reflect on. WFA was framed as a policy response to a number of factors – inadequate range and level of service, poor coordination, problems of access for families, and insufficient adaptability. Whereas organisational or legislative change appeared as the preferred solution earlier on, a change in the 'cultural system' (Boyle et al, 2010: 15–16) setting legitimate goals, and the technology that determines the means available for reaching them, appears more instinctively relevant today. The above approach – of breaking down a work process into elements – contrasts with the more unifying process demonstrated by creating a professional project (see, for example, Macdonald 1995, 187–208).

At the core of Braverman's de-skilling thesis is the unequal relationship between employer and employee, and 'the manner in which the labour force is dominated and shaped by the accumulation of capital' (Braverman, 1974: 53). In the Marxist tradition, Braverman argues that its creative characteristics make human labour exceedingly adaptable, with unlimited potential for production. From the standpoint of the capitalist, this is good news, but in the context of the inherently 'antagonistic relations of production', there is 'the problem of realizing the 'full usefulness' of that labour power' (Braverman, 1974: 57). It is imperative to exert control over the labour process in order to maximise the productive potential of labour (and therefore profits). This applies equally to professionals as providers of labour where the focus is on making full use of their knowledge and skills – productive potential – by controlling the work process. Capitalists turned therefore to developments in management and machinery, which not only enhanced the control of labour but also progressively de-skilled the worker. Braverman summed up Taylor's systematic or scientific approach to management with reference to three related principles (Taylor, 2003): 'the first principle is the gathering and development of knowledge of the labour processes', 'the second is the concentration of this knowledge as the exclusive province of management – together with its essential converse, the absence of such knowledge among the workers', and 'the third is the use of this monopoly over knowledge to control each step of the labour process and its mode of execution' (Braverman, 1974: 119). Implicit in these principles is the separation of conception from execution, namely the transfer of all mental labour from workers to managers while simultaneously simplifying and standardising the tools and tasks that the worker is instructed to use in order to undertake a de-skilled task within a designated time-frame: 'the manager's brains are under "the workman's cap"'(cited by Montgomery, 1987: 45).

Is de-professionalisation part of the neo-liberal extension of marketisation agenda? Table 6.1 outlines one type of analytical framework for examining the professionalisation/de-professionalisation nexus as formulated at the policy to practice interface. Defining this concept in a multidimensional form highlights the corollary of each separate perspective, as taken from Chapters 4 and 5, for understanding the nature of how de-professionalisation becomes gradually embedded within work practices.

Whereas sociological perspectives have played a leading role in contributing theoretical frameworks that help us to understand professions, other disciplines have offered a more contemporary assessment of this topic; for example, political science, economics and management. An added social policy dimension used here as a tool to evaluate professional activity would focus most likely on the role of practices such as partnership-working, inter-professionalism, leadership and managing change along with other aspects of organisational culture. De-professionalisation would then be reflected in the converse of such practices such as a weakening of partnerships leading to ineffective inter-professional working. A leadership vision has become central to most professional practice, where effective leaders require the skills and confidence to shape culture in a positive direction; and in contrast gathering evidence of ineffective leadership has been conventionally used to account for any poor practices revealed. The spatio-temporal framework that forms the context of this process can be considered at various levels, defined by how de-professionalisation becomes part of a phenomenon in which professional workers are substituted, marginalised and professional skills down-graded. Incompetence may equate with acting unprofessionally and may feature also as a result of this process, but such behaviour does not have the same meaning as de-professionalisation.

Viewed as socially and politically contentious, cuts to services, if interrogated, place the notion of de-professionalisation at the heart of assessing the impact of the commercial model within public

Table 6.1: De-professionalism: a theoretical paradigm

Theoretical framework	Perspective on professions	De-professionalisation index
Neo-Durkheimian	Structural, functionalist accounts view professions as static/stable social stratum – a socially cohesive role, a disinterested integrative function; interdependence of professions, bureaucratic administration and the state	Regarded as a function or by-product of a normally hierarchical process where certain jobs become vulnerable, subordinate and professional identity is scapegoated, replaced by lack of belonging, insecurity
Neo-Weberian	Characterised by social closure and professional dominance; professions develop strategies to advance their own social status, persuade clients/ potential clients about the need for the service they offer, and corner the market in that service and exclude competitors	To cause to appear unprofessional, discredit or deprive of professional status, weaken status, respect or tendency away from position of strength/ equal status; measures for lessening need for specialist knowledge and skills
Neo-Marxist	Focus on power relations where professionals fit into a social structure characterised by two main groups: those who work to produce wealth in society, and those who own the means of production and exploit these workers and expropriate surplus value as profits	De-skilling/vassal status; to remove from professional control/ influence, diminution of autonomy at work and a collective powerlessness; destabilisation of mode of professionalisation
Post-structuralist/ Social Constructionism	Power as dispersed, not simply located in any elite group; involves mapping out discourses associated with particular social periods and places; narrative provides an historical account to demonstrate the evolution and direction of a profession represented by an enactment of the principle of 'progress'	As an inversion of a specific mode of professionalisation where 'progress' has been increasingly under threat; originates in a loss of a autonomy/subordination to external supervision
Managerialism	Related to the changing patterns of professional governance embedded in professional practice associated with demands for increased efficiency in provision/delivery of services, and greater responsiveness to user demands	Measures for lessening need for specialist knowledge/ expertise; experienced as a result of a hierarchical process where jobs become vulnerable
Democratic or Collaborative Professionalism	Demystify professional work/forge alliances between professionals and excluded constituencies, e. g. of patients, users, students, voluntary sector and members of wider community to reduce democratic deficit	Imbalance of power between worker-employer, collective powerlessness to regain status

services, in particular the NHS. How have these cuts helped to downsize professional service-inputs in the form of efficiencies, pay cuts, rationing, reduced training and staff development, all of which potentially affect overall economic productivity? Pointing to examples of reported incapacity to deliver along with variations in overall standards nationwide has become a media-driven way of highlighting ineffectiveness (Kitzinger, 2000; Butler and Drakeford, 2005). Because of the austerity measures following the 2008 financial crisis, public services have been subjected to cuts and reorganisation that have brought about significant disruption, manifested for example in governance, labour market, gender and social and territorial cohesion. Within this context there have been numerous examples in the UK of activities, events and public policies that have shaped the notion of de-professionalisation, including the junior doctors contract dispute in England, 2015–16 (Weaver, 2016); the Francis Inquiry Report (2013; the Think Family/Whole Family Approach guide to good practice (DoH and LGA, 2014); and the Nolan Principles on Standards in Public Life (Committee on Standards in Public Life, 1995), which were established earlier in 1994. The Nolan Principles, namely selflessness, integrity, objectivity, accountability, openness, honesty and leadership, were seen as 'revolutionary' at the time (Leading Governance, 2013) because they focused on behaviour and culture rather than processes.

Reviewing UK evidence, it seems axiomatic that de-professionalisation could be defined by reference to a number of fundamentally quantitative pathways, for example through a lens of service cutbacks, by cuts to staff training budgets and by critiquing models of current training. The idea has become a feature of a market-led approach to provision shaped by a what works philosophy and demonstrated through a political economy model of delivering public services. Further examination of available evidence widens the definition to include a lowering of morale, a demoralisation or denigration of the workforce, and other behavioural impacts such as abuse of power or institutional abuse. Progressive de-skilling (Braverman, 1974; Edgell, 2012) equates to low productivity, and this may occur within an organisation where the acquisition of new skills by individual employees ceases to be regarded as essential by those in management or positions of authority.

Summary

There are a number of ideological reference points from where the notion of de-professionalisation takes shape, including critiques of neo-liberalism, Taylorism/Post-Fordism and the ideology of lifelong learning. The argument is that any theoretical definition of de-professionalisation centres around a specific narrative and most likely includes the notion of de-skilling, drawn from Marx's theory of work in industrial capitalism. An analytical framework then begins to evolve for examining the professionalisation/de-professionalisation nexus, which highlights the corollary of different perspectives drawn from a range of academic disciplines – such as sociology, political science, economics and management. The theoretical translation emphasises the contribution of a loss of autonomy, vulnerability of identity, the imposition of external control and lessening a requirement for specialist knowledge, along with other factors identified as causally associated with patterns of unprofessional behaviour.

The spatio-temporal framework that forms the context of this process can be considered at various 'impact' levels – macro-, meso- or micro- – depending on whether one is referring to public policies, organisational change or daily work routines. The result may be anything from workforce destabilisation to a form of collective powerlessness, and may be associated with interrupted career progression, job insecurity or a lack of belonging. At a practice level it was suggested that the effects of de-professionalisation can be measured through objective indicators or else expressed experientially. The first covers organisational metrics such as staff shortages, increased workloads, pay restraint, unfilled posts and a lowering of employment standards. The second includes feelings of low morale and exploitation, being undervalued by management and/or colleagues, unfair/unequal treatment, being blamed for a reduction in service standards and/ or being forced to step up to senior roles without extra training. In the context of the present era of austerity, an organisational impact is symptomatic of a presence of continued uncertainty and lacks an evidential commitment to rebuilding public services. The question of whether de-professionalisation has become part of the neo-liberal extension of the marketisation agenda is addressed more fully in Chapters 7–10.

PART III

De-professionalism in the public sector: output indicators

7

The impact of service cutbacks, job insecurity and globalisation

Introduction

Cuts to services across health, social care and education have embodied de-professionalisation in terms of reducing the number, type and range of professional staff employed: for example, fewer qualified teachers employed in free schools, more use made of teaching assistants; more health support workers as opposed to fully-trained nurses employed in both hospital and community settings (Siddique, 2015). The impact of service cuts has resulted in reduced professional influence, for example by curtailing local authority responsibilities in relation to child protection, children in need, care leavers and disabled children. Professional influence can be removed further following a children's social care policy objective that places greater reliance on the need to strengthen capacity for developing local authority adoption services and uses new and enhanced powers of an Ofsted inspection regime to regulate child and adult care homes. This model of working appears to value disproportionately the idea of having in post an effective manager over and above any results achieved from the one-to-one intervention of single professionals. There is ample evidence that service cuts have been shaped by an ideological adherence to managerialist methods (see, for example, Rogowski, 2016). De-professionalisation as a consequence of managerialism has become evident in the process of carrying out legal aid work, an activity protected not only for the highest priority cases and that increasingly uses para-legal staff rather than social welfare lawyers. A priority case is defined as 'where there is a risk of serious physical harm or loss of home, or where children may be removed from a family' (Howard, 2016: 20). Within local authority child protection services it is clear that, partly owing to the number of Sure Start children's centre closures, there has been a soaring number of children being removed from their families and placed in care.

Because of the dominant market ideology, National Health Service (NHS) services and assets, including blood supplies, nurses and other care professionals, scanning and diagnostic services, ambulances, care homes, hospital beds and buildings – which the British public own – are being handed over to British and foreign private companies. Privatised services cost the NHS and taxpayer far more than a publicly owned and publicly run NHS. That is because public health systems do not need to pay dividends to shareholders, enjoy lower rates of interest compared with private sector loans, and do not have privatisation's heavy and unnecessary marketising costs of contracts, billings and all the extra administration involved (Klein, 2010; Demello and Furseth, 2016; Greer et al, 2016). One example of the impact of cuts – and its association with a de-professionalisation – is that fewer fully qualified professional staff are employed to work outside hospitals. This is reflected in a diminution in the number of district nurses, community psychiatric nurses and care workers. In parallel, NHS data show that the number of general practitioners (GPs) in England rose only by just 108 in 2015, despite the Conservative government's high-profile pledge to expand the family doctor workforce by 5,000 by 2020 (Clay, 2016).

De-professionalisation in health care?

Cuts to services have been evidenced through extended waiting lists for NHS hospital care (Campbell, 2017h) and by ward closures; for example, some maternity wards in England closed their doors almost 400 times in 2016, according to figures released, triggering claims of pregnant women being 'pushed from pillar to post in the throes of labour' (Asthana, 2017: 9). The closures, often the result of hospitals not having enough staff or money, occurred when the NHS had been under unprecedented pressure and struggling to cope with demand. Chronic staff shortages and the NHS budget squeezes forced hospitals to shut beds: in one English foundation trust a lack of staff meant that it had nine wards comprising 270 beds lying empty in 2014, 2015, 2016 and 2017. It would therefore seem illogical for hospitals to have extra beds available but also unavailable, because they had been taken out of use (Campbell, 2018a).

Health bosses claimed that shortages of money, staff and care outside hospitals meant that the NHS could not cope with an ongoing historically high rise in demand. NHS Providers, which represents hospital trusts, issued a statement: 'There is simply not enough capacity in the system to assure patient safety in the coming winter' (NHS Providers, 2017) The agreed maximum bed occupancy rate had been 85 per cent, to avoid a greater risk of patients acquiring infections such as MRSA or receiving inadequate care. At the time, however, a group of anonymous hospital trust chief executives declared that 'hospitals are already up to 99% full as the NHS braces itself for the winter and expected major flu outbreak' (Campbell, 2017h: 10). They voiced fears that patients could be harmed and staff left unable to cope with the seasonal surge in demand because of their hospitals running out of spare beds. One year on, it was reported that record numbers of people had needed a hospital admission or waited longer than the maximum 18 weeks for a planned operation. Statistics issued in November 2018 showed how hospitals had missed a host of waiting-time targets as they treated unusually high numbers of patients for the time of year. For example, only 87.6 per cent of patients arriving at Accident and Emergency (A&E) were treated within four hours, far off the 95 per cent target; a total of 10,675 patients had to spend at least 30 minutes with ambulance crews before being handed over to A&E staff, in breach of NHS rules; and almost 55,000 patients had spent at least four hours on a trolley while they waited to get a hospital bed. A conclusion drawn by independent thinktank the King's Fund was that the NHS was already 'operating in the red zone'; and many hospitals were under intense strain as a result of 'sustained funding squeezes and staff shortages' (Anandaciva et al, 2018: 2).

Similarly, the notion of NHS staff shortages became epitomised and shaped through the Conservative government's approach to immigration control. For instance, in early 2018 fears were expressed by the media that such shortages would increase as the visa ceiling had been reached. The United Kingdom (UK) had reached its ceiling on skilled visas for non-European workers for an unprecedented third month in a row, deepening the staffing crisis facing the NHS and other key employers. It was reported that the Home Office had sent out hundreds of emails to UK employers and businesses, telling them that their applications for the certificates of sponsorship required to recruit workers from outside the European Union (EU), who are mostly highly skilled, had been refused because they did not meet the minimum points score set for the monthly quota (Travis, 2018). The Home Office subsequently confirmed that the minimum salary for a job to qualify for a skilled work visa was normally £30,000, or £20,800 for a graduate recruit. However, in December 2017, after the quota had been exceeded, the minimum qualifying salary was raised to £55,000, and in the following January visa applications for jobs paying less than £46,000 a year were refused unless they were PhD-level roles or were for jobs on the official shortage occupation lists (MAC, 2019a).

The Labour opposition called for a relaxation of visa rules for NHS staff, complaining about foreign doctors being refused visas to work in Britain; and ministers were urged to remove all health professionals from the cap on skilled workers in order to tackle the NHS's growing staffing crisis. In an effort to relax migration rules to enable more overseas doctors to move to the UK to fill the NHS's growing number of rota gaps, the Shadow Health Secretary, Jonathan Ashworth, in a letter to the Home Secretary, warned that the ban on at least 400 doctors – since December 2017 – taking up posts had demonstrated that 'the government's "hostile environment" policy [was] now directly damaging NHS patient care' (Labour, 2018a). Ashworth requested that doctors, nurses and other health care staff should start being treated separately from the other types of foreign skilled workers covered by the cap, so that more of them might come to the UK (Campbell and Stewart, 2018). In June 2018 the Home Secretary confirmed that the number of qualified family doctors (GPs) was being reviewed – there were 41,877 in September 2015 and the number had barely increased by the same month two years later. Figures from NHS England showed that there had been 179 closures of contracts to run GP practices in 2017–18, compared with 107 the year before. Some health professionals were already on the shortage occupation list because they were in short supply in the UK, including nurses, paramedics, psychiatrists and radiographers. The Brexit controversy had rapidly become a euphemism for de-professionalisation, manifested by a brain-drain of health workers from the EU27 countries that was exacerbating the NHS's chronic staffing crisis.

This politicisation of staff shortages within the NHS was still expressed as a nebulous grievance and was not being advanced in terms of valuing the true contribution of professional workers and their skill-sets. The argument was sustained through several key players, most notably Simon Stevens, Chief Executive of the NHS, speaking out against the cash squeeze over NHS care. Stevens confronted government ministers with the fact that the NHS's budget was rising at about 1 per cent a year when demand for care was growing at 4 per cent. The chair of one of the NHS's biggest trusts, Lord Kerslake, resigned in protest at what he claimed was such serious government underfunding that hospitals could not perform their key role properly. He was stepping down 'because hospitals were being asked to agree to unrealistically demanding savings targets' (Campbell, 2017b: 7). Professor Anita Charlesworth, the director of research at the Health Foundation thinktank and a former head of public spending at the Treasury, backed the claim that the NHS's financial problems were due to underfunding.

Hospitals in the NHS are caught between a rock and a hard-place. Emergency admissions have increased by 3.4% in the first half of this year, there is a shortage of 30,000 nurses and it has proved really hard to free up beds occupied by people who are medically fit to leave but need social care support. (Charlesworth, 2018: 4; The Health Foundation/King's Fund Centre, 2018)

The 2 per cent reduction in funding imposed on the NHS by the Conservative government since 2010 had given rise to reports that there were now people on hospital trolleys waiting for a bed who were not the worried well accused of blocking up A&E departments but individuals who had already been assessed as needing beds. It was suggested that these beds continued to be full not just because people could not be moved out of hospital but because the number of hospital beds had been steadily reduced over the last 20 or more years, so that the UK now had approximately 2.8 beds per 1,000 of population, compared with 8.6 in Germany and 6.2 in France. The Office of Budget Responsibility's prediction was that the NHS's budget would need to increase by £88 billion over the next 50 years to keep pace with the rising demand for health care (King's Fund Centre, 2018a, b).

Problems in accessing health care within rural communities have been particularly heightened during austerity. De-professionalism in this context is evidenced through a reduction of professional influence across all aspects of health and social care provision. In medicine, rural health comprises the interdisciplinary study of health and health care delivery in rural environments, incorporating many fields, including geography, midwifery, nursing, sociology and economics. A cross-party parliamentary inquiry into rural health and social care was established in 2018 alongside the setting up of a national research centre for rural health and care based at the University of Lincoln, in part to compensate for the limited evidence-base covering data on issues such as rural well-being, workforce and learning, mental health and innovation practice (United Lincolnshire Hospitals NHS Trust, 2018). It has been demonstrated that the health care needs of individuals living in rural areas are different from those in urban areas, and rural areas often suffer from a lack of access to health care as a result of socio-economic, workplace and demographic factors. Many rural communities in the UK have a large proportion of elderly people and children, with relatively few people of working age (20–50 years of age). Such communities have a high dependency ratio, also higher mortality rates, less education and poor socio-economic conditions when compared with their urban counterparts.

Rural areas have fewer medical practitioners, mental health programmes, and health and social care facilities, meaning less preventative care and longer response times in emergencies (Rourke, 2008). This lack of health care workers has resulted in unconventional ways of delivering health care to rural dwellers, including medical consultations by phone or internet as well as mobile preventative care and treatment programmes. In the UK there have been increased efforts to attract health and social care professionals to isolated locations, such as increasing the number of medical students from rural areas and improving financial incentives for rural practices (DEFRA, 2013; Cervero et al, 2015). However, running a GP surgery has been described as 'being dependent on the odd locum and goodwill of other practitioners who may need to be a "jack of all trades"' (BBC News interview, 2019). In other countries there have been similar reported problems stemming from inadequate services, which have been exacerbated during austerity. In the United States, for instance, the federal government has projected a shortage of over 20,000 primary care physicians in rural areas by 2025. These practitioners have been described as not having the support of 'sub-specialists, hospitalists or emergency physicians', and are thus treating a wider range of conditions with limited access to sophisticated technology (Missouri Medicine, 2017: 363).

De-professionalisation in adult social care?

Cutbacks in NHS hospitals have demonstrated that they are so full that patients are discharged too soon and the continued split between health and social care is tantamount to 'political mal-administration', according to a House of Commons Public Administration and Constitutional Affairs Select Committee Report published in September 2015 (p 46). This report asserts that the failure to join up health and social care services means that one in five patients are at risk of either getting stuck in hospital or being released before they are fit to go home, creating so-called 'bed-blocking', which costs the NHS in England about £820 million a year (NAO, 2014). The committee had been responding to earlier revelations by the NHS Ombudsman that patients sent home too soon were at risk of being readmitted as emergencies or even of dying, and that a lack of social care was often behind the delay in the discharge of medically fit patients (NHS Press Association, 2014).

The erosion of social care since austerity began in 2010 meant that people were now afraid of being left without vital support in their old age and that over-65s were being denied dignity and left isolated, warned the outgoing Head of the Care Quality Commission (CQC), Sir David Behan (Campbell, 2018d; NESCHA News, 2018; Care Home Professional, 2019). As a society we may appear to be becoming more tolerant of poor standards in, for instance, delivering adult social care and mental health services. People who are fit for medical discharge are waiting for social care packages, and there has been a £4.6 billion cut in social care funding between 2010 and 2016 (Healthwatch, 2016). Lowly-trained care workers are sometimes paid below the minimum wage, and examples have been reported of companies paying for live-in care at under £4 per hour – that is, the company pays only for the actual care-giving time and not for being on call and availability in the domiciliary setting (Brindle, 2015). According to some recent research, 'flying 15-minute undignified care visits' are still being commissioned by 18 English councils (Leonard Cheshire Disability Organisation, 2016: 17). Cuts to care of the elderly have been reported as taking A&E to a tipping point, according to England's care regulator. Several reports by the CQC have showed that hospitals are ending up dangerously full, and 'bed blocking' has hit record levels because of a widespread failure to give elderly people enough support to keep them healthy at home. A worsening lack of both at-home care services and beds in care homes was described as forcing hospitals to admit more patients as emergencies and deepening their already serious financial problems:

> The difficulties in adult social care are already affecting hospitals. Bed occupancy rates exceeded 91% in January to March 2016, the highest quarterly rate for at least six years. And in 2015/16 we saw an increase in the number of people having to wait to be discharged from hospital, in part due to a lack of suitable care options. (CQC, 2016b)

The CQC disclosed in the same report that about 800,000 patients were registered with a GP practice that its inspectors judged to be 'inadequate' on safety grounds. Such safety failings included poor management of medicines, inappropriately trained staff and premises that were unsuitable. A further report published around the same time by Age UK bemoaned the fact that annually thousands of older people end up in hospital with potentially life-threatening infections because GPs and other community -based NHS services do too little to keep them well (Age UK, 2016). It is widely recognised that there has been under-funding of social care for both care homes and home care. A continual dispute has reigned over the actual depth of the cuts in adult social care. The above Age UK report claimed that £470 million is equivalent to the expected fall in the social care budget by the end of 2016. However, the Department of Health (in 2018 renamed Health and Social Care) disputed this claim, but Age UK went on to state that the social care budget had shrank by £1.85 billion since 2010. The Local Government Association, King's Fund health thinktank and Age UK have all consistently been critical of the 2 per cent levy on council tax as unlikely to raise the sums required, asserting that this is no substitute for central government funding for such key care (LGA, 2017).

Simon Stevens, chief executive officer (CEO) to the NHS, urged political parties to find a 'settled and durable new political consensus' on social care funding before 2020 (Clay, 2016), having identified that around 185,000 hospital beds had been lost since 2010 because a lack of social care prevented patients being discharged, up 70 per cent since 2012. In England it is estimated that roughly two fifths of care homes' residents are private, with another two fifths funded by the state. The remaining residents include those who pay fees but have these topped up by local authorities and residents who are funded by the NHS. Some local authorities are paying just £330 a week for residents, the equivalent of less than £2 per hour. Industry research has shown that private residents now pay 40 per cent more on average than publicly funded residents for like-for-like service (Kelly, 2015).

Another report, published by Age UK in February 2018, showed that one third of dementia patients were not getting the right care. More than one in three people in England diagnosed with dementia were not getting the follow-up care they were entitled to. Out of 458,461 dementia patients recorded in 2017, only 282,573 had a new care plan or review during that year. The NHS had specified that everyone diagnosed with the condition should receive an individual care plan, which should be reviewed at least once a year; but Age UK's charity director, Caroline Abrahams asserted: 'Our analysis suggests that many people with dementia are losing out on the NHS follow-up support they need and are supposed always to be offered once they have received their diagnosis' (Saddique, 2018).

Cuts to adult social care budgets have been translated into home closures, along with workers receiving poor pay and conditions. The parlous state of social care has become manifested through de-professionalisation, resulting in negative impacts on the quality of care provided and on the poor socio-economic status of employees. For example, it was reported that one of the UK's biggest providers of agency care workers had been fining staff who phoned in sick £50, raising concerns that frontline employees are being forced to turn up for shifts when they are not fit for work and risk spreading illness to vulnerable patients (Adu, 2018). An investigation by *The Guardian* uncovered evidence of cases where Newcross Healthcare Solutions had not only been failing to pay employees if they cancel shifts because of illness without 24 hours notice, but had also docked money from their pay (Murphy, 2018b). It was reported that the firm – which employed 7,000 staff across 63 branches providing temporary nurses and care workers for residential and nursing homes – made a pre-tax profit of £21 million and paid directors an equity dividend of £17 million in 2017. In the investigation the firm had stated that nine of its 11 branches regulated by the CQC were rated 'good' or 'outstanding'.

Mid-2017 saw yet another care homes sell-off as Britain's biggest provider, HC-One, went up for sale with 369 care homes, reported columnist Polly Toynbee. She had already reported that the Four Seasons care home group had been taken over after making a £450 million loss for its private equity owner; and that another company was selling off Care-UK's 114 care homes (Toynbee, 2017). Care homes have been closing and the number of beds falling since 2015, despite soaring need. Costs rising far faster than inflation have made them unsustainable as local authority fees have fallen rapidly, the minimum wage has risen and immigration rules have been tightened, with social care consuming at least one third of council funds. A report from the King's Fund, Ipsos MORI, the Institute of Fiscal Studies and the Health Foundation warned that many care homes now refused to take state-funded residents. Despite a million more old people, social care cuts of £1.1 billion meant that 400,000 of those frail enough to qualify were now getting no care at all, making them the responsibility of the NHS (Bottery et al, 2018).

The poor investment in care home staff was highlighted in a further *Guardian* investigation based upon the findings from a number of CQC reports. This revealed that some of the country's worst care homes were owned by companies that had made a total profit of £113 million, despite some of the vulnerable people they were supposed to look after being neglected. An analysis of 220 homes rated 'inadequate' by the CQC, according to the most recent inspection report, showed at least 44 – many of which were receiving taxpayer funds to look after residents – were owned by companies making millions of pounds in pre-tax profits.

The firms' total pre-tax profits for the year 2017–2018 amounted to £113m, according to their most recently available accounts, although this figure is likely to be higher … CQC reports from some of the homes rated 'inadequate' record appalling standards of care including how: elderly residents soiled themselves after being left neglected because there were too few staff; patients were left waiting long periods for under-pressure carers to attend when they rang their call bells; carers failed to treat elderly residents with dignity, with underwear exposed and faeces left on a bedrail cushion; and residents were at risk of abuse by other patients, and staff failed to safely manage medicines. (Murphy, 2018c)

The Shadow Minister for Social Care, Barbara Keeley said that such cases were:

symptomatic of our broken care system. This Government has empowered irresponsible providers that are driving down workers' conditions and at the same time damaging the quality of care … [the investigation] has exposed the appalling standards of care being provided by some of the largest providers of outsourced residential care which has left large numbers of vulnerable people in need of care suffering terrible indignity and neglect. (Labour, 2018b)

It is true that outsourcing has led to a host of serious challenges in the UK adult social care sector during austerity years, which appear to include staff exploitation and under-provision of services. One council, Northamptonshire, declared itself bankrupt in 2018 following an inspectors' report into widespread financial and management failures. This report rejected the council leadership's claim that it had been disadvantaged by government funding cuts and underfunded given the pressure of a growing and elderly population. It excoriated the council's 'disastrous attempt' (Butler, 2018a: 11) to restructure services by outsourcing them to private companies and charities, stating that poor design, chaotic management and a lack of controls and oversight were responsible.

De-professionalism has become a term used to unify the characteristics surrounding a loss of autonomy and status, and this has been singularly embodied in a narrative alluding to developments in the social care workforce. Defined as an inversion of a specific mode of professionalisation, producing a loss of autonomy in the practice of a profession and subordination to external supervision and control, the paid labour of social care workers remains deeply devalued, most often with those with limited options entering the profession. The cultural and political foundations of the very inequalities experienced by care workers have been highlighted (Romero and Pérez, 2016); alongside possibly a more pressing claim that the future workforce for the NHS and social care is at risk without urgent action to establish a sustainable and joined up workforce strategy (Health Foundation/King's Fund, 2017). The latter report briefing argued that with more than 900 social care workers estimated to be leaving the profession every day, the sustainability of the sector was under threat. For example 27 per cent of staff left the social care sector in 2015/16, up from 23 per cent in 2012/13; and compounding the issue has been a lack of new workers entering the sector. The report observed that at any one time there are over 80,000 vacancies for social care jobs in England (Health Foundation/King's Fund, 2017).

Key workforce challenges across the health and social care sector have been identified, pointing to a combination of issues around recruitment, retention and morale (Gershlick et al, 2017). In particular, these included pay restraint, the National Living Wage and rising staff shortages. As regards the first, average earnings fell by 6 per cent for health and social care staff in real terms between 2010 and 2017 when adjusted for inflation. If current pay policy continues up to 2020/1, NHS pay at some Agenda for Change bands will have been reduced by up to 12 per cent in real terms in the decades since 2010/11 (NHS Employers, 2019). As for the National Living Wage, in April 2016 this increased for people aged 25 years and over from £6.70 an hour to £7.20 an hour, with a further increase to £7.50 in April 2017, representing a real terms increase of 8 per cent in the hourly rate in two years. An additional increase occurred in April 2019 of 4.9 per cent, from £7.83 to £8.21. The social care workforce continues to be one of the biggest challenges facing NHS leaders in England, this stemming from a conflation of piecemeal workforce planning, a long period of capped pay increases and a lack of attention to long-standing morale issues. For instance, in an NHS staff survey undertaken in 2016, 47 per cent said current staffing levels were insufficient to allow them to do their job properly and 37 per cent had reported ill in the past 12 months owing to stress.

A Government Green Paper on Social Care promised by the summer of 2017 was postponed by another year, only to be delayed again until 2019. Care solutions being put forward included ways to improve integrated care development programmes by Chris Ham, CEO at the King's Fund (Ham and Charles, 2018), and the need for more data on the effectiveness of different professional interventions, prioritised by Nigel Edwards, CEO of the Nuffield Trust (Nuffield Trust, 2018b). The latter included secondary data sharing, collating information about the efficacy of treatments and health professionals on a massive scale and a focus on measurable outcomes, such as improving care by a certain amount or cutting costs by a specified sum. The most urgent problem to be tackled, however, is the shortage of staff, which has been caused by years of underfunding, and plugging the 'dangerous recruitment gaps', along with designing an effective strategic policy to attract new recruits and train existing employees – 'the right numbers of staff with the right skills' (Bagot, 2019: 7).

Can de-professionalisation be reversed by curbing privatisation of care? The Conservative government's Long Term Plan was published in January 2019 and mapped out the NHS's future over the next ten years. In acknowledging his support for this Plan, Simon Stevens, CEO for the NHS, demanded that it should repeal significant sections of the 2012 Health and Social Care Act. This would spell the end of automatic tendering, meaning that large private firms could no longer mount legal challenges to decisions going against them, resulting therefore in some ebbing way of private sector powers. The 2012 Act obliged NHS clinical commissioning groups in England to offer out to tender any contract worth £615,278 or more. This has led to a huge increase in the number of NHS contracts awarded to profit-driven firms such as Virgin Care and Care UK. An estimated £8.7 billion of the service's budget had gone to non-NHS providers of care in 2017–18, most of which were private firms, though that also included some charities and social enterprises. In the context of launching the 2019 Plan, NHS bosses drew up a provisional list of potential legislative changes intended to remove the counterproductive effect that general competition rules and powers can have on the integration of health and social care.

De-professionalisation in education?

De-professionalisation can be seen in the cuts to services experienced in many schools across the UK. A greater onus on solving society's ills has been placed on schools, while they have simultaneously been granted institutional autonomy. Labour Party Shadow Education spokesperson Tristram Hunt argued that the Conservative government had created a 'schools can-fix it narrative', where labour market changes, housing problems and catchment areas all appeared to have been ignored (Hunt, 2016: 27). The Harvard sociologist Robert Putnam expresses similar sentiments: 'Schools work as part of a much broader social ecology of churches, clubs, sports leagues and work placements. A rich network of civic capital ... used to be offered to our kids, trusting interactions with non-parental adults that socialised them and ensured failure did not have to be fatal' (Putnam, 2015: 135–90).

Funding for schools in England has continued to drop in real terms as it fails to match increased need from a fast-growing population of school-age children. In particular, cuts to school support include mental health services and specialist teacher input for children and young people with special needs (Weale, 2015a). Instead, relentless forced academisation and the burgeoning of free schools, unaccountable locally and of hugely variable quality, have resulted in some employing no qualified staff (Millar, 2016). In a similar way, supply teaching is currently dominated by cost-cutting private supply agencies that pay up to £60 a day less than the national rates, often with nothing paid into a teacher's pension scheme. Agencies send in teachers who may lack professional development opportunities and possess few if any professional rights, such as in-house training. 'We need to re-professionalise the teaching profession', asserted Conservative government minister Nick Boles, recognising that some aspects of professionalism are no longer valued and recognised (Lightfoot, 2016: 22).

The UK educational landscape has witnessed a slow growth of school academy trusts, which are at liberty to employ people to teach with as many or as few qualifications as the new 'executive heads' deem fit, so long as such individuals have the 'right skills' (BBC News, 2012). As their business model demands innovation and creativity in continually finding ways to cut costs and save money, as the supply from central government is reduced, employing fewer teachers on lower salaries and employing more poorly paid teaching assistants becomes likely. It has been reported that more than 300 primary schools across England were forced to become academies between 2016 and 2019, causing long-term disruption, increasing instability and high staff turnover (McIntyre and Weale, 2019). Analysis of government data has shown that the Department for Education (DfE) has paid out at least £18.4 million over this period to academy trusts to take on 314 schools 'forcibly removed from local authority control' after being rated inadequate by Ofsted (McIntyre and Weale, 2019: 20). Primary schools have found themselves being passed from one trust to another after conversion, effectively being 'rebrokered' – a phenomenon that Angela Rayner, Shadow Education Secretary, referred to as one of 'zombie schools' being abandoned by failing academy chains. The concept of de-professionalism as being identified with a removal from professional control, influence, and marked by a weakening of professional ties and collective powerlessness (Demailly and De La Broise, 2009) encapsulates neatly this turn of events.

> As each day goes by, the government's academy programme is further exposed to be built on quicksand. Billions of pounds of taxpayers' money has been spent on forcing schools into academy status, only to see those same schools being rebrokered as they are failed by their sponsors ... Some have had to endure multiple rebrokerings and a number of different sponsors, each bringing a change of ethos and approach, new school uniforms, a turnover of staff and a rise in exclusions and off-rolling. (Kevin Courtney, Joint General Secretary of The National Education Union, July 10th 2019)

It has been authentically reported that all schools across England will suffer steep budget cuts at least up to 2020 despite the Conservative government's 'fair funding' scheme, according to an analysis released by teaching unions including the National Association of Head Teachers and the National Union of Teachers (NUT) (Adams 2017). This study suggested that 98 per cent of schools faced a real-terms reduction in funding by 2019, with an average loss for each primary pupil of £339 and £477 for every secondary pupil. The funding formula redistributes funds between urban and more rural schools, a postcode lottery in effect, where in some areas the DfE data found an average loss of £655 for every pupil by 2019/20, some even higher – up to £834 in real terms. The result is that heads have been forced to cut staff, cut the curriculum and cut specialist support; in addition to overcrowded classrooms and teaching assistants not being replaced.

According to published DfE data, teacher numbers have fallen for the first time since 2013 amid complaints that low staff morale and inadequate pay are putting people off the profession. Figures showed that the number has fallen by 1.2 per cent between 2016 and 2017 – the latest year for which data is available (Harding, 2019). Although this decline may seem small, it is likely to cause alarm because teacher numbers need to rise to keep up with the growing pupil population. Between 2017 and 2026 it has been estimated (BBC

News, 2017b) that the number of secondary school pupils is expected to increase by 534,000 – almost 20 per cent. Another group of DfE figures indicated that almost a third of teachers who began teaching in 2010 quit the classroom within five years of qualifying. Of the 21,400 teachers who began their teaching careers in English state schools in 2010, 30 per cent had left by 2015. A joint report by the NUT and the Association of Teachers and Lecturers concluded that staffing problems meant schools are relying on supply teacher agencies and teachers covering roles outside their specialism. It also suggested that the quality of provision had being lowered, with growing teacher workload being blamed for the flight from the profession (Weale, 2016b). This undermining of the integrity of the teaching profession has been accompanied by transformative managerial changes to schools following the introduction of single academies. Such school academies now form a bedrock of government policy, along with grammar schools; they continue to be set up and are largely unaccountable. This represents a pursuit of the neo-liberal model, which seemingly fails to respect adequately the democratic wishes of voters by taking away local authority control, thereby emasculating the notion of the public sphere. Putting schools in the hands of others mainly with business interests, and as a replacement for parent governors, may allow such schools to indulge their own prejudices as long as high test scores are achieved. However, it may not be the case that a public service ethos will vanish entirely, as there remains ample evidence that, where school governance and leadership are strong, such independent features strengthen community interest, as, for example, many schools 'buy excellent HR, financial and school improvement advice … [and] are able to call on the support of a network of experienced, expert advisers' (Rustin, 2016).

Does a rise in the number of teaching assistants represent a possible threat to the professionalism of fully trained teachers? While the number of teachers in mainstream schools in England has remained relatively steady over the last decade or so, the number of full-time equivalent teaching assistants has more than trebled since 2000: from 79,000 to 243,000 (EEF, 2016). Teaching assistants comprise over a quarter of the workforce in mainstream schools in England: 35 per cent of the primary workforce and 14 per cent of the secondary school workforce. The number of full-time equivalent teaching assistants has more than trebled since 2000: from 79,000 to 262,800. About 7 per cent of teaching assistants in state-funded schools have 'higher-level' teaching assistant status. A key reason for increasing the number of teaching assistants was to help deal with problems with teacher workloads. In 2003, the then Labour government introduced the National Agreement to help raise pupil standards and tackle excessive teacher workload, in large part via new and expanded support roles and responsibilities for teaching assistants and other support staff. The growth in the number of teaching assistants has also been driven by the push for greater inclusion of pupils with special educational needs and disabilities into mainstream schools, with teaching assistants often providing the key means by which inclusion is facilitated. Key research studies on the role of teaching assistants have recommended that they should be used to add value to what teachers do, not replace them; that their role should be to help pupils develop independent learning skills and manage their own learning; and notably that they should *not* be used as an informal teaching resource for low-attaining pupils (EEF, 2016; Weale, 2016b; Tickle, 2017).

Summary

The austerity agenda links deficit reduction to cuts in public service budgets. The main argument is that de-professionalisation lies at the heart of assessing the impact of the commercial model in the form of efficiencies, pay cuts, rationing, reducing training/staff development and potentially affecting overall economic productivity. This chapter begins to shape an analytical framework for understanding the UK context in which a process of de-professionalisation exists within an employment culture dominated by inequality, precarity, globalisation and declining solidarity.

Professions offer democratic and legitimate solutions to social problems – scourges of poverty, inequality, homelessness and environmental degradation that threaten the well-being of us all. The crisis in democracy created by an increasingly neo-liberal direction within the EU concerned with austerity and social control, the lack of response to societal problems and the downplaying of individual participation have combined to weaken the progressive and integrative potential of social policy. Since it joined the EU in 1973, the UK has offered strong support for the EU as a market project with a secondary role for social policy. It can as a consequence claim some success in imprinting its neo-liberal orientation on EU policy (Daly, 2019: 107). The EU discourse on social policy thus supports domestic actors who are pushing for a neo-liberal restructuring of economy and society, with fewer human rights and just neo-liberal domination (Lux, 2019: 124). The UK government has promised, however, not to undercut EU businesses on workers' rights and environmental protections in its enthusiasm to form new trade links in a post–Brexit Britain. Brexit in the UK has become seen as reinforcing this neo–liberal model, and as such acts as a kind of metaphor for retrenchment of professionalism. Instead of celebrating the virtues of professional expertise, in contrast this model tends to view professions as raw material within a general commodification process. Part of the success of the UK Leave campaign was to extend the 'austerity logic' of recent governments with the argument that 'we cannot afford the European Union', encapsulated by the infamous red bus NHS funding claim.

8

De-professionalism as defined by services deemed unconventional, under-performing or ineffectual

Introduction

Reducing the number, type and range of professional staff employed particularly within community and social services, for example more health support workers, poorly paid care workers, more teaching assistants, puts a premium on professional displacement. The bigger picture from an economic standpoint shows that uncertainty over the Brexit outcome in the United Kingdom (UK) has led to some fallen investment, productivity stagnation and a flatlining in consumer spending (Eaton, 2018). Restricting immigration from Europe after Brexit would likely lead to lower growth in total jobs and in the output of the UK economy, according to the government's Migration Advisory Committee (MAC, 2018). This report claims that employers, challenged over the role of wages in their decision to hire migrant workers, often appear in denial that low wages are part of their 'image problem' among UK-born workers. Instead, the argument is that businesses employ EU migrants not because they are prepared to accept lower pay and worse conditions but because they are prepared to do work that British workers will not do – providing good quality social care would be a case in point (MAC, 2018).

Children's services have become a prominent example of a rather nebulous policy area as regards interpreting the Conservative government's action and strategy (Narey, 2016). There has been a general consensus among professional bodies that it must provide greater clarity on how it intends to maintain the provision of children's centres (Pre-Learning Alliance/CPAG, 2017). In one major respect a prevailing absence of children's services has become worthy of the term 'ineffectual', raising questions about whether local authorities have been meeting their duties to ensure adequate children's centre provision in their area. Sustained funding cuts have forced local councils to undo much of the pioneering work of the previous Labour governments and have forced local councils to shrink their provision to the extent that many remaining centres now offer little more than a skeleton service. In this sense some services may be regarded as 'ineffective' if judged against original Sure Start objectives. De-professionalism becomes a filter that resonates, for the reason that although this programme was designed to boost the educational and life chances of socially and economically disadvantaged children, a 62 per cent cut in local council early years spending since 2010 has meant that between 500 and 1,000 Sure Start Centres in England have closed since then (Butler, 2019b). According to Naomi Eisenstadt, an expert on child poverty and the inaugural director of the Sure Start Unit, provision for children has become 'hollowed out', sweeping away outreach services designed to encourage the most disadvantaged and hard to reach' families to come to the centres (Butler, 2019e).

Marketisation has led to local councils being reinvented as seeking a lowest cost placement for children requiring residential care – at the end of 2018 there were approximately 8,000 children in England being cared for in a children's home. And between 2012 and 2017, 'out-of-borough placements' rose from 2,250 to 3,680, with children's homes increasingly concentrated in coastal areas and the north–west, where property is cheap (Weale, 2018b). Across the country there has been a huge rise in children being taken into care, a service that has become heavily reliant on expensive agency social workers. The gap between available resources and demand, about £3 billion by 2025 on current estimates, seems to be growing, and spending is concentrated on crisis services, not preventive ones (Butler, 2019d).

Alternative types of intervention in place of professional services

The Conservative government's 'life chances strategy', intended to focus on supporting children during the early years and improving parenting, was expected to be published in 2016, acknowledging that parenting support programmes have become a growing feature of changes to service direction and a substitute for other professional services. It emerged since that, with a change of prime minister, the Department for Work and Pensions (DWP) was to drop this important strategy in favour of a wider scheme on social justice to be outlined in a government Green Paper in early 2017. The outlined intention was to focus not just on the very poor but also on Prime Minister Theresa May's favoured demographic – the 'just about managing' households. A major plank of the strategy would be addressing joblessness in families, as part of how the government views effective parenting, and which it believes would be the biggest step towards improving social mobility for children (Mason, 2016). The philosophical or theoretical underpinnings of parenting support as a policy field serves to reveal its dominant professional orientation, becoming 'either a benign project of support or part of a more controlling educative or retraining exercise' (Daly, 2015: 602). As a form of intervention, it throws the net wider than the truly troubled families where professional child protection intervention is needed.

Some countries tend to regard parenting support as the province of professionals. For example, in the Netherlands parenting support is delivered by pedagogues and/or people trained in social work or youth work. However, the degree of professionalisation of parenting support is lower in England, especially because parenting programmes, which can be delivered by people with relatively little training, have been so predominant there (Daly, 2015: 602–3). Parenting classes were advocated by Prime Minister David Cameron, who suggested that all parents should be offered them as a measure to help alleviate child poverty, often replacing professionals who may currently provide family support. Parenting support is multidimensional and has capacity to play host to varying objectives. Daly and Bray (2015: 633–44) argue that it has become a popular policy solution as it has the advantage of being relatively easily generalisable – especially in the form of programmes, and aligns with current developments of the welfare state towards activation, provision of support through services and interest in localism.

To take the case of the Coalition (and Conservative) government's Troubled Families programme (TFP), the content and form of parenting support offered varied considerably. Local authorities across England were enlisted to deliver the programme, which, although it carried no new legislation or statutory guidance, was expected to be delivered using a family intervention approach. This advocates using a single key worker who can 'grip' the family, their problems and the surrounding agencies' (DCLG, 2012: 18) to work with them in a 'persistent, assertive and challenging' (DCLG, 2012: 23) way that will encourage them to take responsibility for their behaviour and change their ways. These workers are expected to be 'dedicated to the family' and able to 'look at the family from the inside out, to understand its dynamics as a whole; and to offer practical help and support' (DCLG, 2012: 4). Where families did not engage with the programme, workers were encouraged by the government to, in some circumstances, ask 'other agencies to accelerate threat of a sanction to exert maximum pressure on families to change' (DCLG, 2012: 28). The TFP, then, was positioned as a central government programme that would not only 'sort out' troublesome families but would also 'sort out' the public services that were currently working with the families (Crossley and Lambert, 2017). Troubled families were officially defined as those who met three of the four following criteria: involved in youth crime or anti-social behaviour; have children who are regularly truanting or not in school; have an adult on out-of-work benefits; cause high costs to the taxpayer (DCLG, 2012: 9). It represented a deliberate critique by the Conservative government of social work's professionalism, its values and its status as an organised group of workers advocating on behalf of children and families. The use of key workers remains in keeping with the wide body of literature on the role of street-level bureaucrats (Lipsky, 1980, 2010). However, it was acknowledged in an unpublished Whitehall report (see Savage and Wright, 2016) that the TFP, as an interconnected government-controlled intervention, as part of an 'underclass' discourse to tackle entrenched social problems, has to date had no discernible effect on unemployment, truancy or criminality. The proven ineffectiveness of this programme appears alongside a backdrop of cuts to benefits, soaring levels of food bank use and lower funding for all public services.

The increased use of foster carers has characterised current policy, and the de-professionalisation question emerges when it becomes legitimate to ask whether foster carers should be treated as professionals and receive a fee for their service, given the public demand for a high level of life experience, knowledge and skill on the part of those fostering children. The term 'foster carer' has replaced the term 'foster parent' in the UK, in order to signal that this is a professional role (Ribbens McCarthy and Edwards, 2011: 18). Debate continues as to whether foster carers are employed principally as substitute parents or as paid professionals with a legal status. Specialist fostering, involving for example groups of older/younger children, own race and transracial placements, and the viewing of foster carers as professionals, opened new dimensions to the practice of foster care. There has been a paucity of formal research around this subject, particularly relating to its outcomes. The evolutionary history of adoption and fostering has been one of overlaps, leading sometimes to ambiguities and confusion about purpose, expectations, roles and relationships (see, for example, Triseliotis, 1997: 331–6). The early 1970s witnessed a form of fostering used either to divert children from institutions or to get them out and place them with families. The philosophy that informed it was associated with the notions of community care and normalisation that were new at the time (Wolfensberger et al, 1972;

Wolfensberger, 1998; Malin et al, 1999). Besides viewing specialist fostering as being for the most troubled and troublesome children, its other key features were its contractual nature, time-limited with an average of two years, payment of a fee to foster carers, the training and preparation of carers, the preparation of children before placement and the provision of post-placement support to foster carers and children alike (Triseliotis, 1997: 332). Over the years there have been unresolved issues about the role fostering should play, in spite of signs of a slow drift towards professionalisation. It was reported that the number of those fostering in England remained roughly constant for 25 years, around 32,000 (Triseliotis, 1995), but recent evidence shows that by 2016 there had been a marked increase to between 45,000 and 55,000 (Bawden, 2016).

Re-adjusting the ratio of professionals to non-professionals delivering public services

De-professionalisation is also reflected in the way that health support workers are employed by NHS England in proportion to professionally trained nurses (CQC, 2015a, 2015b; Campbell, 2015a, 2015b, 2015d). 'Bed-blocking' costs between £800 and £900 million annually (Campbell, 2015a, 2015b, 2015d; RCN, 2016a), indicating that many chronically ill patients remain in hospital unnecessarily. The need to employ large numbers of temporary and more expensive agency nurses to care for those who remain in hospital unnecessarily has resulted in ballooning financial deficits in hospital budgets. Employment agencies charge exorbitant fees, and official figures show that the £2.72 billion spent on agency and contract staff in the financial year 2015/16 was £1 billion more than planned. Most hospitals now have an increased reliance on temporary staff, including locums, because of personnel shortages: £4 billion was spent on agency staff in 2015 compared to £2.6 billion in 2013/14 and £3.4 billion in 2014 (McVeigh, 2016). Private companies appear to be being awarded huge health contracts at an ever-increasing rate.

The decline in professional advocacy on behalf of youth services, including Connexions, and women's refuge services has likely contributed to difficult outcomes that they currently face, as both have felt the effect of severe cuts (Brignall, 2016). A survey by UNISON of 180 local authorities providing youth services in the UK estimated that cuts in youth service spending, including on staff, between April 2010 and May 2016 stood at £387 million, despite huge disparities in youth unemployment across the UK (for example, 18.3 per cent in 2015 in the north-east region). Other services now more reliant on volunteers and non-professional staff as a result of unwelcome financial cuts include women's refuges, which have been put at risk by benefit changes. For example, it has been claimed that 17 per cent have been shut down over the last five years and two thirds are facing closure because of a change in the way that housing benefit is paid to supported and sheltered housing (Gayle, 2016). There was an intention to cap the amount of rent that housing benefit would cover in the social sector at the same level offered to private landlords in the same area. Nevertheless, the DWP concluded that a deferral of the reforms until 2019 would give women's refuges a period of grace while officials conducted a review into funding for the supported housing sector.

The central argument, however, is not just about the paucity of numbers of professionals employed by public services but a seeming disregard for increasing the number of specialist professionals – for example, hospitals have been reported as being short of transplant surgeons and specialist nurses, and transplant centres are understaffed and struggle to keep up with demand (Campbell, 2018e). Other schemes have reportedly elected to employ a dedicated practitioner in preference to a social work professional in order that they may 'work differently', but one suspects that a chief reason may be to cut corners over financial arrangements and/or to absorb staff more conveniently into the managerial model. This has been the approach adopted by, for example, the Pause pilot project, which is a national scheme to reduce pregnancy, mental health problems and drug addiction and is designed to 'step into the lives of women made fragile by layers of accumulated anguish' and to work intensively alongside them for 18 months on the practical and emotional challenges they face (Tickle, 2017: 36). It is alleged that some prisons, for example those run by G4S, have set about reducing the number of higher paid, experienced, senior professionals and replacing them with cheaper officers, in order to make them profit-making after their takeover in 2011.

Rebalancing the ratio of professional to non-professional staff becomes clearly evident around current funding to deliver public health services across England. A BMA report (2018) claimed that this has reduced significantly over recent years, and planned cuts to the public health grant to local authorities now average 3.9 per cent a year to 2020/1 (BMA, 2018). This report also interrogated the notion that the number of health care practitioners has been reduced compared to that of health advisors or health care assistants in order to reduce costs. It aimed to highlight the impact of cuts to public health budgets at a local level, with key findings that include the observation that changes to public health spending in local areas do not reflect the needs of local populations and that many areas with poor health outcomes are seeing substantial cuts to funding for a range of key public health services.

From a social science perspective, Barry and Yuill (2016: 226–40) place the idea of challenging the professional contribution within a contextual ideological framework towards public health policy as it has developed in the UK, using a model taken from Hanlon et al (2011). In this model, entitled 'The Five Waves of Public Health', a significant watershed (or wave) is marked by the inauguration of the British welfare state following the Second World War. As discussed in Chapter 4, this oversaw, for example, the provision of health care, social security, council housing and education available to all. It was followed by another 'wave of developments 1960–2000', "marked by substantial changes that occurred in the UK and a move towards an increasingly complex and changing society. Emphasis shift[ed] towards tackling risk behaviours (smoking, drinking and diet), alongside a concern that social inequalities lead to health inequalities' (Barry and Yuill, 2016: 237).

Here the argument is that the cause of health problems today is therefore to be found in where one is located in an unequal society; also that in relation to public services the emphasis is moving away from professional activity as such towards the resources and responsibilities of individuals themselves for their own self-care, for becoming self-taught and ultimately a form of self-actualisation, based on Maslow's theory of human development psychology (Maslow, 1943; 1954). The authors review the evidence of Wilkinson and Pickett (2010), who assert the following: 'Rather than providing ever more prisons, doctors, health promoters, social workers, educational psychologists, and drug rehabilitation units, in expensive and at best only partially effective attempts to offset the problems of relative deprivation, it may be cheaper and more rewarding to tackle the underlying inequalities themselves.'

Instead of focusing ultimately on achieving good outcomes as a result of any intervention, professional or otherwise, it may be better to focus on the deeper causes of the problems that give rise to ill health. Marmot (2015) endorses this policy direction when he says that both the government and practitioners should be focused on the 'causes of the causes' – 'building resilient communities' (p 228) and 'promoting a just distribution of health' (p 256) – if we want a fairer society. This is Hanlon et al's (2011: 34) point too, in their call for a new form of health policy that is quite different from what we may be used to thinking of as being health policy.

The budget reductions in the UK have provided evidence that cuts to public health services and support have had a deep impact, as many rely on the specialist expertise of paid professional workers, where the service is known to be cost-effective. Areas affected include substance misuse, sexual health and smoking cessation services, the conclusion being that such constraints impede the ability to develop a comprehensive, responsive approach to public health prevention (see, for example, Buchan et al, 2017; DHSC, 2017; Longevity Science Panel, 2018).

> This can be seen starkly in cuts to drug treatment and prevention services that have occurred, despite increasing harms, and arise in deaths associated with drug misuse in England over recent years. Cuts to obesity services ... we are now seeing unacceptable variation in the quality and quantity of public health services available to the public throughout England with some data indicating a widening of health inequalities across England over recent years. (BMA, 2018: 18)

Sexual health services in England, for example, have been described as 'stretched to the limit' as a record 3.3 million people visited clinics during 2017 (Hargreaves, 2018: 17). This rise in demand comes alongside a move away from NHS-funded provision towards that by local authorities across England, whose budgets have been slashed by hundreds of millions of pounds, according to a Local Government Association report (LGA, 2018b). Of relevance to the main argument is that such transformation signals a reduced opportunity for the service to be led by health care practitioners. This report revealed that in 2017 there were 3,323,000 visits to sexual health clinics in England, up 13 per cent from 2,941,000 in 2013, and that the increased number of visits was equivalent to an extra 210 a day. In 2017 almost half a million of cases of sexually transmitted diseases were recorded in England and Wales, while clinic attendance rose by 13 per cent. The most common diagnosis was chlamydia – easily cured with antibiotics, although it can cause pelvic pain and infertility if left untreated. But what has caused most alarm appears to be a rise in cases of gonorrhoea, up tenfold since 2008, and syphilis, an infection that had virtually been wiped out in Britain but is now running at levels not seen since the Second World War. The rise is mainly among men who have sex with men, but not entirely (Hinsliff, 2018b).

This argument centres not only on the access, availability and funding of professionally trained practitioners to meet demand but on whether it might ever be desirable for these services to be replaced either by an alternative less professional, generic/non-specialist equivalent or by no service at all. The Conservative government's long-awaited NHS strategic plan, issued in January 2019, promises to look for new ways to increase the number of staff in the workforce and to improve mental health provision. At the end of 2018, however, there is still in place an austerity policy-led trend to cut alcohol and drug addiction services by a further £34 million and community smoking cessation services by £3.1 million. The NHS plan suggests that these services would be replaced by new 'specialist alcohol care teams' and 'prescription drugs or counselling', together with encouraging patients to take 'control of their habits' (Borland, 2019: 6).

The plan also heralds the introduction of innovative provision to deal with the reported crisis in child mental health. This service would appear now to offer significant career opportunities as regards bringing about a culture change within a national workforce. For instance, mental health training is currently offered through both a professional route, where the student pays fees and there is no government subsidy, and a non-professional route, where the student is paid by government and where there is a subsidy. The latter programme content to date has been limited in scope and has a claimed aspiration to create 'equivalence', whereby non-professionals receive training to undertake a professional job. Professionals already operating in this field may, however, differ in their support for the rapid expansion of approaches such as whole-school well-being programmes, cognitive behavioural therapy and mindfulness to tackle underlying anxieties, along with other evidence-based psychological, talking, physical, art and family therapies to identify the mental distress caused possibly by earlier life trauma.

Until austerity measures were implemented from 2010 onwards, the term 'youth services' referred to a wide range of provision, including community and adolescent mental health services, professional youth services, drug and alcohol outreach programmes, and all -year-round activities, including diversionary programmes that help young people to build up confidence, resilience and access to multi-agency support. This seems to have represented the tip of the iceberg as regards inadequate child mental health provision, and it is probably the more structured, formalised types of professional services that have now become residualised, only meaningfully to be addressed by reinvestment in youth services as a whole. Young people with mental health difficulties have been described as profoundly distressed at being held on paediatric wards, because of a national shortage of child and adolescent psychiatric inpatient beds (Jones, 2018). Mental health hospital trusts in particular rely heavily on locum doctors and agency and bank staff to cover vacancies, and this is not conducive to effective patient care, evidence showing that continuity of care in this specialty is essential in building trust between patients and practitioners.

A decline in professional advocacy surfaced through research carried out for the Children's Commissioner for England, which found children were often unable to get appropriate support at school and in the community (Children's Commissioner, 2019). This had been contributing to children ending up in costly institutional placements, sometimes for months or years, and often based many miles away from their home. The review gathered data available about some of the most vulnerable children – those living in secure children's homes, youth justice settings, mental health wards and other residential placements. It showed that there were 250 children identified as having a learning disability or autism residing in mental health hospitals in England in February 2019, compared with 110 in March 2015; and it was claimed that the latter figure had been recorded because of 'under-identification' of these children in the past. The advocacy organisation Coram Voice questioned whether such children needed to be locked up, given the lack of appropriate community services available (Coram Voice, 2019). It claimed that children locked away were 'invisible' in the system, and that they deserved to be given a voice as regards the care they received: 'Ready access to advocacy helps them understand their rights and entitlements and gives them a professional who can work alongside them to ensure that they are heard by those that work with them' (Coram Voice, 2019)

As a final point, the process of outsourcing can reduce access to professional services by its lack of focus on individual need. The outsourcing group Capita, it was alleged, put patients at risk of serious harm after taking over the NHS's administration service, according to a National Audit Office (NAO) report (NAO, 2018). Failures resulted in 87 women being notified incorrectly that they were no longer part of the cervical screening programme, and this may have comprised patient safety. This report, released in March 2018, said that patients may also have been harmed by a failure to update the official list of 37,000 qualified general practitioners (GPs), dentists and opticians. Capita's performance and NHS England's decision to outsource administration services resulted in continuing problems for primary care practitioners, said the NAO. In August 2015, NHS England entered into a seven-year, £330 million contract with Capita for primary care support services covering payments to GP practices, opticians and pharmacies, pensions and changes to the lists of qualified practitioners. At the same time the Ministry claimed that £60 million equalled the sum saved for taxpayers by NHS England's decision to outsource administration services. Capita proposed an overall reduction in staff numbers and closed 35 out of 38 support offices, cutting staff from 1,300 to 650. The NAO report said that patients could potentially have been put at risk owing to problems with the 'performers list' – a list of GPs, dentists and opticians practising in the NHS, including whether they are suitably qualified and have passed other relevant checks.

Is de-professionalisation associated with 'under-performing' services?

The headline 'hospitals under-performing due to a lack of health care professionals' was quoted from evidence following Care Quality Commission (CQC) inspections placing some hospitals in special measures, for example Addenbrookes (Cambridge), where the CQC report highlighted 'serious concerns' (Campbell, 2015a, 2015b, 2015d; CQC, 2015a). These included 'a significant shortage of staff in a number of key areas, including critical care; staff having been moved from ward to ward to cover gaps in rotas, even though some lacked the necessary training … [and] too few midwives, coupled with a high use of agency and bank staff' (p 8). This form of what amounted to hospital 'blacklisting' may cause damage by contamination to the reputation of individual professional staff employed there, albeit undeserved. The CQC report suggested the need for an 'improvement director', but in the confusion it was not clear what exactly merited 'inadequate' patient care or indeed 'special measures'.

An earlier scandal in the UK in the mid-2000s in the Stafford hospital run by the mid-Staffordshire NHS Foundation Trust concerned the level of poor-quality health care and emphasised the role of staff malpractice in 'under-performing' medical services. Recommendations of the Francis Report (2013) included: to make all those who provide care for patients accountable for what they do; to enhance recruitment, education, training and support of all contributors to the provision of health care; and, most importantly, to integrate the essential shared values of a common culture that needed to be fostered by leaders of the organisation. By mid-2016 it was reported that the tough inspection regime for hospitals introduced to prevent a repeat of the Mid-Staffordshire care scandal had been relaxed as the NHS regulator adjusted to budget cuts brought in by the Secretary of State for Health. The CQC would now undertake 'fewer and smaller inspections of hospitals in England and rely more on information provided by patients and NHS trusts under a new five-year strategy' (Campbell and Johnson, 2016: 9). This change will likely see a rolling-back of the in-depth approach to assessing the quality and safety of hospital services; the Mid-Staffordshire Report required scores of CQC inspectors spending up to a week examining how hospitals operate. As part of the new CQC strategy, inspectors would be expected to concentrate on core services, such as Accident and Emergency (A&E) and critical care, and no longer examine in detail how a wide range of departments were doing. The CQC admitted it was having to scale back and rethink because it would be receiving 'fewer resources' – £32 million less by 2019 than the £249 million it received in 2016 from the Department of Health. The likely result is that fewer inspections will be carried out: this is saddening in a situation where CQC rates just 1 per cent of care homes as outstanding and 40 per cent as either requiring improvement or inadequate (Quinn, 2016).

A number of 'serious incidents' were uncovered according to a further report from the CQC into Brighton and Sussex University Hospitals NHS Trust (CQC, 2016a), including so-called 'never-events' where surgeons operated on the wrong part of patients' bodies and where it was suggested that not enough staff were available to ensure that patients were receiving safe care. A later substantive inquiry at the Shrewsbury and Telford Hospitals Trust into dozens of baby deaths and injuries declared its A&E and maternity care 'inadequate' according to the NHS Care Regulator. This CQC report addressed the fact that this particular Trust had been under pressure over a growing catalogue of alleged breaches of care standards. The Trust runs two hospitals and provides care for 420,000 people; at the time it had 715 beds and employed 5,000 staff. This 'under-performing' hospital service was put under 'special measures' in November 2018 and ordered:

> to review and improve midwifery staffing levels to meet the needs of women and keep women and babies safe... Patients were deemed to be at risk of malnutrition and bedsores were not properly assessed, (there was) a lack of children's doctors in its A & E units and a general lack of doctors and nurses. (Borland et al, 2018)

The CQC report did not seek to apportion blame directly to staff but, as with previous interventions, focused instead on management processes, recommending a response almost counterintuitive to what the overwhelming body of evidence seemed to demonstrate; that is, a need to hire more professionally-trained staff with the right kind of expertise. Professor Ted Baker, the CQC's chief inspector of hospitals, said he was 'particularly concerned about the emergency department and maternity service ... while we found staff to be caring and dedicated, there is clearly much work needed at the Trust to ensure care is delivered in a way that ensures people are safe' (CQC, 2018c).

Other well-publicised reports, for example from the Nuffield Trust and Health Foundation thinktanks, continued to stress fears over standards of care, including one from NHS England that examined a range of data and attributed new ratings, claiming that almost nine in ten NHS groups were failing cancer patients with low rates of diagnosis and treatment:

> The fact that so many clinical commissioning groups (CCGs) in England have been identified as providing inadequate care to cancer patients through delayed diagnosis, first treatments and referrals is very concerning ... The data shows that of 209 CCGs only 22 have been 'performing well', for example in the last 2 years the target to start treatment (for cancer) within 62 days has only been met once, with 2,000 cancer patients now waiting longer to start treatment. (NHS England, 2017: 12–13)

The argument for underperforming services was supported by evidence from the Social Mobility Commission in relationship to two-year olds who were not having their health and education needs routinely reviewed by a professional. This report indicated that the number of full-time equivalent health visitors in England fell by 1,000 in one year between 2015 and 2016, with the result that one in four babies born in the UK was not receiving mandatory check-ups from health visitors during their first two years:

> Despite this being a crucial period for families, there is still too little support for parents in the earliest stage of their child's life. With the socio-economic gap in outcomes emerging early, providing support to parents at this point

could reap divisions for social mobility later on in life. (Social Mobility Commission, 2016)

A process of de-professionalisation characterised by a reduction in service standards has become intensified as a result of depleted staff numbers. A report by neo-natal experts at Oxford and Leicester universities, namely the MBRRACE-UK coalition, estimated that around 180 full-term babies had died in childbirth annually owing to mistakes, staff shortages and delays in delivering the infant. Four out of five (80 per cent) of the 225 full-term stillbirths and neo-natal deaths a year in the UK could have been prevented if mothers had received better care and maternity units were better staffed. This report claimed that about 180 babies a year were dying during childbirth because of midwife shortages, mistakes by maternity staff and delays in delivering the infant (NPEU-MBRRACE, 2018). There have also been serious fears raised over standards of care as more patients have been readmitted to hospital. The number of patients who have had to be taken back into hospital in England within 30 days rose 19.2 per cent from 1,158 in 2010/11 to 2016/17, according to a report by the Nuffield Trust and Health Foundation thinktanks (Nuffield Trust, 2018b).

A growing number of patients have been reported as being readmitted as emergency cases within days of being discharged, raising fears that hospitals are so busy and understaffed that they are providing inadequate care (Campbell, 2018a). In a similar vein, evidence has emerged of a sharp rise in unexpected deaths of ambulance patients, leading to warnings that NHS ambulance services have been under 'excessive pressure'. Figures for England obtained under freedom of information rules showed that 'serious incidents' resulting in death more than doubled from 31 in 2012 to 72 in 2016, rising annually (Marsh, 2017). NHS Providers now say that the policy of giving the NHS only small budget increases, under the implementation of austerity in 2010, has damaged patient care, created serious staffing problems and has led to key targets being routinely missed (Campbell et al, 2018).

De-professionalism as defined by deprivation of professional intervention has characterised a 'cancelling of operations and cancer scans going unread' across the NHS because consultant doctors began working to rule in a standoff over NHS pensions (Campbell, 2019c). As a consequence, waiting times for treatment, already too lengthy, have also worsened as hospitals have struggled to find senior doctors prepared to work more than their planned shifts. Changes to pension rules in 2016 have meant that rising numbers of consultants receive large bills linked to the value of their pension, providing them with a disincentive to work extra hours. The impact of higher taxes has been described by some consultants as an existential threat to parts of the NHS (Campbell, 2019c). Consultants' decisions also mean hospitals are struggling to find enough doctors to ensure shifts in their A&E or acute units are staffed, including emergency care and out-of hours rotas. Evidence taken from practitioners and NHS providers has indicated that this situation will continue to pose a real risk to the quality or safety of care of patients; and coming a decade into austerity might be read as offering little if any reassurance that any continuation of this era will not stem the tide of deepening further health inequalities.

As regards efforts to improve state provision to support children and families, the term 'under-performing' became a commonplace through several serious case reviews (SCRs) that have been undertaken. These have highlighted, for instance, key misjudgements by child protection workers, police and other professionals who may have missed opportunities to intervene to protect children. Arguably this situation has worsened through years of government cuts to the services that are there to prevent tragedies from happening. The SCR investigating two child deaths in Northamptonshire criticised 'poor quality decision-making and inadequate practice; unqualified staff making key decisions; hundreds of cases left unassessed for weeks and a chronic shortage of experienced social workers' (Butler, 2019c: 18). An NHS internal inquiry into potentially suicidal autistic children with mental health problems found that health professionals dealing with the young people did not carry out proper risk assessments, and did not record risky behaviour that meant they were in danger of harming themselves. This example, described as illustrating flaws in care, arose from the fact that several staff had been found breaching safety guidelines and had been responsible for some poor judgements in making decisions relating to patient safety (Campbell, 2019a: 9). Although it has long been a criticism of the Conservative government that it has failed to protect mental health budgets, Prime Minister Theresa May in the final weeks of her premiership announced a package of staff training measures. These measures were seen, however, as open-ended as they were not intended to be signed off before a Treasury Spending Review occurring later in 2019, almost certainly involving a new chancellor. They included a goal of training teachers to spot the early signs of mental health issues in children, and of encouraging NHS staff to learn about suicide prevention. There would also be updated professional guidance for social workers to oblige them to take relevant training around children's mental health.

Is de-professionalisation defined by a lack of efficiency as regards some treatment interventions – the example of mental health services

The professional dominance model that underpins aspects of this discourse has been encapsulated by the neo-Weberian framework (Rogers and Pilgrim, 2014: 141–2). It focuses, for example, on the relationship between the status of psychiatry as a medical specialty and the role of physical treatment, its treatment role being seen to remain in a precarious state of legitimacy. The model refers to the way by which professionals exercise power over others, including a context where they may seek to establish a dominant relationship over other occupational groups working with the same clients. Such a professional group may seek to exclude existing equal competitors or it may seek to usurp the role of existing superiors. It may subordinate them, an example being obstetricians directing the work of midwives, or limit their therapeutic powers to one part of the body. Historically there has always been a problem of legitimacy about the effectiveness of psychiatric treatment, including doubts about efficacy and acceptability; whereas there is mixed evidence about the effectiveness of psychotherapy – an overall estimate is that it is only of marginal utility (McQueen and Henwood, 2002; Rogers and Pilgrim, 2014: 134–5): 'Thus this professionalisation of narratives could be criticised for undermining the legitimacy and effectiveness of ordinary relationships, which when working well contain elements of clarification, reflection and social support' (Rogers and Pilgrim, 2014: 135).

The increasing use of evidenced-based research questions the efficacy of any psychiatric drug within the discourse of 'treatment' or 'cure', whether it is biological or psychological, along with questioning the impact of evidence-based practice (EBP) on treatment. The extent of its formal academic impact in the field of mental health is shown by the appearance in 1997 of a dedicated journal, *Evidence-Based Mental Health*. The rising popularity of EBP was linked to the imperatives of health policy-makers to control service costs, and was overlain by a discourse of concern to assess the health benefits and risks of technology and treatments (Faulkner, 2008; Pilgrim, 1997). These concerns can be seen as rhetorical devices, which include the purported strengths of multidisciplinarity and benefits to users of cost-effective treatments; for instance, a user perspective on treatment effectiveness can challenge professional definitions of EBP. It is common now for all parties to accept, in principle, evidence as a basis for clinically effective and cost-effective interventions.

The argument for characterising this competing discourse in terms of de-professionalisation arises for instance from the different narratives used by professionals towards assessing risk in mental health care; and ensuring risks to health and safety of adults who self-harm or are in receipt of protection are mitigated (see Brown et al, 2015; Godefroy, 2015). Understanding of mental illness and of the role of those charged with their care (or control) play a key role in resolving tensions concerning the outcomes of post-incident inquiries, such as Serious Case Reviews (SCRs); whereas understanding of the probability and prediction is generally very poor among both professionals and the public. Unrealistic expectations for risk assessment and management in general psychiatric practice carry a variety of significant costs, taking a number of forms, to those with a mental illness, to mental health professionals and to services. Especially important are changes in professional practice and accountabilities that are significantly divorced from traditional practice. These include implications for trust in patient–clinician relationships and the organisations in which mental health professionals work and practise that often breach the ethical principle of justice (fairness) and heighten discrimination against people with mental illness (Szmukler and Rose, 2013).

Risk assessment has become a primary focus of almost all CQC reviews covering mental health provision, and was central to the narrative of a report covering Norfolk and Suffolk NHS Foundation Trust that placed this mental health service provider in special measures as a result of a lengthy inspection in 2017 (CQC, 2018a). Its recommendations covered a need for learning from previous SCRs to be shared and actions implemented:

> suitably qualified and experienced staff must be available to meet people's care and treatment needs ... the Trust leadership team (needs to take) action at the pace required to resolve failings in safety. Staff did not assess and manage the risks they posed to patients ... [they] did not manage medicines and equipment safely, they did not undertake proper reviews of patients who were in seclusion and there were insufficient staff to meet patients' needs in some community services ... Staff (in community teams) did not meet targets for assessment or respond appropriately to emergency or urgent referrals. Inspectors found that staff

were often downgrading referrals from urgent to routine without ensuring that it was safe to do so. There was a paucity of evidence as regards records of people who had been denied a service and records showed some patients harmed themselves while waiting for contact from clinical staff. (CQC, 2018b: 28)

This report recognised 'failures' of staff but preferred not to engage with the background surrounding this conclusion. The CQC Report of this 'under-performing' service may unwittingly have glossed over the fact that there often exists a profound level of ambivalence over the correct forms of treatment that mental health service users should receive. A contemporary media outcry of too little funding for mental health services (Campbell, 2018e; O'Hara, 2018) may have resulted partially from such ambiguity, the relative absence of an effective professional lobby group(s) in support of service users and even a visceral lack of consensus over what are seen to be the right kind of services and support deserving funding priority. Professions may have been seen as in competition with one another and thus could be accused of not fully getting their act together.

The CQC NHS England vowed to transform mental health services with an extra £1 billion a year, although there have since been some doubts that this sum was being ring-fenced (Quinn and Campbell, 2016). The present Conservative government along with the previous Coalition have presided over the decimation of mental health services – 'a car crash' according to Professor Sue Bailey, former president of the Royal College of Psychiatrists (Allan, 2017: 39). Department of Health figures indicate (Campbell, 2016c) that the number of mental health nurses working in the NHS have dropped by almost a sixth since the Conservatives came to power in 2010. While there were 45,384 mental health nurses working in England in 2010, there were just 38,774 in July 2016. The government's national plan originally had a number of targets; for example, people facing a mental health crisis would be able to get community care such as psychological treatments 24 hours a day.

In addition, each area should have a multi-agency suicide prevention plan, yet local plans would not be specifically required to recruit additional trained professional staff; for example, nurses or social workers. From 2017 there has been a call for urgent action to improve mental health services for students. With suicide rates among students on the rise and a sharp increase in demand for mental health support, universities have acknowledged that current services are letting students down (Weale, 2018a). The Universities UK (UUK) Report Minding Our Future (UUK, 2018) stated that the number of students dropping out with mental health problems has more than trebled in recent years, and several universities in the UK have seen a number of student suicides over a short period of time. This particular report calls for a partnership arrangement at local level to assess needs and to design and deliver services, involving national and local government, schools, colleges, the NHS and universities to 'join up mental health care services around students' (Weale, 2018b).

Additionally, there has been renewed evidence that more women than men have taken their own lives in mental health units. For instance, data collected by the CQC shows that 224 people died of self-inflicted injuries between 2010 and 2016 in mental health hospitals in England (CQC, 2018e). Deborah Coles, director of the charity Inquest, which investigates deaths involving detained people, stated in this report: 'Critical to this is the need for greater oversight, accountability and learning. The lack of an independent investigation system for deaths in mental health settings, unlike that for deaths in police or prison custody, undermines this necessary scrutiny' (Campbell, 2019d).

The size and nature of responsibility facing mental health professionals may at times appear almost overwhelming, yet there are now some signs of an earnest transformation towards developing a more cohesive workforce. For example, the 'Think Ahead' approved mental health training is a government-subsidised route for recruiting and training staff to work in and lead future services:

> We're looking for remarkable people to do remarkable things. You'll need to show leadership potential and other attributes – build relationships with people, and support them through care, talking therapies, community action and standing up for legal rights, empower individuals, and their families, carers, communities, to lead fulfilling independent lives. (Think Ahead Mental Health Training website www.i-act.co.uk/)

Currently, a scenario of de-professionalisation becomes signified by an ever-increasing workload assigned to community care teams along with an inadequate number of skilled, qualified professionals to provide expert assistance. The precarious and challenging nature of some mental health interventions may have left a legacy that has had impacts on the manner in which some professionals and mental health workers are perceived within wider society. An example can be taken from the system of application for detention retained by the Mental Health Act 2007, which amended the previous 1983 Act. This role became widened to include nurses, occupational therapists and psychologists, as well as social workers, and renamed the Approved Mental Health Professional. The four categories of mental disorder left over from the 1959 Act were replaced by a single broader definition of mental disorder. When considering if a person needs to be detained owing to their mental disorder, there are now medical and non-medical professionals involved in that decision. There are benefits stemming from this amendment to the process, namely that since the 1959 Act the importance of the social perspective as a counterpoint to the medical perspective has continued to gain ground. This is not because of the increasing independence of Approved Social Workers under the 1983 Act, but more contemporarily because of the increasing voice of the service user/survivor movements. It has been suggested that social workers are uniquely placed to hear the views of service users, to give weight to them and champion the need to uphold their human rights when considering the use of the Mental Health Act 1983 or Mental Capacity Act 2005 (Godefroy, 2015: 25).

A similar approach towards reconfiguring the nature of professional intervention in mental health care arises when a person has been arrested in connection with an offence and brought to a police station, where they come within the provisions of the Police and Criminal Evidence Act 1984. This provides special protection for mentally disordered or mentally vulnerable persons whilst they are in police custody. Following the Bradley Report (2009), there has been an increase in the number of mental health professionals available in police stations. The role of these professionals is to ensure that the mental health needs of detainees are met, and to advise police on appropriate action if they are of the view that the person is acutely mentally disordered. The police also have access to doctors, namely forensic medical examiners, who are usually GPs who are on call to attend the police station when required. They are expected to deal with all the medical needs of detainees, and not all have any specialist skills or training in mental health (Godefroy, 2015: 117).

The trend towards reversing the pattern of insufficient mental health services has been led by outpourings of government rhetoric along with some earmarked funding. For example, all CCGs have been required to ensure they raise spending on mental health by more than the size of the overall annual budget increase they received for the financial year 2018/19, thereby meeting the mental health investment standard (Campbell, 2018e). This has become the policy that NHS chiefs are using to increase funding for psychological and psychiatric services after concern over years of under-investment. The government's 2019 NHS Long Term Plan seeks to halt the 'crisis' (O'Hara, 2018: 36) in mental health care by its promise to fund mental health teams, including staff based in schools and colleges to provide ongoing support after referral, whereas the NHS therapy service for people with milder mental health problems is to be expanded to ensure more people receive psychological help.

Summary

CQC reports show that some hospitals and primary care services are 'under-performing' owing to a lack of health and social care professionals – some professionals lack the necessary training, for example for critical care, long-term and chronic illness, such as Alzheimer's Disease. There has been a rolling back of rigorous inspectorate following the Francis Report (2013), and it is hard to avoid the conclusion that de-professionalisation has led to a reduction in service standards owing to fewer staff in post. For example, NHS bosses have stood accused of endangering patients over a controversial privatisation of cancer scanning services (Campbell, 2019b), and a firm supplying home carers has been accused of failing to pay social care staff for travel time appointments, meaning they earn less than the minimum wage (Murphy, 2019). Similarly, a former Ofsted head claimed that funding for schools was 'an issue', and that regional and ethnic differences were affecting educational success, as they were struggling to get and keep enough teachers, let alone good teachers, and standards were threatened as a result (Dodd, 2019).

Austerity is an extension of the neo-liberal logic to characterise any form of public spending as 'unproductive' (Mendoza, 2015: 83). Chancellor Philip Hammond said that his priority had been to tackle 'Britain's chronically low productivity' (Politics Home, 2019), yet admitted having been hampered by the lack of investment. However, with interest rates already extremely low in 2019 and the public sector ailing, there would appear to be a strong case for a future expansionary budget. This austerity period has been characterised not only by a continuation of the downplaying of traditional social policy values but also by an increased disillusionment with and mistrust of democratic politics and institutions (Corbett and Walker, 2019: 101). In an effort to address one particular social policy failure, the NHS Long-Term Plan unveiled in early 2019 offered the beginnings of a progressive and coherent strategy for modernisation, including a redistribution of resources to the poorest areas and least healthy people. Evidence suggests that risks of fragmentation and marketisation had not disappeared, but there was a strong call for the regime of competitive tendering introduced by 2013's Health and Social Care Act to be scrapped (Campbell, 2019d). Resolving the staffing crisis in health and social care has now become a main government priority, with a 'workforce strategy' expected in due course along with a training budget. Social care continues to be the unaddressed social policy problem of the age, with councils unable to meet their obligations to a rapidly ageing population and an explosion of need predicted over the next 20 years. The £2.3 billion additional funding promised for mental health is another positive step, though targets in this area, particularly with regard to young people, appear to remain somewhat opaque.

The situation may be defined as a perfect realisation of the unrealised, profoundly compromised. There is a view that UK public services rely far too much on the commitment of inadequately trained staff given the depleted nature of large sectors of provision; this is due to financial pressures. Both in modern health and social care and for instance in law enforcement, related occupations require highly sophisticated skills based on advanced levels of education; and restricting training opportunities inevitably leads to an individual's incapacity to cope with growing job demands. For instance, today's nurses need the knowledge and skills to carry out complex technical and behavioural assessments and interventions. Police are dealing with cyber crime and the immense subtleties of terrorism and sexual abuse. Neither occupation can now be practised with a training based on hanging out with experienced practitioners, picking up tips, tricks and manoeuvres. That inflexible model just perpetuates poor habits and bad science. Graduate jobs are not fixed for all time but evolve with the rest of society and economy (Dingwall, 2016).

9

Professional training programmes: financial cuts and content critique

Introduction

There has been a noticeable withdrawal of local authority, hospital trust and in-house funding support for higher-level, clinical and specialist training. Yet most professions now recognise that learning and professional development are lifelong, to be acquired with the aid of continuing professional development programmes (CPD). Led by the Royal College of Nursing, the British Medical Association, the Royal College of General Practitioners and the Patients Association, a coalition of more than 20 charities, medical and professional bodies, and trade unions released an open letter to Prime Minister David Cameron in June 2016, saying that moves to drop funding for student nurses and midwives represented an 'untested gamble' (Johnston, 2016). The proposals included stopping bursaries to support nurses during their training and switching them to student loans. Previously, nursing training had been treated differently from other higher and further education courses precisely to help reverse the shortages. The organisations highlighted the 'worrying lack of clarity or consultation about the effect that funding changes could have on those who need to train for more advanced or specialist roles, such as health visitors or district nurses' (RCN, 2016b; *The Telegraph*, 2019). Simultaneously, an RCN survey pointed to a dramatic fall in the number of school nurses, with almost a third working unpaid overtime every day to keep up with their workload. The research showed the number of school nursing posts had fallen by 10 per cent since 2010, leaving 2,700 school nurses now caring for more than 9 million pupils, despite a rising incidence in issues, especially in mental health among children (McVeigh, 2016).

De-professionalisation as a market-led critique of social work training

De-professionalisation may be demonstrated through the trajectory of a political economy model of delivering public services, where, for example, education policy has been progressively shaped by the needs or demands of a market economy. It aims to cut employers' costs and leads to the gradual marketisation of all services. Such a model comes close to the theory of elite control, in which the National Health Service (NHS) can be thought of as the product of conflict and power struggles between a political and a medical elite and arguably will remain so in the light of policy changes brought about by the Health and Social Care Act 2012 (see, for example, Greer et al 2016: 3–26). The political economy model therefore suggests that most major policy decisions are subject to the backing of big business' or capitalist interests. This perspective falls in line with Marxist views of class-structured society in which a ruling class controls policy and makes most of, if not all, the big decisions, particularly where policies affect the quality of the labour force (Blakemore and Warwick-Booth, 2013: 165).

As regards the social work profession, Tunstill (2016) asserts that 'there is a new and dangerously comprehensive quality to the current scope of (training) proposals under debate in the United Kingdom (UK) which makes them almost invulnerable to evidence-based critique, let alone revision', and goes on to describe a political party consensus about new developments, such as the introduction of an elite social work training route, Frontline (largely independent of the UK university sector). In excess of £100 million of extra funding has between 2013 and 2016 been given for fast-track training to expand the successful Frontline and Step Up schemes to help attract top-calibre graduates into social work, so that by 2018 one in four children's social workers would be qualifying in this way. Up to £20 million will be provided for a new What Works Centre to disseminate best practice (Taylor, 2016).

The ability of social workers to offer and provide a range of child and family support services was threatened by proposed clauses in the 2017 Children and Social Work Act, which exempts local authorities from meeting key existing statutory duties. Privatisation seems to pass for innovation. Considering the professional credentials of social work, the Conservative government at the time of writing is being advised on how to implement a preferred definition of the social work task, through a Knowledge and Skills Statement. Independent reviews of aspects of professional social work training were set up to explore the form of training that was 'ideally structured' to serve the profession, namely Croisdale-Appleby (2014) and Narey (2014). It is now an almost compulsory requirement of local authorities to buy in franchised packages, such as Signs of Safety and Attachment Measuring packages, with large sums being spent on this 'effectively privatised knowledge' (Tunstill, 2016: 3). Some social workers may come to view this as a threat to the integrity of existing training programmes, which have been validated and overseen by the profession's own association and have shaped their own professional lives.

Here the de-professionalisation process threatens professional knowledge per se, in a move to a professional/post-professional environment where organisations privatise knowledge and charge would-be professionals. The introduction of a quasi-professional qualification system, outside HE – examples being Frontline and Teach First – symbolises a major change in this direction. This may include a threat to rigorous regulation, where a central argument is that the commodification of knowledge by neo-liberal economic strategy becomes identified with the transfer of a publicly funded good, knowledge – with no cost – into the private sector, where it is used to generate profit.

Reviewing the viability and completeness of current training for health-care professionals

The critique of the basic direction of training as a component of de-professionalisation operates similarly within health care, where we have only to point to the high number of national and local reviews of nurse and paramedical training over the last 40 years since the political economy model of delivering public services took hold (see, for example, DHSS, 1972, 1986; Jay, 1979; DoH, 1988; Nursing and Midwifery Council UK, 2010, 2015). This may appear intrusive to professions if the action becomes part of a strategy to remove clinical tasks from professional control or influence. What about our reliance on overseas nurses and cuts to the number of UK nurses in training? More than 55,000 EU nationals work as doctors and nurses in a health service that would collapse without them, argues journalist Polly Toynbee (2016). The reason we need so many foreign nurses is that after 2010 the number of UK nurse training places was cut, with the gap filled from abroad. The Secretary of State declared that the 10,000 extra nurses employed under the present Conservative government had been as a result of importing nurses to cover for training cuts. In 2015 Health Education England was training 3,100 fewer nurses than a decade previously, a 19 per cent cut. Yet only 60 per cent of the newly trained entered the NHS, as the long-enforced 1 per cent pay cap meant that they could earn more in other occupations. Furthermore, the Conservative government removed nursing bursaries with the intention of widening access to nurse training, whilst at the same time blocking visas to non-EU nurses. This means that, like other students, they will have to take out loans and accumulate large debts. The Department of Health claimed that this would allow universities to create some 10,000 more training places: currently they are turning away 37,000 applicants, according to available Universities UK (UUK) figures (King's Fund, 2018a, 2018b).

This somewhat nuanced version of de-professionalisation has been characterised as witnessing a trend towards tolerance of incomplete or deficient training. For example, it has been reported that there have been deep cuts – up to 45 per cent – in nurses' post-registration specialist training, signifying that closure of courses will create acute shortages in specialisms, such as Accident and Emergency, intensive care, diabetes and cancer and palliative nursing (Mulholland, 2016). There is some evidence that in the NHS trained foreign nurses are prepared to work for less than professional wages, although this is not consistent with occupying a professional role and responsibilities.

The treatment of patients being held in mental health wards in England has frequently been placed under the microscope, in particular by the Care Quality Commission (CQC), who have critiqued not only the appropriateness of the type of care patients receive but also the fact that staff have often lacked the relevant skills and training required to deal with a range of complex behavioural problems posed by some patients. In order to escalate the introduction of more viable and complete modes of professional training, the CQC recommended a change in safety culture across the NHS to reduce the number of patients who experience avoidable harm. The claim was made that 'too many people [were] being injured or suffering unnecessary harm because NHS staff are not supported by sufficient training' (CQC, 2019: 21). Despite an outpouring of several reports and reviews from the CQC, for example alleging that harm has been caused 'because of the complexity of the current patient safety system', others based outside the government's regulatory framework have pointed to 'systemic failures' in the 'system of care' that has caused the problem. 'Why are we imprisoning and torturing people, blocking their human rights?' (Legal Voice, 2017) asks Sarah Ryan, activist and mother of Connor Sparrow Hawk, who alongside Roger Colvin campaigned successfully to prosecute an NHS trust for breaching health and safety laws following the deaths of their relatives in care. This has been seen not only as an organisational and professional failure but as a significant breach of an individual's human rights. 'By placing individuals with autism in cells, using prone unnatural restraint techniques and forced medication…or by segregating people in hospitals as there are no adequate community placements, we are in effect breaking the law. We can't recommend hospital closures as there is nowhere else for people to go'.

Education in schools and reconfiguring approaches to funding staff training in line with workforce remodelling

De-professionalisation points to a lack of commonality of standards, including wide differences in the number and availability of specialist trained teachers in schools. The UK lacks a standardised approach towards central planning of teacher supply along with benchmarked ratio requirements as regards the number of teachers to pupils. Also lacking is a methodology for how this might translate into a demand for additional teacher training or up-skilling. Reduction in teacher training opportunities has been reflected in a narrowing of the curriculum through academicisation – focusing on academic over vocational. This has been manifested partially, for example, by a lowering of the number of specialist staff trained to support children with special educational needs and disabilities who, it is alleged, have been failed by a system that is on the verge of crisis as demand for specialist support soars and threatens to bankrupt local authorities (Weale and McIntyre, 2018). The lack of financial support for training teachers in specialist subjects and its impact on reducing the capacity of many teachers to teach specific subjects has evolved alongside what might be regarded as a direct attack on the integrity of teaching as a profession. This has resulted, for example, in a repositioning of early childhood education and care and in the professionalisation of those working in these settings (Wingrave and McMahon, 2016). Various professional identities have therefore become reconstructed and the sector professionalised through academicisation, which has resulted in a number of challenges in the wider education workforce, creating issues of perception and parity for teachers.

National education reforms most associated with the remodelling of the workforce arose directly from New Labour's political agenda, which involved making the public sector more 'middle-class friendly – by reconceptualising a comprehensive education system designed to meet the needs of its new individualistic voter base. It involved a new discourse of leadership [to] enhance the roles of public sector managers, crucial agents of change in the reform process' (Ball, 2008: 137). This policy agenda required the remodelling of the teaching workforce as part of a more general strategy of flexibilisation and skill mix across the public services. There would also be a dual process of re-professionalisation (the construction of a new cadre of qualified and trained school leaders) and aspects of de-professionalisation (a much closer specification of the work of school practitioners, particularly in primary schools, and the introduction of new kinds of workers – such as classroom assistants – into schools). Various 'policy experiments', such as Education Action Zones and academies, allowed the employment of non-registered, non-qualified teachers. In 2007 a Report by PricewaterhouseCoopers (PWC), commissioned by the Department for Education and Skills, recommended that 'Schools should be led by chief executives who may not necessarily be teachers' (PWC website).

Academy schools are state-funded schools in England that are directly funded by the Department of Education (DfE) and independent of local authority control (Academies Act 2010). The terms of the arrangements are set out in individual academy funding agreements, and most are self-governing non-profitable charitable trusts that may receive additional support from personal or corporate sponsors, either financially or in kind. Most academies are secondary schools and most secondary schools are academies. However, slightly more than 25 per cent of primary schools, as well as some of the remaining first, middle and secondary schools, are also academies. Academies do not have to follow the National Curriculum but do have to ensure that their curriculum is broad and balanced and that it includes the core subjects of Maths and English. They also have the opportunity to set aside existing national agreements on pay, conditions and certification of teachers; that is to say, they can employ non-qualified individuals. The academies programme contracts out publicly funded schools to a huge array of third-party providers. However, some critics claim that the programme has bred fragmentation and segregation instead of a coherent, intelligible and equitable system (Donnelly et al, 2017). Additionally, there are long-standing criticisms that it is heavily influenced by politician-driven curriculums, an obsession with standards, league tables and Ofsted surveillance, and that it is embedded in an audit and accountability culture.

The idea of intellectualising our entire education system from top to bottom is one that has taken hold in recent times. The relegation and degradation of those subjects considered of less value by the powers that be, art, design and technology, drama and so on, has accelerated. The most telling example of this trend, very much inspired by Michael Gove and many before him, is the introduction of the English Baccalaureate (EBacc), where purely academic subjects are placed above others in the hierarchy of curriculum value and school performance indicators (Rogers, 2016). One feature of this modernising approach has been a concern expressed by many parents and teachers about the impact of the EBacc and its lack of breadth and balance frustrating the full potential of students and teachers. It has been described as a school performance indicator linked to the General Certificate of Secondary Education (GCSE) which measures the percentage of students in a school who achieve five or more 5–9 (formerly A–C) grades in traditional academic GCSE subjects. The reason for its introduction by the Conservative government was to combat the perceived fall in the number of students studying foreign languages and science. The government declared that under its office it would make the EBacc a compulsory qualification for students in secondary schools in the UK (Vaughan, 2017).

The EBacc has arguably narrowed the curriculum in many schools in a manner that does not consider young people's varied aspirations and educational needs, precluding vocational and arts subjects. Funding constraints in schools have halted teacher up-skilling and training opportunities and pedagogical approaches, for example group-work and problem-solving, no longer in the school curriculum. Such rigorous activities might offer students opportunities to interact, hypothesise, interpret, imagine, debate, disagree and give opinions – all essential for developing cooperation and successful work with colleagues in future workplaces. Inappropriate notions of distinctively academic or vocational pathways in education have sidelined developing enthusiasm and aptitudes that lie in the range of creative and technical subjects that underpin the UK's arts and creative industries. Schools need professionally trained teachers who are able to offer flexibility and skill transfer in subjects that will actually be needed by employers.

Aspects of this debate widened when the Conservative government announced its preference to extend the number of grammar schools in England and to offer better training opportunities to those qualified teachers who chose to work in grammar schools. Despite having excluded the vast majority of schools from any extra funding, in May 2018 Education Secretary Damian Hinds signalled that grammar schools would be given more than £50 million to expand as he unveiled a fund for selective schools that agreed to improve applications from disadvantaged children (Adams, 2018a). A further related controversy seemed set to begin when it was stated that Prince Charles had been lobbying on behalf of a charity he patronised for looser rules on teacher training. The main point was that he had founded a charity, Teach First, in 2002, which fast-tracks university graduates through three months of training, which entails a six-week training course following by a further six weeks of supervised training in the classroom. The alleged aim of the charity had been to recruit teachers for inner-city schools that were struggling to find teachers, with the charity receiving a fee for each teacher placement. In England, where the charity bids for contracts to supply teachers, it was reported that more than 10,000 teachers for state schools and academies had been recruited and trained by the organisation (Carrell and McEnaney, 2018). The need for teacher professionalism allied with 'real world' training is highlighted by an example from the fast-growing trend in the UK towards home schooling. The number of children that this involves is thought to be around 50,000 – a number that has increased sharply in recent years; and local authorities have a duty to ensure that all such children receive a 'suitable' education. It is understood that in 2018 the government sought to tighten and clarify the rules surrounding home education, where at present there is no mandatory register, little formal monitoring or local authority support. Some concerns have also been expressed around safeguarding, and what happens when children disappear from the view of professionals who might otherwise support them (Ray, 2017; Issimdar, 2018).

Early childhood education and care workforce: deregulation, low training and low pay?

The pursuit of quality tends to conflict with ensuring a rapid expansion of places for early education and nursery care for children and making provision more affordable within a market system. It is also a contested concept. The childcare market in England relies on consumer choice, but even when information is good parents are likely to have to prioritise affordability and covering their own working hours (Lewis and West, 2017). The government's approach to the issue of quality has changed since 2010, with the deregulation of the early years sector set as a stated aim (Gove, 2012). A major emphasis has been put on freeing providers to offer more high-quality places with more flexible hours, to invest in high-calibre staff and to provide more choice for parents (DfE, 2013a).

The early years workforce in the UK is low paid and low qualified when compared with most other Western European countries (DfE, 2013b; EC et al, 2014). In an independent review of qualifications (commissioned by the government), Professor Cathy Nutbrown (2012) proposed a clear ladder with qualifications at level 3 (upper secondary education) becoming the minimum standard, leading to 'early years teacher' with qualified teacher status. However, she did not recommend a graduate-led workforce (as per French provision for three-, four- and five-year-olds) or the introduction of a substantial post-18 specialised education (as per the three-year qualification in the Netherlands). The Coalition government abolished Labour's earmarked grant to improve workforce training and graduate leadership; instead, it strengthened the entry requirements for those seeking a level 3 childcare qualification and accepted the idea of early years teachers in 2013, albeit without granting crucial parity with schoolteachers. In 2013, while 87 per cent of staff in formal settings were qualified to level 3, the figure for childminders was only 66 per cent (Brind et al, 2014).

As a measure of de-professionalisation, it can be taken as acknowledged that since 2010 there has been only qualified support by central government for intervention to further improve qualifications. The first major Coalition document on the early years stated that 'employers have primary responsibility for the quality and effectiveness of their staff' (DfE/DH, 2011: 64), a position in harmony with the hands-off approach to regulation (Lewis and West, 2017). The 2012 survey of provider finances noted that providers felt that there was some need for staff training, but this was not seen as 'a massively pressing concern' (Brind et al, 2012: 4). In marked contrast to nursery and primary schools, which have qualified teachers, only 13 per cent of paid staff in mainly for-profit, full-day care settings employ a teacher (DfE, 2015). Most staff are low qualified (especially in poor areas), earning little above the minimum wage (Gambaro, 2012).

The debate about deregulation and quality came to a head over the issue of staff-to-child ratios, which had been clearly specified by Labour. A key government document (DfE, 2013c) set out the minister's wish to relax the ratios for all ages of pre-school children and to encourage providers to hire a qualified teacher, which would enable them to move from a 1:8 to a 1:13 ratio for three and four year-olds. The minister also wanted childminders to be able to look after up to four, rather than three, children under five. Relaxing ratios in a country with a low qualified and low paid workforce posed difficulties and aroused opposition from Nutbrown, as well as private sector providers' organisations and groups such as Mumsnet and Netmums, who backed the Rewind on Ratios campaign (House of Commons, 2013). Most damagingly, the Liberal Democrat Coalition partners withdrew their support (House of Commons, 2013), and this dimension of deregulation was dropped.

The higher ratio permitted by the presence of a teacher would make it possible to take more children, which in turn would financially benefit providers; and hence, it was hoped, parents (by lowering fees) and staff (by raising pay), while also securing better quality childcare (DfE, 2013c; 2015a). However, the different dimensions of policy being pursued by the government during this period lacked consistency in relation to promoting quality; for example, there was as much encouragement and more practical support for childminders than for increasing the proportion of graduates in the workforce. In conclusion, while the central issue – for quality – of the low qualifications held by the childcare workforce was addressed in part, reforms did not lead to a graduate-led workforce being established, even though evidence pointed to positive impacts where staff are highly qualified, as in Denmark and France (West, 2016). Deregulation has been key to Conservative government thinking on quality, which has centred on the promotion of the childcare market first and foremost and, alongside that, the restriction of government intervention actively to promote quality at both central and local levels. Austerity politics have not ruled out state intervention (Farnsworth and Irving, 2015); rather, the Coalition and Conservative governments have shown little enthusiasm for positive intervention of the kind designed to secure a better regulatory framework benefiting children or to raise the skills of the workforce (Lewis and West, 2017).

Modernising staff training approaches to maximise workforce capacity

The health and social care system is not only struggling to meet the care needs of our ageing population, but it is completely unprepared for the consequences of looking after growing numbers of older people with extremely complex health problems (Lowton et al, 2017). Specialist health and social care services, currently in short supply on a national scale, along with a need for more knowledge and skills training for both professionals and carers, are unable to respond to the increased demand and increasing complexity that, for example, adult mental health conditions such as depression and anxiety will bring.

> I think the key difficulty for providing proper health services for these 'new' ageing populations in adulthood is that our definition of success in this context is so focused on the short-term. The current crisis in the NHS reflects our concerns about patients' immediate care needs rather

than considering what our health and social care services will also require in the future in order to care for patients. We are unwilling or, perhaps, incapable – due to our parliamentary cycles and the current government's ethos of austerity – of looking ahead to see what type of support, intervention and care these 'new' ageing populations will need, and how we, as a society, can provide it. (quotation from Professor Karen Lowton in an article by Amelia Hill, 16 January 2017)

This not only taps into the austerity agenda, given that local councils are unable to fund the increased demand from older people requiring the highest levels of care, and where evidence shows that this number has risen by 50 per cent in the last five years in some authorities, but also underlines the high value placed on social care services in terms of how a responsible government needs to act. Given that the rate is repeated over the next five years and that further funding would be required, national solidarity suggests that the health care demands of ageing populations are regarded as of major importance and therefore receive the kind of broad vision and diverse expertise that only well-resourced professionals are able to provide.

De-professionalisation defined by financial cuts to staff training is highlighted in circumstances where it appears that a virtual absence of bespoke training available in a given speciality becomes accepted as a kind of norm. For example, a relevant report commissioned by the British Medical Association (BMA, 2016), using a sample of interviewees – 237 doctors and 269 members of the public – concerned the adequacy of health professionals' training as regards end of life care. The findings indicated a postcode lottery variation in the quality of care received, and specifically that doctors needed training to help them handle difficult conversations with dying patients and their relatives about the inevitability of death. This report reviewed the viability of current training for health care professionals within this practice domain and urged doctors to be guided by their clinical judgement, and to resist pressure from relatives or a fear of failure to continue treatment that would bring no benefit.

A second example may be taken from the area of learning disabilities. Research has indicated that lack of training for health professionals could be contributing to 1,200 avoidable deaths of people with a learning disability in England each year. A poll of health-care professionals for Mencap found 23 per cent had received no training on meeting the needs of patients with a learning disability and 45 per cent thought the lack of training might contribute to avoidable deaths. Almost half (47 per cent) of hospitals did not include information on learning disabilities in their induction training for clinical staff. Almost a quarter (22 per cent) of universities did not include training on making reasonable adjustments to the care of someone with a learning disability (which is a legal duty under the Equality Act 2010) in their undergraduate medicine degree (Mencap, 2018; Siddique, 2018).

In pursuance of an effective skill transfer strategy as part of the Conservative government's Long-Term Plan for the NHS, most chief executive officers would now prefer to follow a laid-down plan of action that supports interventions based on delivering a multidisciplinary, flexible approach to both health and social care. This offers opportunities for deploying a range of staff acting in different roles. As an example of interprofessional working a focus then would be on a 'trans-disciplinary approach' (Lacey, 2001: 15–16), where sharing or transferring information and skills across traditional professional boundaries enables one, two or more members to be primary workers supported by others working as consultants. There is some evidence that this pragmatism was applied during the junior doctors strike action between 2015 and 2016, when health professionals from several disciplines 'stood in' to fill the gap left by doctors' absences (Campbell, 2016c).

Summary

Restricting training opportunities inevitably leads to an individual's incapacity to cope with growing job demands. A withdrawal of local authority, hospital trust and in-house funding support for higher-level, clinical, pedagogic and specialist training, along with dropped funding for student nursing bursaries, represents a stance where the effect is to weaken or discredit the notion of professionalism through distancing practitioners from learning about new developments within their field of expertise. Most professions now recognise that learning and professional development are lifelong through CPD despite the fact that a majority of pathways to progress along with other opportunities have become self-funded. A research study by the Children's Services Funding Alliance has demonstrated that there are examples of exceptionally highly trained staff being lost to the system through restructures or because of their constant worry about an uncertain future (Butler, 2018b; LGA, 2018a). This represents a devaluing of professional training as a preferred method in enhancing the quality of public services against a background, for example in the early years sector, where much provision has become deprived of long-term funding – overall councils have suffered a 30 per cent cut in government funding for children's departments in England between 2010 and 2017/18. It was reported that this was despite rising demand for services from trained staff, from family crisis support to child protection. In marked contrast there are examples of innovative services within adult social care, such as homecare providers recruiting people from outside the domiciliary care sector, particularly from customer service and retail, believing the priority was to find people with the right values who could acquire the skills needed to help older people to live well at home (Williams, 2018). One such Well-being Team manager commented: 'Our stance is that if we recruit great people for their values, we can teach them what they need to know to be skilled at caring for people, with compassion at the top of the list' (Williams, 2018: 34)

This chapter has demonstrated how de-professionalisation has been shaped through the application of a political economy model of delivering public services – in the health, education and social care sectors. For example, many children's services have become taken over by 'high –performing' local authorities and 'teams of experts', where they have been granted academy-style freedoms, in some cases choosing to rely less on the expertise of trained professionals, preferring to train their own staff. This political economy model places renewed emphasis on a multidisciplinary flexible approach with more joint working, transfer of skills, workload-sharing, displacement and mentoring across disciplines, maybe resulting in some individuals becoming less indispensable. An overall training gap creates a lack of commonality of standards, with a reduction in the number of specialist trained teachers in schools or paramedics working in primary care and hospital trusts. Others lower down the hierarchy, such as teaching assistants, instead of being valued for their experience and skills gained on the job, have often become victims of service cuts, or else have been manipulated into transferring their contribution to other areas – 'collective powerlessness to conceive of any positive reconstitution of a lost professionalism' (Demailly and De La Broise, 2009: 10).

PART IV

De-professionalism in the public sector: subjective or experiential indicators

10

A demoralisation or disparagement of the workforce?

Introduction

The professions represent independent sources of power in our society as they are located within the welfare state, according to the Durkheimian framework described in Chapter 4. This is one reason why they are under such swingeing attack from the neo-liberals, with their dogmatic assertion of the power of the 'market' over all else. If you can prevail with employing cheaper, untrained, lesser or differently trained staff, then an employer will go there. As for the professions, the problem is not so much with restrictive practices as with restricted access, as recent governments increasingly seek to shift power away from the professions and to monetise all relationships.

De-professionalisation as displacement

There is a mysterious gap between the welcome and widely shared concern that disabled and older people should receive good quality care and the lack of action to ensure this becomes a reality (Williams, 2012; Elliott, 2015b). The decision in 2016 to postpone the funding gap in the 2014 Care Act underlines the low priority policy-makers attach to work with older and vulnerable younger people. This lack of funding for a professionalised version of social care is symbolic of the core problem, namely commodification, the fragmentation of the care relationship into standardised tasks that objectify the client. There is perhaps an underlying assumption by central government that, since social care will not contribute to export-led growth, it deserves to remain a low-status, low-paid activity. Professor Ruth Lister has drawn on feminist theorising around an ethic of care to uncover 'gendered moral rationalities', in which economic rationality itself can take second place to different forms of rationality that prioritise caring over economic success (Lister, 1997). For instance, social policies that recognised the dignity of people living in poverty and the value of care-giving could represent small steps towards accepting a role for the state in acknowledging the psychological need for respect of one's dignity as a human being.

The vulnerability – or displacement – of social care professionals can be seen in the Coalition and Conservative governments' approach to troubled families, which 'use[d] family support workers, family intervention workers or key workers from a range of backgrounds. Some are from social work and youth work, some are nursery staff and some are teachers, some are police officers and housing officers. Their background is not as important as their skills and their tenacity' (Casey, 2014: 60; DCLG, 2012, 2013). Set up after the riots in 2011, the government's £1.3 billion scheme to help Britain's most troubled families was designed to give intensive support to 120,000 of Britain's most challenging families – Prime Minister David Cameron later announced an expansion to help 400,000 more families until 2020, costing an extra £900 million. All families were identified by local authorities, and each was given a dedicated key-worker responsible for ensuring that they received appropriate help. The idea was to provide coordinated help to people who in the past would have been dealt with by a variety of government bodies, such as the police, social services and Jobcentre Plus. Success was to be judged by different measures, including reductions in truancy, criminal convictions and benefit dependency. Councils who took part in the initial £400 million scheme were paid when set goals were reached.

However, a government-commissioned analysis by the National Institute of Economic and Social Research reporting in 2016 could find no evidence that the programme was having 'any significant or systematic impact' on employment prospects, performance at school, crime and anti-social behaviour or dependency on benefits (NIESR, 2016b). Similarly, the Conservative government's rather over-enthusiastic support for the third-sector agency Kids Company, widely reported in the media, was for an organisation founded on an unorthodox approach of dealing with troubled young people through psychotherapy, and for some represented a displacement of traditional helping professions. Here was an ethos that clinical phenomena are viewed behaviourally (gangs) or emotionally (depression) and understood not as failings of particular individuals or families. This perspective may have disturbed the world view of the political class but in practical terms resulted in denigrating the efforts of cash-strapped social service, health and youth workers (Weale, 2015b; Butler, 2016). The Conservative government chose to fund a virtually non-professional service whose reported outcomes had always been questionable; and agreed to provide a £3 million rescue package plus a further special grant of £4.5 million in 2014. Kids Company was funded regardless of officials repeatedly expressing concerns over financial sustainability and poor management practices.

De-professionalisation as reducing self-esteem

Such a shifting of authority or autonomy away from professional groups will likely have an insidious effect on morale, defined existentially as how an individual feels about job, status and position, centring strategically on building confidence, enthusiasm and discipline within the workforce. Bourdieu's notion of cultural and symbolic capital may be relevant here, as he claims that this can exist in the objectified state in the form of cultural goods, and in the institutionalised state such as educational qualifications (Bourdieu, 1984). When such values decline, the social dynamic depends on people possessing these qualities and valuing them. His concept of habitus can work in a way to explain how an individual becomes part of a recognised group; but it aligns embodied actions with social locations, and centres on how an individual feels about their sense of belonging (McKenzie, 2016: 31–2). De-professionalisation encompasses a lowering expectation of performance within an organisation's workforce, often contrasting with how one might have been valued previously.

'What you've got is a profession that is exhausted, battered and demoralised and this has come from an awful lot of changes from the DfE that were supposed to improve standards for children...(and) they wonder why people don't want to come into the profession,' asserts a headteacher from a large inner-city comprehensive school who blames the growth of testing, children's mental health issues, compulsory academisation and the narrowing of the national curriculum as main reasons for teachers choosing to leave the profession.

> The sacrifices that we as nurses make for minimal pay and appreciation are demoralising. It will pain me to leave but ultimately I believe it will be better for my mental health. Giving up valuable time with my family and friends for £23,500 a year and experiencing what I can only describe as chronic fatigue, starts to seem like too big of a sacrifice. (Bianca, a nurse working in the paediatric intensive care unit of a hospital, BBC News, 2017a)

To illustrate the point about lowering morale, take the example of a schoolteacher who was highly valued for a specific subject. Once this subject becomes redundant or no longer in fashion, the teacher might experience difficulty in moving to an alternative and equally valued activity. There is a counter-argument that it should be a person's ability to transfer their teaching skills to another subject and to engage an audience that provides an essential professional quality (Dearing Report, 1997; Freidson, 2001). Confronting adversarial circumstances may not bring out the best in individuals, and indeed can become corrosive of professional identity.

The Conservative government appears to have ignored the views of teaching professionals through its 'forced academicisation of schools' policy (Boffey, 2015: 15). Local schools had been run by democratically elected local bodies since the school boards were created by the 1870 Education Act. That Act required the state, for the first time, to provide a school place for every child; and it is this aspect of democratic accountability that sustains the school system to uphold high standards, judged in part by teacher quality. The plan to force all schools into academy status can be seen as a ploy to hasten the unravelling of local democracy begun by Margaret Thatcher's Conservative government and pursued with varying degrees of enthusiasm by subsequent governments – both right and left – and not least by the present government's (2019) squeeze on local financing. The choice concerns decision-making and power vested in Whitehall, especially funding, and the role that should be given to individual school representatives whether teachers or parents when it comes to understanding what schools and local communities want and need. Current proposals are to exclude those without specialist skills and knowledge from being parent governors, underpinned by the fallacious idea that local people don't share a strong interest in the direction of the school (Coughlan, 2016; Moorhead, 2016a). 'In 10 years people will say academies should be locally accountable, and LEAs will be reinvented' (Wilby, 2016: 80, quoting the Provost of Eton).

This type of unidimensional policy narrative impacts on morale, viewing teacher professionals as outsiders alongside, if not in competition with, business and employer interests. In England it has been reported that teacher numbers have fallen for the first time in six years amid complaints that low staff morale and inadequate pay are putting people off the profession (NFER, 2018). Figures show the number fell by 1.2 per cent between 2016 and 2017 – the latest year for which data is available (Harding, 2019). The number of teachers leaving the profession has been increasing since 2010 – highlighting a chronic problem with teacher retention. This report, entitled 'Teacher Workforce Dynamics in England', called for the government to place a greater emphasis on improving teacher retention in order to ease supply pressures. Between 2010/11 and 2014/15, the rate of working age teachers quitting rose from 8.9 per cent to 10.3 per cent in primary schools. For secondary schools, it rose from 10.8 per cent to 11.8 per cent, the analysis of school workforce census data by the National Foundation for Educational Research (NFER) shows. The study concluded that this, alongside rising pupil numbers and shortfalls in trainee teachers, made retaining teachers all the more important.

Morale related to an ability to empathise

Assuming an ability to empathise as being linked to morale, it is fundamental that the former is relevant to helping relationships and therefore is given primacy in all the varied counselling and psychotherapy theories and schools of training. It is often stated, implicitly or explicitly, that the more empathetic a person can be, the better the outcomes and levels of satisfaction will be in terms of helping relationships (Rogers et al, 2015: 18–19). However, it is important to note that empathy is, in fact, a multidimensional entity with different emotional and cognitive facets. Davis (1980) identifies at least three key components: perspective taking – the ability to imagine and adopt the perspective of other people; empathetic concern – the ability to experience feelings of warmth, compassion and concern for others; and empathic distress – the experience of feeling anxiety and discomfort when hearing about the difficult experiences of others. Empathy is all about imagining other minds, appreciating that different people have different perspectives, and responding to their thoughts and feelings with an appropriate emotion. It is one of our most valuable natural resources, and a necessary step in rebuilding trust so that other difficult steps can follow (Baron–Cohen, 2019).

Is there a relationship between over-empathy and morale? A number of authors have highlighted the risks of being emotionally over-involved with others in terms of compassion fatigue and burnout, and empathic distress may be a significant element of this. Research by Grant and Kinman (2013, 2014) provided some useful insights into the ways in which the different facets of empathy demonstrated by social workers impacted on their own well-being. They noted that the demonstration of both empathic concern and perspective taking appears to enhance resilience and well-being, while the experience of empathic distress has the opposite effect, with negative consequences for the psychological well-being of the practitioner (Grant and

Kinman, 2014: 28). For instance social workers need to go into a job with a realistic view of the challenges it will bring, but then need the right support as they progress. They become demoralised possibly because they are working with families at the extreme end of tension, family stress and breakdown. Demoralised feelings may be addressed through professional development and reflective practice and are considered key to continuing professional development (CPD). 'As we move to a profession that acknowledges lifelong learning as a way of keeping up to date, ensuring that research informs practice and striving continually to improve skills and values for practice...much emphasis becomes placed on the Professional Capabilities Framework – see HCFC 2012' (Parker and Bradley, 2014: xvi–xvii).

As with the concept of empathy, morale is multidimensional, defined by a family of relevant components. Most research to date, however, has treated morale in unidimensional terms, making it impossible to address what we consider basic questions about morale. Do different types of groups have different morale profiles? What are the components of morale? A definitive answer would require extensive linguistic analyses and discussions with focus groups of different types. A tentative set of dimensions is confidence, enthusiasm, optimism, resilience, leadership, loyalty, social cohesion and a common purpose (Peterson et al, 2008).

Demoralisation and workload

De-professionalisation defined by a lowering of workforce morale has for example come from a survey of general practitioner (GP) workloads:

> An overworked, overstretched GP workforce is being buried under an avalanche of workload including pointless paperwork. Poor morale affects a majority of GPs who report that their services have worsened in the past year. From a survey of 2,837 GPs 55% expressed the view that there has been a deterioration of service in the past year claiming 'workload as unmanageable' or being 'starved of resources and staff' meaning that many patients can't get the appointments, treatment and services they deserve. (Campbell, 2015b: 8)

It was further revealed that the number of GPs retiring early had doubled since 2010. A Guardian Healthcare Professionals Network survey showed that four out of five health-care workers had considered leaving their job in the NHS and an overwhelming majority (84 per cent) of those had thought about it more in the past year – 'I worry about the long days … I'm so scared of making a mistake' (Campbell and Siddique, 2016: 12). Increasing workloads, cuts to the health service, unreasonable expectations and long working hours were some of the factors said to be damaging the lives of NHS professionals at a time of escalated pressure. Surging stress, longer hours and poor pay have helped drive 159,134 nurses out of the NHS in five years was the *Daily Mirror* strapline in April 2018, remarking that the annual exodus had risen 17 per cent in that period. Government data showed that 33,530 nurses quit in England in the year to September 2017; and the number of EU nurses coming to work in the UK also fell 90 per cent during the same year. As a result of axing the nursing bursary, applications for nursing degrees had fallen by 10 per cent – with a knock-on effect for the higher education sector – while those signing up faced huge debt. The RCN Lead Janet Davies said: 'This paints a bleak picture. After years of pay cuts and under-investment, we are haemorrhaging the best professionals' (RCN Magazines, 2018).

'If anyone says to you that staff morale is at an all-time low, you know you are doing something right' was an alleged claim made by the ex-Chief Inspector of Schools Michael Wilshaw. Doubts were subsequently expressed vehemently about the extent to which Wilshaw had been responsible for the alleged 'improvement' in Ofsted; but there had been none when it came to his reported role in 'the demoralisation of the teaching profession' (Culverhouse, 2016: 34). His attribution of the improved rating of primary schools to 'Ofsted's hard work' was claimed as both too generalised and insulting to teachers. Teachers began to make a case for proportionate inspections based on dialogue and mutual trust to promote school improvement as opposed to the current audit-style approach of 18 criteria for judging leadership, nine for governance, nine for teaching, learning and assessment, and three for learning outcomes from 20 different groups of learners (boys, girls, ethnic groups and so on). Additionally, the lengthy Ofsted inspection handbook contained criteria for evaluating provision for pupils' spiritual, moral, social and cultural development. Certainly the burdensome and ever-changing demands that some inspections imposed on teachers continued to play their part in lowering morale. A survey of teachers in schools showed that nearly half of teachers planned to leave in the next five years as a result of 'reaching breaking-point' over their workload:

> We are in the midst of a teacher recruitment and retention crisis brought on in large part by a culture of unmanageable workload. The biggest generator of workload, say teachers, is constant change caused by government policy. What is destroying our schools is ambitious politicians who have little concern for children's education or welfare. (Lightfoot, 2016: 30)

Also demonstrated in this survey was a widening gulf between teacher morale within the two sectors, state and independent, with teachers in the latter much more likely to say they were happy in their work and much less likely to complain of unmanageable workloads. For instance, class size was viewed as an important factor:

> I was teaching classes of 31, now I have 11. That makes a big difference but it isn't the main reason why I am much happier now. In the state schools I was coming to see children as data walking round, they no longer seemed human. Here the teachers are nurturing each individual child and developing them not just academically but as people. You're doing everything for the sake of the child, not to tick a box for the school. I'm treated as a professional, my opinions are listened to and I feel much more appreciated. (Lightfoot, 2016: 30)

One teaching union stated that Ofsted was 'wasting about £150 million annually of taxpayers' money by creating a climate of fear in schools and colleges (National Education Union, 2018). The pressure group Reclaiming Education in a conference report concluded: 'Our children are the most unhappy in the developed world while their teachers face a higher workload than practically anywhere else' (Reclaiming Education, 2018; House of Commons Committee of Public Accounts, 2018: 390–2).

In a similar vein, a document entitled a 'New education programme for Labour' revealed the Opposition Party's ten-point draft charter to evolve a 'national education service'. It stated that the party would 'tackle all barriers to learning', that teachers would be 'valued as highly-skilled professionals' and that there would be a focus on reducing workload (George, 2017: 3).

A decline in teacher morale has been evidenced by schools' reduced capacity to provide inclusive and high-quality education, represented through increased 'off-rolling', observed as having a parlous and detrimental impact. This is the practice whereby schools remove difficult or low-achieving pupils from their rolls so that they are not included in their GCSE results or in order to reduce their costs. Data taken from research conducted by the Education Policy Institute revealed that one in 12 schoolchildren in 2012–17 were removed from rolls without explanation (Hutchinson and Crenna-Jennings, 2019; Weale, 2019a). This investigation into the true scale of off-rolling from schools in England found that more than 49,000 pupils from a single cohort disappeared from the school rolls – some of whom will have been moved more than once – and that the numbers appeared to have gone up in recent years. The research took into account pupils removed from school rolls owing to family reasons, such as moving house, or to a higher-performing school, so the figures represented pupil exits that were likely to have been instigated by schools.

Increased workload, poor pay and pupil discipline have been cited consistently as key reasons for a decline in teacher morale, according to Mary Bousted, General Secretary of the National Education Union. Unlike formal exclusions, there has been to date no requirement to record the reason why pupils have been removed from a school roll, which may have left a sense of covering over the cracks when a school was asked to account for any individual departure (Long and Danechi, 2019). However in March 2018 the Conservative government established a review of school exclusions practice, led by former Children's Minister Edward Timpson, 'to consider how schools use exclusion overall and how this impacts their pupils, and in particular, why some groups of pupils are more likely to be excluded from school. It (would) also consider practice in relation to behaviour management and alternative interventions schools take in place of exclusion' (gov.uk, 2018).

The Timpson Review was published in May 2019 (DfE, 2019a) and it set out recommendations, including measures related to off-rolling, such as that 'the DfE should make schools responsible for the children they exclude and accountable for their educational outcomes, and consult on how to do this'; also, 'when Ofsted finds off-rolling, this should always be reflected in inspection reports and in all but exceptional cases should result in a judgement that the school's leadership and management is inadequate'. Of relevance to the construct of teacher morale, the Review recommended that 'The DfE should ensure that accessible, meaningful and substantive training on behaviour is a mandatory part of initial teacher training embedded in the Early Career framework' (gov.uk, 2019: 5–15).

De-professionalisation as an attack on social status or position. A contemporary case-study: the 2015–16 strike by junior doctors

In the Weberian tradition (Rogers and Pilgrim, 2014: 108), professions develop strategies to advance their own social status. Collective social advancement rests upon social closure, and it is clear for example that the medical profession in its strike action led by junior doctors tried to use its special status as a profession to persuade the world at large, including the media, of their deserving case. De-professionalisation exists in this case as a metaphor to caricature in media representation both the action and its response, as follows:

1. The strike action was viewed through the lens of cuts to services, for instance by the use of arguments that the new contract proposed by the Conservative government for a seven-day NHS would mean over-stretched services, and would allegedly affect patient safety deleteriously, contravening values and ethics of medical professionals.
2. Both the action and confrontations between junior doctors and the government had a demoralising personal impact on doctors as professionals in carrying out their existing duties.
3. Junior doctors might have become scapegoated through government and/or management failings arising out of the operation of the internal market, which elects to spend large sums on governance – procurement and competitive bidding, inspectorates, performance measurement – rather than clinical and diagnostic expertise.
4. The image of junior doctors became negatively encapsulated following reporting of British Medical Association (BMA) negotiations as 'politically motivated' or 'politically expedient' – as opposed to 'principled action' – which is 'sometimes incompetent', primarily seen to be about status and pay and resulting in a potential loss of public trust (Newell and Donnelly, 2016).

The link between declining morale, status and professional well-being and how this became acted out politically was all too evident where the stand-off on pay and working conditions between the Secretary of State for Health, Jeremy Hunt, and the BMA in England become the main story; that is, a personality clash. The argument was presented thus: does the Conservative government value junior doctors? Apparently not. 'It is simply unacceptable to devalue and denigrate doctors and the medical profession to the point where medicine in the UK is no longer a profession that the majority of doctors would recommend' (Roberts, 2016).

Professionals tarnished by conflict: the seven-day NHS and the imposed contract

A continuing drama of alleged service deficiency or shortage associated with the impact of a series of strikes led by junior doctors created a confrontation with the government following the imposition of a new contract. Much of the reported narrative of this dispute was rooted in the fact that there would be threats to existing services. Doctors argued that proposed reforms were equivalent to patient safety compromise, loss of earnings and cuts to services, whereas the government asserted that staff needed to reorganise in order to get medical cover in NHS hospitals onto a more cost-effective footing and thereby fulfil their party manifesto promise to achieve delivery of a seven-day NHS. Prior to the two-day unprecedented strike, which included emergency services (26–7 April 2016), the BMA claimed that junior doctors would be considering strike action indefinitely, a mass resignation and the possibility of seeking alternative employment; the organisation recommended that trainees should pursue careers outside medicine, and also spoke about unspecified 'alternative forms of permanent action' (Campbell and Siddique, 2016: 8).

The Department of Health responded by accusing the BMA of risking patients' safety. Health Minister Ben Gummer said:

> This is evidence of an organisation in total disarray and the action proposed shows a regrettable disregard for patient care ... for the JDC (junior doctors committee) this dispute is now clearly political, which makes it all the worse that by their actions the BMA are putting patients in harm's way. (Campbell, 2016b: 913)

For the junior doctors, it would seem that a precondition of meeting ministers was for the notion of an imposed contract to be dropped, claiming that no patients would be at risk as senior consultants would provide full cover during strike periods. It was their overwhelming view that senior figures in the medical profession should stand up to the government because the dispute was a 'key battleground' in the service's future (Sparrow, 2016: 16). An alternative perspective suggests that it was the doctors themselves who had failed to live up to the demands of their profession and were letting their profession down with their actions. 'When someone is paid a high salary, that comes with the responsibilities of a profession' (Stone, 2016).

'So demoralised, so alienated and so angry' are the junior doctors, remarked Nick Robinson (BBC Radio 4, 2016), 'that they are willing to walk-off the job. Their reaction may be neither proportionate or appropriate, but is reminiscent of the miners' strike of 1980s in which the government refused to back down.' The argument went that if the government let the doctors win, then others similarly dissatisfied would go out on strike, for example fire-workers, teachers and lecturers who were balloting for strike action at the same time. Ministers seemed to fear that capitulation to BMA demands to change the terms and conditions that England's 45,000 junior doctors worked under from August 2016 might encourage other public sector trade unions (Clarke, 2016; Elgot and Campbell, 2016). The government's utopian plan for a seven-day NHS would require existing doctors to work longer hours – 'doomed to failure owing to a lack of doctors, finance and diagnostic-testing services' warned Professor Jane Dacre, leader of England's hospital doctors. 'Worsening shortages of NHS medics and the inadequacy of support services vital to allow patients to be discharged, meant the promise is unrealistic, especially with the NHS's £2 billion deficit' (Campbell, 2015a: 8).

The affront to the medical profession was demonstrated by the fact that the Conservative government tried to introduce a seven-day NHS without properly defining what it meant by this. The position throughout the majority of the strike was that an unbroken emergency service had been provided by various grades of NHS staff, including both consultants and junior doctors, who worked unsocial hours, often staying on well beyond the ends of their shifts. In January and February 2016 the country saw the first walkouts since November 1975 as many of the NHS's junior doctors – defined as medics below the level of consultant – went on strike.

Figures released by NHS England showed that on 26 April 2016, 21,608 junior doctors – 78 per cent of those due to work – participated in the industrial action. It was stated that this was down from the 88 per cent who did so on each day during the previous strike action from 6 to 8 April. Such an unresolved dispute around junior doctor contracts that imposed unsafe hours inevitably distracts from the perceptible crisis in the NHS – around cuts to services – including the overall lack of doctors. One interpretation is that de-professionalisation represents a cover or compromise of the doctors' relationship with the public, for example by carrying out strike action that undermines trust and ultimately impacts on how doctors are perceived by the public. A GP registrar stated:

> This is the saddest day of my professional life. The strike is now wholly unfortunate, regrettable and damaging. I would like to hope that all parties wish it had never come to this. No one will come out of it well. I don't support withholding emergency care. I don't think that it directly causes harm, or affects safety, but it affects our relationship with the people we serve. Our profession has to have trust with the society we serve at its heart, and while I agree there is a longer-term view in all-out striking, for me a line is crossed. (Roberts, 2016a)

Studies of the effects of doctors' strikes have shown that they can be made safe with appropriate safeguards, as their roles will be taken over by consultants, fully trained and the most experienced doctors. Was the Secretary of State stating that the consultant workforce was not up to the task? (Gani, 2015). Much reporting of the doctors' strike in the media described it as a 48-hour withdrawal of emergency care by junior doctors, but in fact the withdrawal was mainly restricted to between the hours of 8am and 5pm. On those days the clinical care of patients and the emergency provision through Accident and Emergency services was, to all intents and purposes, provided by consultants. It was argued that the medical care would be of at least the standard usually provided, or even a higher standard since, by definition, consultants have more experience than junior doctors. What may have suffered, it was claimed, was administration work, meetings and routine planned out-patient care where normally these were provided by junior doctors.

Co-operation not confrontation: harm is one thing, but are patients getting the best possible treatment?

One obvious effect of the strike action was that the growing confrontation left junior doctors feeling devalued, a further signifier of de-professionalisation. Employee health can have a profound impact on productivity, retention, workplace engagement and morale; and research has demonstrated that well-being has been shown to act as an indirect driver of employee morale and productivity (Peterson et al, 2008). The initial ballot for strike action in January 2016 suggested that the proposed changes would lead to a limited service, poor conditions and long hours, and cuts in pay for weekend antisocial hours, resulting possibly in an overall indictment of their professionalism. For junior doctors, safety was declared to be the main issue, as they were expected to work longer hours given staff shortages. 'Each one needs to work 1–3 hours extra daily because of staffing problems and under-staffing' (Toynbee, 2015). Overtime payments had to be fought for and were only paid when hours exceeded 87 hours per week. The government required junior doctors to work more nights and weekends. From the perspective of some junior doctors and consultants, the Conservative government continued to refuse to negotiate, and it appears that this became a personal issue for the Secretary of State, which he seemed intent on winning irrespective of the effect it had on the public. Doctors claimed that the BMA had been painted as a militant body trying to bring the government down. Whatever the eventual outcome, this dispute represented a prime example of a left–right confrontation between a professional narrative: a determination to provide a high-quality service to patients and the public versus the government's public sector market reform narrative, which included asset-stripping, with a barely hidden agenda of handing hospitals over to corporate interests. This was backed by a grim scenario whereby various ministers became seemingly indifferent to reasonable grievance among public sector workers, seeing trade unions as guardians of a mediocre and financially unsustainable status quo (Boffey, 2011; Doward, 2017).

In August 2016, the BMA announced a new wave of strikes by junior doctors in England over their contract, beginning with an unprecedented five-day walkout in September followed by similar five-day walkouts in the ensuing months up until the end of the year. Hospitals began to make contingency plans for strikes each month but admitted to having had little notice to prepare. The BMA stated that it had made repeated attempts over the past two months to work constructively with the Conservative government to address the outstanding areas of concern, including the impact on those junior doctors not working full time, a majority of whom were women, and on those working the most weekends, typically in specialties where there was already a shortage of doctors. There was clear evidence of a growing frustration across the NHS that this employment dispute had not been resolved effectively, particularly bearing in mind that there was a lack of unanimous support for taking strike action among BMA members. Junior doctors were advised consistently by the General Medical Council that they should call off their five-day strikes and that putting patients at risk of significant harm could lead to them being struck off. This statement was issued to doctors under the authority of the 1983 Medical Act, suggesting that doctors could face sanctions if they acted unprofessionally: 'Given the scale and nature of what is proposed, we believe patients will suffer' (GMC's Chief Executive).

The Patients Association also expressed concern over the strike action, saying it was 'gravely troubled' at the 'catastrophic impact this will have on so many patients' as winter approached (Boseley and Weaver, 2016). NHS Lead Simon Stevens repeatedly asked the BMA to call off its series of planned week-long strikes, warning that hospitals could not cope without 50,000 junior doctors and that seriously ill patients would be put at risk. However, throughout 2016 BMA leaders appeared to be continuing to back the walkouts partly because they wished to avoid junior doctors breaking away and forming their own union (Campbell, 2016c). In a scenario characterised by murky and messy industrial relations there arose a lack of cooperation and instead confrontation, where the junior doctors eventually may have lost some public support. Until the late summer of 2016 the doctors enjoyed public backing in their fight with the government, but they could have risked squandering that support and angering patients by escalating the dispute. In this instance the argument for de-professionalisation resonates where a major part of the workforce continues to withdraw its labour and the quality of the service therefore must have become affected.

Was there any real hope of this dispute being satisfactorily resolved? The government showed no signs of backing down on its determination to force through the doctors' contract, declaring that it would take 18 months before all 45,000 trainee medics were on it. The BMA said that it would only call off strikes if the imposition of the new contract was halted. In September 2016 Conservative Health Secretary Jeremy Hunt claimed to be surprised at the need for continued strike action and accused (ITV National News, 2016) the BMA and junior doctors of 'playing politics', describing their response as 'disproportionate' given that they appeared to have accepted the new contract back in May. For his part, Hunt hoped to exploit divisions in the BMA over the wisdom of the strike action to force the junior doctors to back down. In turn, doctors claimed (PULSE, 2016) that they were 'demoralised' and that their trade union had been 'demonised'; yet the dispute seemed to have become intractable as both sides continued to claim that it had all been the other side's fault.

In May 2016 the then chair of the BMA's junior doctors committee endorsed a revised version of the contract, but members rejected it by 58 per cent to 42 per cent. In August the union threatened a series of five-day walkouts between then and Christmas, but abandoned the plans in the face of huge opposition, both internal and external. Junior doctors began moving onto the contract in October. Speaking on the BBC's Radio 4 'The World at One' in the same month, the BMA's representative Dr Mark Porter stated that 'it is now time to address the real issues of demoralisation and alienation that doctors face today' (11 October). So, who won? 'They did', said Nadia Masood, a hospital registrar and one of five junior doctors who in September 2016 challenged in the high court the legality of Jeremy Hunt's decision to impose the contract. That action ended in defeat too. 'The Government have won in the short-term and I'm worried that they will now do the same thing to nurses, consultants – to all NHS staff. But in the long-term, I fear that more people will decide not to train to be NHS consultants, burned out mentally and physically' (quoting from interview with Nadia Masood, Campbell, 2017c).

De-professionalisation as an attack on social status: an example of the foster carer workforce

De-professionalisation defined as an attack on social status creating low morale reached a watershed moment in late 2016 in the case of foster carers (foster parents), where it was reported that despite many being both highly experienced and qualified in the care of children over the years they had not been valued as such. For instance, unlike caring professions such as nursing, foster carers cannot challenge decisions to cut fees or change working conditions because they lack any formal employment status. 'They are self-employed , but by statute can only work for one provider. It's not a normal employment situation' (Chief Executive of UK Fostering Network Charity, www.thefosteringnetwork.org.uk/advice-information/finances/tax-and-national-insurance).

A fundamental disadvantage that they experience as substitute parents performing a professional role is that they receive no sick pay, no holiday pay and no pension rights. Around 60 foster carers voted to unionise and join the Independent Workers' Union of Great Britain in a bid to improve their working conditions. In addition to anger over welfare cuts, foster carers were said to have become increasingly fed up at their precarious legal status. Many felt that an attempt to challenge a decision or make a complaint would be ignored and could lead to them being de-registered by the local authority because they were not protected by whistle-blowing legislation.

Foster carers are rarely, if ever, informed about why a child is moved from their care and it can happen out of the blue … No explanations are given. The council then subjects the foster carer to another 'official' review. The foster carer cannot be accompanied by a legal representative, to speak up for him or her, and is not allowed to see any evidence presented at the hearing. The foster carer can then be de-registered and banned from working with children or vulnerable people again. (5RB, 2018)

Because they have no employment rights, foster carers cannot claim unfair dismissal. The current legal situation in the UK may leave them highly vulnerable, and as such children could be put at risk because of fear of the consequences of speaking out. Issues of accountability, complaints and low social status appear to have undermined the effectiveness of foster carers working in a professional capacity.

Foster carers should not have to continue working without any rights or protections. Carrying out the vital, often difficult, work we do on behalf of the state, and the communities in which we live, all foster carers deserve to be working under fair terms and conditions, with fair remuneration and support. (quote from an experienced foster carer; Anderson, 2019)

De-professionalisation as an attack on social status: an example of university teachers

A lack of morale can become evident from increased regulation in the workplace. Marketisation now means that too much funding is diverted from core tasks, teaching and research, into gaming ratings and rankings. Marketisation has also become a threat to the gold standard represented by UK degrees. The more the 'top universities' preen themselves as premier league, consigning the rest to the depths, the more alternative providers, with unchecked standards, crowd into the market, and the more the question will be asked about whatever happened to the trusted UK academic brand (Scott, 2018). For example, current regimes of performance measurement in the UK's higher education sector are said not only to lead to decreased professional autonomy (Frostenson, 2015) but also are unlikely to deliver any real improvement, according to some research:

The most likely outcomes will be further increases in the de-professionalisation of academic staff and commodification of the work they carry out. Why? Firstly, this is because the regimes of measurement reflect the triumph of a flawed postmodern philosophy which privileges and emphasises system deconstruction and economic functionality. Secondly, the regimes reflect a further instalment in the two-decade old story of New Public Management (NPM) and the transformation of the public sector through the importance of private sector practices and philosophies. Thirdly, the regimes will not deliver on their objectives because they are fundamentally flawed in terms of management process. (Adcroft and Willis, 2006: 58)

De-professionalisation of the professoriate – hiring policies based on tokenised identity politics and cronyism, the increasing intellectual and ideological conformity expected from faculty and students, and the subsequent curtailment of academic freedom – have become endemic. It has been alleged that some appointments to academic and managerial positions within universities are made when their fields of study have been unrelated to the courses that they teach (Southwell, 2017). This would underscore any threat posed to academic integrity and institutional legitimacy, where fairness and intellectual rigour have been eroded, with the implicit endorsement of administration and faculty alike.

In addition to depriving students of scholarly and pedagogic expertise, this sort of staffing sends a clear message to students: university accomplishments are relatively unimportant. Students might rightfully begin to ask why they should pursue advanced degrees or even undergraduate degrees when the university itself apparently deems such qualifications unnecessary for teaching (Southwell, 2017: 3).

An argument levelled against the effects of the knowledge economy discourse as it works in and through national education policies is that it constructs a narrow, instrumental approach to the economics of knowledge and to intellectual culture in general; in other words, that knowledge is commodified. What that means is, in fetishising commodities, we are denying the primacy of human relationships in the production of value, in effect erasing the social (Ball and Olmedo,

2011). Our understanding of the world shifts from social values created by people to one in which 'everything is viewed in terms of quantities; everything is simply a sum of value realised or hoped for' (Slater and Tonkiss, 2001: 162). This shift is neatly captured in the title of a book by Slaughter and Leslie (1997), *Academic Capitalism*. The term describes the phenomenon of universities' and their staff's increasing attention to market potential as the impetus for research funding income to the marketability of the knowledge they produce from research, and they see this trend being exploited by governments as grants are replaced with 'market money', which is linked to performance indicators.

Performance and morale in higher education has been the focus of evaluation in terms of a systems approach, specifically to examine how innovation attempts to improve quality and efficiency of education along with its impact on morale. This might explain unintended consequences of faculty hiring decisions and salary inequities and how this has led to performance and financial problems (Kim and Rehg, 2018). The authors of this research suggest that such mapping would be valuable to higher education managers seeking ways to enhance their strategic planning. Britain has now developed the most rigorous, costly and time-consuming system of assessments of any country in the world, and indeed one author commenting on universities several years ago claimed 'to an outsider, the [UK] seems obsessed by evaluations of every kind' (Smith, 2001: 170). Performance measurement may enable greater transparency and, coupled with targets and self-evaluation, equally may produce characteristics of role models to aspire to. At the same time such measures have the capacity to undermine or threaten the position or status of employees and place them on the defensive. This process can be used for self-improvement and professional development but also as part of a management stick and carrot. Where some targets may be unrealistic, with the dominant narrative defined by attributes of the 'consummate professional', then a simulated reality may reflect also the status of the 'nearly-man' – someone who narrowly fails to achieve the success or position expected of them in their particular field of endeavour.

Has managerialism in UK higher education led to the lowering of morale and status of academics?

There is a gulf between academics and university management, and it is growing. This may account for issues of morale within the university teaching sector. As higher education has grown in size and complexity, so institutions have felt the need to strengthen their management arrangements. Executive management teams now rule, populated by an expanding cadre of career track deputy and Pro-VCs (PVCs). Until recently, these career track managers were only seen in post-1992 universities where PVCs have always been permanent management positions. In contrast, in pre-1992 universities PVCs have traditionally been hybrid academic managers assuming the role on a part-time basis, whilst maintaining an underlying academic career. But now that being a PVC has become a full-time job rather than a part-time role, career track managers are taking over in pre-1992s too. So, what does this new breed of PVCs look like, asked the author of one survey (Shepherd, 2017). By and large they are not ex-academics; instead they have made a conscious decision to take a management path. Typically, they have become PVCs by climbing the academic management hierarchy from head of department to dean and are motivated by a 'desire for a seat at the top table', 'to change things strategically' (Shepherd, 2017). Most would seem happy to assert their right to manage other academics; hence what we're seeing is a shift of power from rank-and-file academics to this new professional elite, whose number and influence has grown.

There was a 55 per cent increase in numbers of PVCs in pre-1992 English universities between 2005 and 2016, from 148 to 229. The role itself has become more managerial with executive variants, such as provosts or PVCs/deans, being created. Furthermore, the range of PVC portfolios has expanded beyond traditional areas of teaching, learning and research to external relations, internationalisation, planning and strategic development. Hence career track mangers have not only colonised the top jobs, but also extended their collective management remit. Divorced from day-to-day academic activities, specialist knowledge rapidly becomes out of date and professional credibility increasingly difficult to maintain (Shepherd, 2017). The ladder of academic career opportunities for lecturers, teachers and researchers has therefore become overshadowed by a culture of management cadre domination. This influx of management strength has meant that academic managers sometimes tend to value academics differently, ignoring aspects of meritocratic achievement. They may celebrate the success of those who earn large external funding through research or alternative entrepreneurial ventures, and those classed as 'senior academics' who give well-attended public lectures on the national stage, seen as raising the profile of the university in some esteemed way. This may be presented either as a morale booster or as a subversive attack on others who 'fail' to perform at this high level. Morale of university academics may be affected negatively when managers appoint them and then de-appoint them to posts fairly arbitrarily, depending on the university's latest fashionable trend. A given reason may be that when a manager decides that a faculty cannot afford a certain number of professors, one or two must go to balance the books; or when a manager wishes to appoint one of their friends/ allies to lead a specialist department, even if the person concerned lacks either a teaching or research portfolio in that particular specialty.

Universities across the UK have warned staff to prepare for redundancies in 2019, because of deteriorating balance sheets and lowered forecasts for student numbers, coupled with the uncertainty of Brexit (the potential impact on international students of a no-deal Brexit) and cuts to tuition fees in England as a result of the review of university funding ordered by Prime Minister Theresa May that is due to report in 2019 (Adams, 2019).

> Knee-jerk cuts to staff will harm universities' ability to deliver high-quality teaching and research and provide the support students need. Staff are already overstretched and asking those who remain to do even more is not a sustainable strategy. Students repeatedly say they want greater investment in their staff as a top priority, yet the proportion of expenditure spent on staff has fallen. Cutting staff will send out entirely the wrong signal to potential students. (Matt Waddup, University and College Union; Adams, 2018c)

Summary

Recent governments have increasingly sought to shift power away from the professions and to give them restricted access. For example, a lack of funding for professional social care is symbolic of commodification, the fragmentation of the care relationship into standardised tasks that objectify the client. In universities the commodification of academic labour represents its use value, in the forms of its contribution to the development of the student as a person, as a citizen or at least as a depository and carrier of culturally valued knowledge. This becomes a form of displacement addressed by a preoccupation with doing those things that will increase the exchange value of academic labour in terms of the resources that flow, directly or indirectly, from a strong performance on the measures of research output and teaching quality. De-professionalisation encompasses a lowering recognition of performance within an organisation's workforce, often contrasting with previous valuations. Any major organisational upheaval may tend to have a negative impact on morale, for example changes to school curricula, health service fragmentation plans; and particularly when professional groups see their views/voices being side-lined or ignored. Different surveys have revealed evidence of poor morale among, for example, GPs, teachers in schools and health-care workers.

Is there a gender difference? Feminisation of parts of the workforce, for example home care services, residential care and health support workers, has over a long period established a toxic culture associated with poor working conditions, leading to low morale that may impact on a person's ability to empathise with vulnerable clients. The risks of being emotionally over-involved with others in terms of compassion and burnout, and empathetic distress, may impact on a professional's own well-being. Many women have been forced to take poorly paid jobs in the social care sector, and this is tantamount to a waste of women's skills and experience. 'Teachers on charity' was a headline in mid-2018 describing a local charity awarding grants to 'homeless and hungry professionals', after it had been claimed that such charities are seeing an increase in the number of teachers who are themselves struggling to make ends meet, with twice as many education workers applying for financial assistance grants in 2017 compared with 2010 (Ferguson, 2018: 32; Education Support Partnership, UK charity publication: Education Support Partnership/BBC Teach). When some teachers are in dire financial circumstances themselves, how can they help their pupils? An argument is made – and developed in Chapter 11 – for an industrial strategy to encourage innovation, higher productivity and better wages. Demoralised feelings may be addressed through professional development and reflective practice as a key component of CPD training.

De-professionalisation was represented through an attack on the social status and position of doctors' groups. Perceptions of too much political intervention were made in a long-standing confrontation between the Conservative government and junior doctors over working conditions, which allegedly resulted in inflicting lasting damage on the latter's morale. De-professionalisation has been characterised, in this and in other cases, as embodied in increasing workloads and a loss of autonomy in the practice and boundaries of a profession. Sometimes this may involve subordination to external supervision accompanied by unreasonable expectations applying lower down in the pecking order of hierarchy. Take the case of foster care workers (or foster parents) who have experienced devaluing of status, no legal rights as such and cannot challenge decisions to cut their fees or change their working conditions because they have no official employment status – they have no employment rights and therefore cannot claim unfair dismissal.

A further caricaturing of demoralisation has highlighted a reporting of the growing number of incidents, for example of NHS personnel suffering violent attacks at work, with understaffing and delays in patients accessing services being blamed for the rise. It has been claimed that the trade union UNISON reported more than 56,000 physical assaults on staff in 2016/17, up almost 10 per cent on the year before – nurses, paramedics and mental health staff were among those most likely to be assaulted (Campbell, 2018b). In a similar vein NHS figures revealed an almost annual trebling between 2012 and 2018 of the rising number of sexual assaults on ambulance staff, detailing how patients have subjected them to sexual harassment, indecent exposure and sexual assault, leaving them traumatised and in fear (Health Business, 2018). 'These figures show there is a national problem, with disgusting attacks on emergency workers, and it is getting worse' (GMB Union Secretary). 'Across the entire NHS, staff shortages are harming patient care and helping to create a hostile environment where health workers are increasingly at risk of being assaulted' (Public Health Agency, 2019; UNISON, 2018b).

Finally, it has been reported through the Office of National Statistics that 305 'overworked' NHS nurses took their own lives between 2012 and 2019, sparking calls for a government inquiry (Cole, 2019). This surprising statistic has been associated with the notion of a toxic culture in parts of the NHS, where victims' families have called for vital mental health training and support and an end to a culture that has left many feeling alone. It has also prompted one RCN chief to comment: 'Nursing staff experience high levels of stress, a shortage of colleagues and long working hours; and that [some] employers ignore or disregard mental health issues in the workplace. They feel they "should cope". We must all redouble our efforts to support nursing staff' (Cole, 2019: 18).

11

Professional abuse of power: discreditation or a lowering of productivity?

Introduction

De-professionalisation as defined by abuse of power implies a discrediting or deprivation of professional status, resulting in a weakening of respect or tendency away from a position of strength or equal rights. Similarly, the concept may be defined through a perception of low productivity, where low economic value becomes associated with low status. In both cases a person's work situation may become vulnerable and subordinate, and professional identity scapegoated (Demailly, 2003; Kuhlmann and Saks, 2008). Here the context might be abuse of power through incidents of physical and verbal abuse, or alternatively may involve an act of sexual abuse and invasion of personal privacy. In the case of the former, examples include such as those that have taken place in care homes or within institutional contexts. It is assumed that different dimensions, for example the physical environment, lack of client privacy, isolation and loss of occupation, may have an impact on the power differentials between individuals involved. However, the characteristics of that relationship that are rooted in social inequality and power imbalances have gained far less attention (Repper and Perkins, 2009). Institutional abuse can be defined as the maltreatment of a person – often children or older adults – by a system of power. This can range from acts similar to home-based child abuse, such as neglect, physical and sexual abuse, to the effects of 'helping' interventions working below acceptable service standards or relying on harsh or unfair ways to modify behaviour (Powers et al, 1990). De-professionalisation defined as working below acceptable standards may include failing to fulfil objectives set by the organisation, for example 'minding' patients instead of providing care, nurturing or treatment.

Definitions and terms of reference

There are several definitions for professional abuse, and their distinctions are usually pronounced according to professional fields. One of the general descriptions, however, that sought to bridge the variations was put forward by the National Council of Psychotherapists, which explained professional abuse as a violation of an organisation's code of ethics (O'Sullivan, 2018). Some sources refer to this as standards of behaviour, which include the maintenance of professional boundaries and the treatment of people with respect and dignity (Mind, 2017). A more comprehensive version of this description states that this type of abuse is 'a pattern of conduct in which a person abuses, violates or takes advantage of a victim within the context of the abuser's profession' (Khele et al, 2008: 124). For example, certain social scientists working in the field of disability choose to define disability as a form of social oppression involving the social imposition of restrictions of activity on people engendering undermining of their psycho-emotional well-being. This definition (of professional action) becomes widened as 'psycho-emotional disablism involves the intended and unintended hurtful words and social actions of non-disabled people such as parents and professionals in inter-personal engagement with people with impairments' (Thomas, 2007: 72).

> Professional abusers are the individuals who prey on the weaknesses of others in their workplaces or in other places related to economical strands of society. Their fundamental behaviour is based in the following actions: taking advantage of their client or patient's trust; exploiting their vulnerability; not acting in their best interests or failing to keep professional boundaries. (https://en.wikipedia.org/wiki/Professional_abuse, retrieved 7 August 2018)

There are different forms of abuse: discriminatory, financial, physical, psychological and sexual; and professional abuse always involves betrayal, exploitation and violation of professional boundaries. This does not fully cover different dimensions of the abuse of power where a robust legal framework is lacking, for instance where this may relate to the activities of politicians in their role as public servants. Professionals can abuse in three ways: non-feasance – ignore and take no indicated action defined as neglect; misfeasance – take inappropriate action or give intentionally incorrect advice; or malfeasance – hostile, aggressive action taken to injure the client's interests. Abuse of power, in the form of malfeasance in office or official misconduct, is the commission of an unlawful act done in an official capacity that affects the performance of official duties.

A de-professionalisation nuance applies to a range of professional duties, such as teacher abuse towards students in schools, which includes bullying (Hoel and Cooper, 2000) and sexual misconduct (Goldstein, 2000; Knoll, 2010). Health care professionals, for instance, experience much legitimate gratification from their work. They derive feelings of competency by gathering necessary data, skilfully diagnosing and appropriately treating a patient. They gain satisfaction from earning a living while performing humane, complex and vital tasks. However, when a health care professional derives gratification from a manipulative, controlling or threatening relationship with a patient, whether the behaviour is of an intimate or sexual nature, such behaviour is exploitative and thus violates the ethical and legal obligations of the profession (Lundgren et al, 2005). An effect is to weaken a professional person's authority along with doing damage to his/her overall integrity. The Sexual Offences Act 2003 criminalised all sexual activity in England and Wales between teachers and pupils under 18, irrespective of the fact that the general age of consent is 16, and even if the parties concerned were in a consensual relationship. Accounts of pupil–teacher romantic and sexual relationships are usually presented in the media through a discourse of scandal, exploitation and denial (Myers, 2002; Sikes, 2006).

Finding solutions to resolve an organisational issue of abuse of power

As for solutions, there are several strategies available to organisations seeking to address professional abuse. Those who have been subjected to professional abuse could pursue a course of action ranging from lodging a complaint to reporting abuse to the police or taking legal action. A study revealed that this problem often arises when there is an extreme power imbalance between the professional and the victim (Kumar, 2000). A framework based on different grades of client empowerment and ways of strengthening it can help solve the problem. Abuse of authority within the public service domain has characterised a range of functions carried out by public servants, and this has become a leading focus of media interest and scrutiny. In 2018 hundreds of civil servants working in Whitehall made complaints about suffering sexual harassment or bullying at the hands of colleagues, but only a fraction of staff subsequently faced any form of disciplinary action

(Murphy, 2018a). 'It's completely unacceptable that the civil service, which should be the gold standard in training and management, is yet to tackle this issue', claimed Conservative MP Maria Miller, Chair of the Women and Equalities Select Committee (Commons Select Committee, 2018). A report on sexual harassment by the Commons Leader, Andrea Leadsom, published earlier in the same year, was described as 'offer[ing] a promising blueprint for professionalising the entire outfit' (Maltby, 2018: 4). In 2018 the Conservative government introduced a new statutory code of practice to tackle sexual harassment at work and to protect workers, but some campaigners say its response has fallen short of properly tackling the issue (Mohdin, 2018). The Women and Equalities Select Committee's Report (Commons Select Committee, 2018a) had called on the government in October to put sexual harassment at the top of the agenda; to require regulators to take a more active role; to make enforcement processes work better for employees by setting out the statutory code of practice; to clean up the use of non-disclosure agreements; and to publish better government data.

De-professionalisation implies a paucity or absence of appropriate professional or leadership training in matters relating to sexuality and sexual harassment, where in the current climate many working professionals have no choice but to deal with these issues using their own initiative. Educator sexual misconduct has received increasing attention in recent years, and this has exposed a number of concerning issues, including a lack of formal research in the area, such as grooming patterns and warning signs, along with difficulties in recognising and prosecuting cases. Public responses to high-profile cases of sexual misconduct involving female teachers suggest that gender-biased views on sex offenders remain prominent in society (Sanghara and Wilson, 2006; Knoll, 2010; Morris, 2018). In the health and social care field, it has become fairly clear that professional sexual abuse in mental health services has received little attention in the literature on safeguarding, in the quality of mental health services or in the regulation, education and training of staff. Much of the literature on this particular subject has been generated in the United States (USA) with a focus on sexual boundary violations in psychotherapy (Schoener, 1995; Melville-Wiseman, 2008). As regards the violation of professional boundary-keeping, there has been little reference in academic and professional journals serving complementary practitioners – reflexology or massage, where touch is an essential part of the treatment. In a study of homeopaths and HIV-prevention outreach workers, described by Deverell and Sharma, some of the healers interviewed remarked that touch often facilitated the 'opening up' and 'tuning in' processes, assisting the flow of information from patients who might otherwise have found it difficult to talk about themselves (Deverell and Sharma, 2000: 41).

Professional boundary violation has become an issue of considerable concern to health and social care regulators (Fischer et al, 2008; Cronquist, 2011; Benbow, 2013). The General Social Care Council (as it was known until 2012 when it was subsumed into the Health and Social Care Professions Council) commissioned research into professional boundaries (Doel et al, 2009) and produced guidance for practitioners (GSCC, 2011). Such guidance failed to tackle the distinctively challenging problem of preventing or responding to sexual boundary violations. A generally understood definition of professional sexual abuse is of a situation where a professional is working with a person who is vulnerable by virtue of a mental health need, and through that professional relationship engages in some form of sexual contact, by doing so abusing his/her position of authority. Defining what is meant by a professional, a person vulnerable through mental health needs or where sexual contact may begin has presented serious challenges, but for clarity a focus might be on situations that are deemed unambiguously wrong and harmful to victims.

Such scenarios constitute a criminal offence under the United Kingdom (UK) Sexual Offences Act 2003 Sections 38–44 – an amendment to Section 82 of this Act was brought into force by the Violent Crime Reduction Act 2007. Similarly, an action can be prosecuted as a civil offence under the Mental Health Act 1983/2007 Section 127, as it may represent a breach of all regulated health and social care professional codes of conduct, practice or ethics (Melville-Wiseman, 2012: 27). Melville-Wiseman undertook research into practitioner views of professional sexual abuse in mental health services in the UK, concluding that in spite of high-profile cases, and changes to the law and regulation of mental health professionals, it remains a significant problem. The author describes her study as taking a 'social inequalities perspective' and focuses on systemic and institutional dimensions: 'Professional sexual abuse presents particular challenges for colleagues and managers of services when incidents are reported or come to light through everyday practice … (and) even when mental health care is provided in the community it can still become corrupted' (Melville-Wiseman, 2012: 26).

This study tentatively suggests that the problem of abuse of authority is endemic but hidden by ineffective management responses. Recommendations include adopting new approaches to selection, training and support for professionals, which might involve counter-intuitive approaches to policing colleagues and institutional cultures, a mode of whistle-blowing.

Institutional/de-institutionalisation culture and its association with an abuse of power

Institutions label people and pressurise them to act in ways consistent with behaviour imputed by that label (Goodley, 2017: 69). An early scenario analysing an abuse of power in the mental health field was given in Goffman's classic study (Goffman, 1961), where he describes a sense of betrayal and loss of identity afflicting new patients arriving in a psychiatric hospital and where the role of staff in presenting to the inmate their view of his situation is crucial in separating him from ordinary life outside. A related early study by a consultant psychiatrist pointed to 'clusters of factors' (Barton, 1959: 8–21) in the mental health environment causing institutional neurosis to develop: loss of contact with the outside world; enforced idleness; bossiness of medical and nursing staff; loss of friends, personal possessions and personal events; and drugs – the use of sedatives to produce apathy (Barton, 1959). Critiques of institutions had an impact on policy formation in an existential way, as they infiltrated both the humanistic and toxic characteristics relating to the long-term effects of so-called 'care' environments. To quote Goffman, a patient can be reduced from a person with many roles to a cypher with one – the 'inmate role', partly through environmental culture but exacerbated by the attitudes and behaviour of those staff responsible for their care. Goffman invented the notion of the total institution, contending that generally they have four main characteristics: batch living, binary management, the inmate role and the institutional perspective. His contention was that institutions have features in common. Not all features are specific to each institution, but residing in an institution represents the antithesis of living as an individual person, involving a process of disculturation or role-stripping. In some instances the effect was so pernicious that any individual subjected to it was to be rendered incapable of normal living when returned to the community. Goffman permitted analyses of attitude formation and the iterative processes of exclusion, observing that in 'total institutions, territories of the self are violated', and that the 'boundary containing the individual places between his being and the environment is invaded' (Goffman, 1961: 29).

In Wardhaugh and Wilding's (1993) examination of what they termed the 'corruption of care', the authors sought to identify what it was about the nature of institutions that allowed abusive practices to take places within their confines. They drew on earlier work by Foucault (1977a), who along with Goffman had begun to identify the de-personalisation and de-humanisation of individuals residing in institutions. The argument was that specific changes may happen to professionals when they work in services where power imbalances flourish and where clients are routinely de-personalised through medical models that focus on diagnosis and treatment. Within such systems professionals may inadvertently be authorised to apply unusual moral imperatives in their relationships with people in their care, such as putting the rights and interests of others before themselves when such actions may lead to endangering their own being. Inhibitions about mistreating a fellow human being or witnessing another mistreat a fellow human being will not apply, and abuse will flourish. If managers within such systems are overburdened and weak or non-existent chains of accountability have developed, resultant direct or indirect collusion with abusive practices on their part also emerge (Cambridge, 1999; Colton, 2002; Godefroy, 2015: 65–7).

Race (1999, 2007), in a number of books and chapters, has examined the 'value system' – materialism, individualism, sensualism and externalism – underpinning human services focusing on community care, which he claims involves a process characterising services as assessing people in terms of a problem of a material nature:

> Either something is 'wrong' with the person that can be defined in a technical professional way, very often as a 'disease' or a 'syndrome', or a whole class or group of people are categorised as being 'in need' of a technical service, rather than possessing more fundamental needs that they have in common with most other human beings. (Race, 1999: 72–3)

Race's references include both institutional and community forms of care provision, seen as 'masking impersonal rationing by – in the case of community care – joining two words with high appeal, emptying them of content, and filling the hollowed out space with bureaucratic professional activity' (Race, 1999: 69). One conclusion offers an indictment of how most services are delivered, suggesting that professionalism has been successful in using and developing externalism in society, to the point that people are even defining the quality of their lives by the availability of services. Race defines externalism in terms of 'people growing up empty, shallow, superficial, without strength in spiritual values, morality, character and often even personality, dependent on external inputs and supports of an ongoing nature' (Race, 1999: 66). The growth of the human professions has become all-pervasive:

> Beginning with medicine, then nursing, with teaching providing a curious mixture of the moral and the technical, these human professions have come to dominate the twentieth-century world of services ... There is debate as to whether they have all produced fruit, but the presence of psychologists, social workers, therapists of various varieties, and the most recent hybrid, the counsellor (consultores ubicumques) is a significant feature of the service garden. (Race, 1999: 73)

As for contributing towards an ongoing debate around theoretical frameworks used in studying professions, this position might be viewed as occupying a post-structuralist slant – based on headings set out in Chapter 5 – where power needs to be dispersed, not simply located in any elite group. Such a perspective involves mapping out discourses associated with particular social periods and places; and its application to the institutional versus community care controversy, which still exists after 50 or so years, has been characterised through a lens based on discursive practices. This latter notion offers an account without endorsement of any self-conscious collective activity of professionals to advance their own interests or to act, say, on behalf of the state (Rogers and Pilgrim, 2014: 111).

Any claims to professionalism may have been viewed as the triumph not only of the new values system, but also of a multigenerational breeding programme of rational, technical shapers of values, whose key influence has, paradoxically, been largely to deny the need for a consistent set of values to determine how services ought to be carried out. This type of neo-Weberian perspective instead gives credence to understanding how several professions have evolved into bodies solving problems of their own defining, and thus influencing services to become the laboratory where they can test out their technological theories (Saul, 1992; McKnight, 1995).

Disability theorists measure de-professionalisation in terms of one of its possible outcomes, as a disempowering process used to objectify service users. They can take a broader perspective and argue that interactionism – which can technically involve an abuse of power – focuses upon impairments rather than the social and economic environment by which impairments lead to disability (Parrott and Maguinness, 2017: 58–77). It then follows that this can lead to a greater appreciation of power as it is exercised to preserve the functioning of social relations, particularly where in a closed community staff may have a tendency to abuse their position of authority. Tyler (2013) uses the term 'abjection' to explain a process of discrediting others, and this may apply in expressing attitudes towards vulnerable citizens whom the state has a responsibility to protect, such that they become stigmatised and presented as discredited and discreditable. This recognises the importance of subjective interpretations of social actors in a social world, a focus taken up by Erving Goffman, whose work remains an inspiration to disability researchers. He saw disabled people as subjected to stigmatisation and spoilt identities (Goffman, 1959; 1963). His work elaborates on the discrepancy between an individual's actual social identity and virtual one, where he is treated as insane when he knows this is not just. 'But for the ex-mental patient the problem can be quite different; it is not that he must face prejudice against himself, but rather that he must face unwitting acceptance of himself by individuals who are prejudiced against persons of the kind he can be revealed to be' (Goffman, 1963: 58).

In England there remain large numbers of people being kept in so-called rehabilitation wards of mental health hospitals, condemned by the National Health Service (NHS) watchdog as 'outdated and sometimes institutionalised care' (Marsh, 2019: 12). A Care Quality Commission (CQC) report found in 2017 that more than 3,500 patients in 248 mental health wards were being kept locked in (CQC, 2017). This report asserted that the practice left already vulnerable patients feeling isolated and less likely to recover; and here de-professionalisation as an abuse of power becomes expressed as a fundamental breach of people's human rights.

De-professionalisation as defined by abuse of power, a discrediting of professional status

Over recent years there have been difficulties reported by UK health authorities and health trusts when seeking to deal with doctors with performance problems, which demonstrate that their incompetence might be viewed as equivalent to an abuse of authority and status. Momentum for the drive to scrutinise the activities of the medical profession came in January 2000 when a general practitioner, Dr Harold Shipman, was convicted of murdering 15 of his patients. Pressure to identify or deal with inadequate or dangerous doctors increased, and a revolution in medicine was called for to establish a redefinition of professionalism and a more active role in self-regulation, involving appointment of a committee to inquire into the future of professional self-regulation, headed by the Chief Medical Officer, Sir Liam Donaldson. This led to another round of General Medical Council (GMC) reform, with a civil standard of proof replacing the more demanding criminal standard of proof in fitness to practice proceedings (Klein, 2010: 187–208). The case of Shipman illustrated how doctors may abuse their position through wrongly prescribing drugs, to gain compliance, obedience and/or control. Collectively the medical profession was under pressure to strengthen the machinery of accountability. The pressure increased following the report by Sir Ian Kennedy diagnosing a failure in the profession's own system of self-regulation (Secretary of State for Health, 2002). The GMC, pushed by the Labour government, set about reforming its disciplinary procedures and introducing a system of revalidation: the notion that doctors would periodically be required to demonstrate their continued competence to remain on the medical register.

More recently, it has been reported that patients are being put at risk because doctors are giving them drugs they do not need and sending them for unnecessary surgery to avoid a complaint being made against them (Bourne et al, 2015; Campbell, 2017e; Boseley, 2018). This points more to the impact of many doctors becoming overstretched and demoralised rather than their being guilty of performing deliberately abusive acts. Such events have been evaluated in a study covering the impact of complaints procedures on the welfare, health and clinical practice of doctors in the UK, where there are reported examples of a professional group choosing not to perform procedures that involve more risk than usual (Perraudin, 2017). A substantive public inquiry following a scandal at Gosport Hospital, Hampshire, in which the deaths of more than 90 patients and the lives of up to 600 people were cut short by powerful painkillers, focused on the actions of Dr Jane Barton, who described herself as 'a hard-working doctor doing her best in an under-resourced part of the NHS' (ITV National News, 2018). In this case an over-prescription of opioids had been institutional and routine, the inquiry report concluded. This was deeply critical of Barton, the consultants, the nurses and the pharmacist who dispensed them, and also of the NHS management, Department of Health staff and ministers for failing to help the families involved (Gosport War Memorial Hospital, 2018).

Drug misuse, or having the power to prescribe, has sometimes been at the heart of a professional dilemma; it has been argued that by stigmatising drug use we prevent it from having any positive attributes, and this may steer people away from it (Satel, 2007). The suggestion is that we may separate drug use from drug users so that the drug itself is stigmatised but not the user, and therefore any stigma is taken away from the person, along with any potential compliance or labelling by professionals involved. Where a professional abuses power to control another, s/he may be described as performing an action to bad effect or for a bad purpose, may exploit a situation to perpetuate unfair or underhand practice, or simply benefit unjustly or unfairly from another's efforts. Different forms of power may corrupt or encourage dishonesty, and these may include turning a blind eye to corrupt practices.

Other detailed reports into sexual and physical assaults committed by rogue medical personnel concluded that the NHS needed to do more to spot warning signs that staff are using their position in order to abuse patients (CQC, 2018d; Foley and Cummins, 2018). One such report conducted by Verity Investigators described the problem as being particularly acute for doctors who achieve 'superhero' status. The analysis of how health care professionals were able to get away with their misbehaviour for years concluded that the NHS needs to overhaul its procedures to prevent a repeat of such scandals. Examples included breast surgeon Ian Paterson, who was jailed in 2017 for 15 years for carrying out unnecessary cancer operations – this case highlighted a medical doctor's pattern of wounding by intent by carrying out needless surgery on patients. A further case involved specialist Myles Bradbury, who was jailed for 22 years – reduced on appeal – in 2014 for abusing young cancer patients. 'NHS organisations must be much more alert to these patterns of behaviour to identify and stop abuse by staff. The NHS must learn lessons from these cases...' (Campbell, 2017f).

This independent investigation into governance arrangements in the paediatric haemotology and oncology service at Cambridge University Hospitals NHS Foundation Trust identified types of 'devious and deceitful' tactics used by NHS personnel to create opportunities to exploit vulnerable patients (Verita, 2015: 30–43). It focused on identifying patterns of behaviour that bosses, management teams and the NHS workforce as a whole needed to be warned about and told to report if they become suspicious. For example, alarm bells should ring when any member of staff began to act as a 'lone wolf' – creating space and opportunities within the working environment to carry out abuse. One example given involved a convicted medic who practised in a separate location, where he was subject to less stringent assessment and away from the eyes of colleagues who may have challenged his approach; while another was described as having relocated to a specialist eating disorders unit physically separate from the main hospital.

In 2012 the Independent Police Complaints Commission published a report concerning the abuse of police powers to perpetrate sexual violence (IPCC, 2012). It alluded to the fact that in the previous year former Northumbria Police Constable Stephen Mitchell had been jailed for life for a number of serious sex attacks against women he met through his job. The abuse of police powers for purposes of sexual exploitation, or even violence, is something that fundamentally betrays the trust that communities and individuals place in individual officers and the service in general. This report stated:

> It is essential to ensure that systems are in place to prevent, monitor and deal swiftly with any individual who exploits the trust of professional officers. It is not possible to know precisely how many people have been victims of police officers or staff abusing their powers. There is no evidence to suggest it is commonplace, but nor can we be confident that all such cases are reported. (IPCC, 2012: 2)

The report continued that the police service has a formal responsibility to recognise abuse of authority as a 'distinct area of corruption', and to take steps to reduce its occurrence, identify it as soon as possible if it occurs and effectively deal with it. Striking a similar chord to the findings of investigators concerned with reporting the actions of those employed by health care organisations, the IPCC report claimed that the perpetrators of abuse target individuals 'in a vulnerable position' (pp 8–11).

> For a variety of reasons, including alcohol or drug dependency, mental health difficulties or having experienced domestic abuse, this made them vulnerable to a person who wished to abuse them ... and the circumstances in which people fall into contact with police often following traumatic or alarming experiences, may increase that particular vulnerability. (IPCC, 2012: 8–11)

Such behaviour has parallels with similar abuses carried out by other professionals, such as members of the medical and social work professions who are in a position of power and who have trust placed in them. As regards the police service, however, this behaviour is also seen as a form of corruption, and subsequent reporting on such offences has clarified that it should be dealt with as such. This includes cases in which officers or staff may have misused police computer systems in order to target individuals who might be vulnerable to abuse. It also includes any criminal offence or misconduct attributed to undercover officers who may have deceived women into intimate relationships without disclosing their true identities (Evans, 2018).

De-professionalisation as defined by abuse of power, an ebbing away of authority – an example of the clergy

The challenge posed by enterprise culture was briefly considered by a study that looked at the work of the clergy as a profession that was defined as already on the margins of society (Cameron, 2000). This study sought to consider the workplace practices that members of the clergy used to sustain their professional modes of interacting with their clients, focusing on conflict avoidance and safeguarding professional work. Findings suggested that clergy had little alternative but to minimise conflict (with Church members) in their daily activities if they were to sustain a membership organisation with members holding diverse opinions, and also to suppress conflict so as to maximise member activism, thus releasing more time for their preferred pastoral work. The author concluded that this represented a neo-Weberian stance towards theorising professions, defining the concept of authority as power legitimated by a means acceptable to those subject to it, and that authority is the only form of power in organisations (Weber, 1947; Cameron, 2000).

This notion of the Church occupying a moral authority role would appear to have been 'damaged massively' (a term used by the Archbishop of Brisbane in February 2019 (Knaus, 2019)) in recent years by the scale and nature of child sexual abuse that has come to light in both the Catholic and Anglican churches (Independent Inquiry into Child Sexual Abuse (IICSA), 2017). There are few robust primary studies into its prevalence; and the most detailed data on child sexual abuse in the Catholic Church comes from the US John Jay College of Criminal Justice study on the nature and scope of sexual abuse of minors by Catholic priests and deacons, which found that around 4 per cent of US Catholic priests had been the subject of allegations of child sexual abuse (John Jay College of Criminal Justice, 2004). It would appear that no such robust studies into prevalence of child sexual abuse in the Catholic Church exist for England and Wales. A more recent study carried out by the Royal Commission in Australia, employing a similar methodology to the US John Jay study, found that around 7 per cent of Catholic priests in Australia had been the subject of claims of child sexual abuse (Royal Commission into Institutional Responses to Child Sexual Abuse, 2017).

From the English IICSA study, there appear to have been three main factors contributing to the occurrence of abuse by the clergy:

- The structure of the Catholic Church and the authority vested in individual bishops was cited as a factor that allowed child sexual abuse to occur in some dioceses and meant that responses to abuse have been inconsistent (Garrett, 2013; UN Convention on the Rights of the Child, 2014).
- Clericalism, the belief that the clergy is superior to the laity, has been identified in the literature as a factor that may enable child sexual abuse to occur and hinder an effective response to it (Barth, 2010).
- Attitudes to sexuality, for instance a patriarchal dominance, within the Catholic Church have also been suggested as factors explaining the incidence of child sexual abuse in the Church and the Church's response (Hogan, 2011; Keenan, 2011).

The reference to de-professionalisation arises from interpreting the Church's response to these allegations of clerical abuse, which have been characterised by a range of sources as one of 'corrupted leadership' (Reyes, 2018) and secrecy seeking to protect the Church's reputation (Doyle et al, 2006; Truth, Justice and Healing Council, 2014). The Church has become all the more vulnerable precisely because its power has long gone largely unchallenged.

> But what might have happened slowly and gently has instead happened quickly and bitterly. Buddhist monks in Vietnam used to set themselves on fire – the Irish bishops and cardinals have done so metaphorically, but no less shockingly. The petrol they poured over themselves was what Francis, in his open letter (released in August 2018), called 'atrocities perpetrated by consecrated persons'. The flame they set to it was the systematic covering up and effective facilitation of the sexual abuse of children by clergy. (O'Toole, 2018: 4)

Certain alleged practices, such as the relocation of offending priests to new dioceses, have seemed to put the needs of the perpetrator first and prioritise the perpetrator over the needs of victims and survivors and safety of children (UN Convention on the Rights of the Child, 2014). A review of the literature, including some public inquiry reports, concluded that a thorough-going renewal of the priestly ministry and its theology in policy and praxis was needed (Cahill and Wilkinson, 2017). This review also suggested that the response to victims by the Church had not met their needs (Center for Constitutional Rights on behalf of the Survivors Network of those Abused by Priests, 2013; McLellan Commission, 2015).

An overall impression gained was that Catholic bishops had not led the implementation of child protection measures and that 'risk remains very high' (BBC News, 2018c), particularly in Catholic children homes in certain parts of the world. It was reported that bishops of both persuasions, ideological and pastoral, dealt most inappropriately with the problem by the way they covered it up and treated the victim survivors and their families with disrespect, lack of compassion and even contempt (Cahill and Wilkinson, 2017). And to attribute these practices solely to a series of personal failings of individual priests and religious, insinuating that they were 'just a few rotten apples', was simply not credible, 'intellectually dishonest' (p 162), and evidence of 'selective moral disengagement' (p 168) (Cahill and Wilkinson, 2017).

The resultant discreditation and weakening of status of Church professionals implied through allegations that continue to be made to the IICSA would appear to be linked partly to a sense of powerlessness experienced among victims. For example, a portrait painted by one victim in his testimony of bishops 'playing grubby games with legal processes at the expense of victims' makes it difficult to see how such members of the clergy would be capable of articulating an inspiring vision of leadership (Parsons, 2019). A principal allegation has been that the Church, as represented by its own leaders, seemed concerned only to protect itself from moral or financial liability. The Elliott Review was set up in 2016 to recommend safeguarding proposals for the Church of England, particularly in the areas of disclosures and accountability (Church of England, 2017). As regards both the IICSA (Independent Inquiry into Child Sexual Abuse) and the Elliott Review, a continuous flow of allegations have been received from abused victims that the Church failed to act, that victims did not receive a response adequately addressing their needs and/or that complaints were dismissed on the grounds that they had been filed outside a specified time limit (BBC News, 2018d; Parsons, 2019).

In July 2019 the Archbishop of Canterbury, Justin Welby, threw his weight behind calls for the government to make the reporting of sexual abuse of children and vulnerable adults mandatory. He told IICSA): 'I am convinced that we need to move to mandatory reporting for regulated activities' (Sherwood, 2019: 11; Swerling, 2019). Such 'regulated activities' covered areas where professionals came into routine contact with children and vulnerable adults, such as teaching, healthcare and sporting activities – in a Church context this would cover clergy and youth leaders. Survivors of clerical abuse have argued that mandatory reporting of allegations or suspicions of abuse to statutory authorities is a vital component of effective child protection; and that a failure to comply should lead to criminal sanctions.

De-professionalisation as defined by low productivity, low economic value and low status

Increases in productivity, which is output per unit of input employed, result from deploying better raw materials, better trained or educated labour, or better machines, even if no changes in factor qualities or proportions take place. 'New ideas can raise efficiency by being applied to new products: imagination can design a better mousetrap, with no change in the quantity, quality or proportions of factors' (Lipsey, 1979: 232). Productivity was envisaged as the 'main problem' affecting the economy by the then Conservative Chancellor of the Exchequer George Osborne in his budget speech of March 2016 (gov.uk, 2016), in which he highlighted the significance of a national living wage, necessary because the country's growth had been heavily biased towards low-productivity jobs that do not pay very well. For most UK employers, lowering the cost of production may be seen as an obvious benefit, but this usually produces a degrading effect upon the technical capacity of the worker.

In contrast, the Labour Party leader Jeremy Corbyn has pledged to introduce policies to increase work productivity – 'to rebuild and transform Britain so that no one and no community is left behind' (Elliott, 2015a: 40). This would be achieved by introducing sectoral collective bargaining and mandatory collective bargaining for companies with more than 250 employees, thereby demonstrating a commitment to workers' rights, social justice, government investment in the manufacturing sector and public sector, and good quality jobs (Trade Union leader Len McCluskey's speech at the Trade Union Annual Conference 2016 (McCluskey, 2016)). As to the reality, economic growth in the UK has remained slow, and despite bank bailouts, spending cuts, wage freezes and pumping millions into financial markets, ordinary workers have benefited much less from it (Chakrabortty, 2016; Davies, 2017).

A slightly different economic direction was augured in a speech by Conservative Prime Minister Theresa May (Politics Home, 2016) at her first party conference, when she endeavoured to claim the political 'middle ground' by referring to enhancing individual worker productivity with a need for an 'industrial strategy'. She announced this industrial strategy in January 2017 and spoke of a ten-point plan to revive the economy, embracing a more productive, trade-focused strategy, with an emphasis on developing education, training and life-long learning. The industrial strategy emphasised five areas for attention: innovation, infrastructure, skills, spreading prosperity across the country and ensuring that businesses have access to finance. May stated that the strategy would be interventionist in purpose, but the intention was not for the state to become an agent of public reform. She continued: 'businesses would be incentivised to invest in skills in a big way, for example through a lowering of tax rates. As the planned split from the European Union (EU) would make hiring from overseas tougher there would be different sector deals to up-skill groups of workers' (Elliott, 2017: 38). Technological change, it would appear, has shifted the distribution of income from labour to capital, and according to the Organisation for Economic Co-operation and Development (OECD), up to 80 per cent of the decline in labour's share of national income between 1980 and 2010 was the result of the impact of technology (OECD, 2017).

> Digitalisation and globalisation have had many profoundly positive impacts, but policies could and should do better to help those directly affected by the associated changes, thereby mitigating the widening of socio-economic gaps in countries where inequality is very large ... [Technology] provides new ways for people to connect, socialise, collaborate and participate in societies; they enable the production of more and better products and services at cheaper prices, they foster the diffusion of knowledge and technology; they spur innovation, productivity and growth and have allowed millions of people in developing and emerging economies to escape poverty and improve their living standards. (OECD, 2017: 41–73)

An investment in plant, machinery and other efficiency-increasing technology to meet demand has become an aspiration of the

Conservative government's industrial strategy, represented, for example, by incentivising British universities to focus more on technical skills as skills training should be at the heart of the policy. The argument is that skills in the workforce are crucial for firms' ability to put innovative ideas into practice and increase productivity. Focus has traditionally been on high-level skills, but intermediate-skilled technicians and wider workforce skills would also be essential. More 'face time' with tutors would represent a changed culture in vocational education, bringing about, for example, a planned increase in university places for medical education. Furthermore, different sectors of the economy and workforce will be singled out for special treatment, for example automotive engineering. This approach will involve greater investment in infrastructure, in training and skills by setting targets, and by implication will be a concerted effort to stop employers paying low wages through continuing to employ cheap foreign labour. The Chancellor of the Exchequer (2016) Philip Hammond failed to acknowledge the true value of many public sector jobs:

> The problem is not highly skilled and highly paid bankers, brain surgeons, software engineers. You will not find, if you walk around towns in Britain and ask people how they feel about migration, that they have a problem with people with skills and high earnings coming to the UK ... They recognise that those people are a positive contribution to the UK economy. The issue that we have to deal with is people with low skills competing for entry-level jobs, the pressure on wages at the lowest end. (Treanor, 2016: 36)

A different approach for dealing with low workforce productivity was set out in a speech by Shadow Chancellor John McDonnell at the Labour Party conference of 2018, where he demonstrated a stronger interest in addressing the 'failures of the market', in so far as they affect things such as productivity, wages, geographic inequality, intergenerational inequality, house prices and the overall purpose of business. 'The 15–20% loss of productivity over the last decade, with hiring and firing workers in the UK having become much easier, to the point where capital investment is now less attractive, it is unsurprising that productivity is so weak' (O'Neill, 2018: 5). For instance, in the health and social care sector – where approximately 9 per cent of the 4.1 million employees are non-UK nationals – a residential care home employer may choose to employ a majority of cheap, relatively unskilled workers regardless of potential disbenefits and disadvantages to the client group. Could this action be termed de-professionalisation by the back door? If the Conservative government's aspirations are to be taken seriously, then it does not follow that economic growth would be possible if dependent on low-paid, low-skilled migrant labour. For gross domestic product (GDP) per capita to grow, this requires economic expansion emanating from an improvement in productivity, not simply from bringing ever large numbers of low-skilled people into the economy. The national living wage, a policy introduced by the Conservative government, fitted with the Prime Minister May's rhetoric about boosting prospects for the poorest, and was set in relation to median wages targeting 60 per cent of median UK pay by 2020. A small rise in the minimum wage would encourage employers to deploy workers more productively and help boost local economies by more than £1 billion, according to a study by the Smith Institute (Hunter, 2018). Employers need the spur of a higher minimum wage to shake them out of a cycle of low productivity and low growth that depresses company revenues and has trapped about 2 million workers on the current minimum wage of £7.70 an hour, or £8.21 for those aged 25 or older (Inman, 2018).

Low productivity resulting from de-skilling

De-professionalisation as an applied concept within the sociology of work can be linked to 'progressive de-skilling' (Braverman, 1974; Wood, 1982; Garson, 1988), which in turn equates to low productivity as characterised by an organisation where the acquisition of any new skills by individual employees is not conceptualised as of paramount importance by those in management or positions of authority. Despite the centrality of the concept of skill in the sociological analysis of work and its widespread use in everyday discussions of occupations, there is little agreement about how best to define and measure this familiar idea (Vallas, 1990). Braverman's historical account of de-skilling is the leading and most powerful version of the pessimistic position, which tends to use a definition of skill that emphasises the skill content of a job and the amount of task-specific training required to do it, as he argues that much work has been de-skilled. In contrast to this lies an optimistic position, where exercising responsibility and obtaining increased educational qualifications are viewed as salient factors, that is to say up-skilling (Edgell, 2012: 56). For the capitalist there is an imperative to exert control over the labour process in order to maximise the productive potential of labour and therefore profits; such that employers turned to developments in management and technology.

A growth of entrepreneurial activity can be associated with increased productivity and output, and the 'professional as entrepreneur' should not be discounted (see, for example, Bröckling, 2016: 66–80). Here entrepreneurship is defined as:

> To reform or revolutionise the pattern of production by exploiting an invention or, more generally, an untried technological possibility for producing a new commodity or producing an old one in a new way, by opening up a new source of supply of materials or a new outlet for products, by reorganising an industry and so on. (Bröckling, 2016: 70)

Joseph Schumpeter, a leading economist, depicted the entrepreneur as someone breaking loose from familiar routines and blazing trails on their own. The crucial quality for him was not inventiveness but the ability to establish 'new combinations' (Schumpeter, 1942) in production and distribution. For this reason he emphasised the role of power in entrepreneurial activity. Enterprise is a 'special care of the social phenomenon of leadership' (Schumpeter, 1928: 412):

> The leader type is characterised for one thing by a special way of looking at things. Less by intellect than by will, by the power to grasp very particular things and see them as real. Also by the capacity to go it alone and go before the others, to not feel uncertainty and resistance as opposing grounds, and so essentially by his effect on others; what we can call 'authority', 'gravity', 'command' … he is the special trailblazer of the modern human and the capitalist, the individualist way of life. (Schumpeter, 1934: 134)

Through the lens of authoritarian monetarist economics, the current scenario presents a UK economy requiring further stimulus and investment. Low productivity links with low pay and how it interacts with working hours and is reflected in the extent to which staff may fail to take ownership of their work. What brings average productivity down is a higher proportion of people in low-paid work and a long-term failure to invest in capital equipment. Only by analysing the economy sector by sector will it be possible to identify where attention is needed, either by better training or legislation to outlaw poor employment practices. 'As Henry Ford knew, as with an under-performing factory, if you mothball a workforce then a company will lack paying customers for its products' (Edgell, 2012: 91–5). The cause of diminishing opportunities even for skilled work is the concentration of the benefit from automation into the hands of the elite. Business heads' rewards are now disproportionate to those for their workforce. Equalisation in pay levels, coupled with redistributive taxes, could allow provision of a basic income sufficient to permit a shorter working week. As technology advances, we have become much more efficient at producing the goods and food we need, however, these benefits have been retained by an ever-decreasing minority, while the incomes of the majority have stagnated or even regressed.

Has the de-skilled worker an incentive to acquire new skills?

In contrast, we consider de-professionalisation as evoking images of lacking an opportunity to demonstrate initiative, control or authority. For the de-skilled worker – for whom there may be a disincentive to acquire new skills– engaged in an innovative and successful organisation, this feature may become part of the conversation around lower productivity or it may not. It has been claimed that one aspect of globalisation of the workforce has been its contribution to the growth of the 'precariat' – a term describing an emerging class of people facing lives of insecurity, moving in and out of jobs that give little meaning to their lives (Standing, 2014). An epidemic growth of workforce insecurity goes hand in hand with the way companies or organisations have become commodities, to be bought and sold through mergers and acquisitions. The frenzy with which firms are now traded, split up and repackaged is a feature of global capitalism. And corporations have become increasingly owned by foreign shareholders, led by pension and private equity funds. Companies want more flexible labour forces so that they can respond quickly to external threats.

Commodification has also made the division of labour within enterprises more fluid. If activities can be done more cheaply in one location, they are off-shored (within firms) or outsourced (to partner firms or others). This fragments the labour process; internal job structures and bureaucratic careers are disrupted, owing to uncertainty over whether jobs people might have expected to do will be off-shored or outsourced. For example, the care industry in the UK is estimated to employ in excess of 160,000 workers on zero-hours contracts, while the public sector, especially the NHS, has increasingly adopted flexible contracts, indicating that insecure employment has become a permanent and growing feature of the jobs market (Inman, 2016). De-professionalisation in this example can be regarded as a function or by-product of a normally hierarchical process where certain jobs become vulnerable and subordinate, and professional identity is scapegoated, replaced by insecurity and a lack of belonging (transformative – contextual dimension, see Chapter 6). In its 2017 outlook, the Chartered Institute of Personnel and Development, which represents people working in human services, forecasted slower economic growth, fewer new jobs and downward pressure on pay, which would compound challenges from low productivity and uncertainty about Britain's future relationship with the EU.

The argument goes that this disruption feeds into the way skills are developed. The incentive to invest in skills is determined by the cost of acquiring them, the opportunity cost of doing so and the prospective additional income. If the risk increases of not having an opportunity to practise skills, investment in them will decline, as will the psychological commitment to the company. In short, if firms become more fluid, workers will be discouraged from trying to build careers inside them. They will experience a corrosion of identity, as dehumanisation becomes a powerful metaphor for exploitation, low status and low wages.

> Precarious unemployment in the neo-liberal framework has been viewed as a matter of individual responsibility, making it almost 'voluntary'. People came to be regarded as more or less 'employable' and the answer was to make them more employable, upgrading their 'skills' or reforming their 'habits' and 'attitudes' (Standing, 2014: 77)

An alternative suggestion is that businesses would rather employ cheap labour than spend more on new machinery or equipment, which explains why investment in the UK as a share of GDP is still well below where it was before the 2008 recession. The argument for higher investment as the bedrock of a more successful economy is that it boosts productivity, leading to higher wages, a bigger tax take and smaller deficit. Investing in skills and infrastructure, thereby investing in growth and leading to a more competitive market, was suggested as a hallmark of the Conservative government's Productivity Plan, according to the Business Secretary of State, Sajid Javid, in a speech delivered in December 2015. However, evidence from the budget watchdog (Elliott, 2015c) showed that productivity would not get better soon, and this was similarly the case during the political campaign running up to the EU referendum in June 2016. Investment in the UK has been decreasing, job opportunities dwindling and

Britain's reputation abroad diminishing. This was the view taken by Mark Carney, Governor General of the Bank of England, who said in 2016 that the UK economy relies on the 'kindness of strangers' – out of all the 28 members of the EU, the UK is second only to Ireland in its dependence on investment from abroad (Treanor and Watt, 2016: 29).

Unlike the German workforce, where efficiency and training have been highlighted, and unlike Sweden that boasts of its anti-corruption and good industrial relations, the UK economy now relies too much on its cheapness – in taxes, wages and regulation (Chakrabortty, 2018a). According to a report by the Press Association, wages are still worth a third less in some parts of the UK than was the case in 2008; and the average worker has lost £11,800 in real earnings since that time (Press Association, 2019). In defence of workers' rights, Frances O'Grady, TUC General Secretary, stated that wage growth in the UK has been 'stuck in the slow lane' (TUC, 2018) and that the government should put pressure on businesses to pay staff more. One way of doing this is through insisting that workers acquire new skills and qualifications and forcing companies to reward individuals accordingly by acknowledging the attributed value of particular jobs. The argument is that Britain has been paying the price for decades of underinvestment and cut-price competition. It would seem that we have a highly skilled workforce, with almost half of Britain's young people holding a university degree. And yet in 2014, Charlie Mayfield, head of the UK Commission on Employment and Skills, pointed out that over one in five British jobs required only primary-school education (Anderson, 2014; BBC News, 2014). There is a counter-argument that this type of nebulous assertion lacks solid evidence, and for example fails to acknowledge in a meaningful way the real value and demands of the wide range of occupations present in human services.

Funds for local economies and infrastructure to ramp up productivity – where are the solutions?

The Conservative government announced a £1.6 billion funding boost for left-behind towns in England in March 2019. Prime Minister Theresa May said the Stronger Towns Fund, much of it allocated to the north of England and the Midlands, will go over seven years to areas that had not 'shared the proceeds of growth'. She introduced the initiative as follows: 'Communities across the country voted for Brexit as an expression of their desire to see change – that must be a change for the better, with more opportunity and greater control' (Elgot, 2019: 7). James Brokenshire, Secretary of State for Communities, Local Government and Housing, described this funding as 'potentially transformative', with the aim of creating skills and providing opportunities for the public sector to work with the private sector, along with assist deprived areas in the years after Brexit. Labour Shadow Chancellor John McDonnell said the fund 'smacks of desperation from a government reduced to bribing MPs to vote for their damaging flagship Brexit legislation'; whereas the Labour MP for Wigan, Lisa Nandy, said that it 'must represent the start of an overhaul in the government's approach to investment' (Bounds, 2019).

The Labour Opposition's view has remained that relentless cuts have not helped Britain's long-term economic prospects nor produced successful growth; instead they have impacted negatively on the integrity of public services. This view is that between 2010 and 2019 both Conservative chancellors – Osborne and Hammond – have been equally committed to a self-defeating goal of massively reducing the public sector from 43 per cent to below 30 per cent, and pushing forward these plans in the short-term interests of an elite class of tax-avoiding private businesses and multinational corporations. 'The UK's top executives will have made more money over the first two and a half days of 2017 than a typical worker will earn all year, according to an analysis that lays bare the gulf between executives at Britain's biggest companies and the rest of the workforce' (Allen, 2017: 39). It has been claimed also that no economically successful country in modern history has voluntarily reduced its public services as a supposed growth-promotion strategy (Commission on Growth and Development, 2008; Department for Communities and Local Government, 2012). The Office of Budget Responsibility's (OBR) assumption of growth has been underpinned consistently by the belief that labour productivity will grow briskly despite the fact that there has been no increase in productivity since the advent of the 2008 recession.

It has been reported that there are no causal links between the UK's flat productivity since the 2008 crash and particular changes in employment practices. There is as yet no statistical evidence at a national level of a link between lower hours and higher productivity. Equally, there is no evidence that longer working hours achieve better outcomes – they just lead to burnout and stress (Inman and Jolly, 2018). The Labour Party has produced a number of 'big ideas' to boost productivity (Helm, 2018). These include experimenting with a universal basic income and setting up local co-operatives, where the plan would be for Labour councils to favour them when choosing service providers. This has short-term costs, but will aim to support local employers who pay well and to involve staff in decisions that can bring broader benefits. Workers on boards has become rooted as a serious idea, where companies with more than 250 staff would be legally bound to have worker directors elected by the entire workforce. The party has stipulated that the proportion of workers could be as high as a third, and that there would also be a plan to give workers financial shares in their company. A final recommendation is nationalisation – but spurning traditional state ownership in favour of models that involve workers, consumers and other stakeholders, and to nationalise natural monopolies, such as the water industry, electricity and gas suppliers.

Summary

This chapter has considered the idea of de-professionalisation in the context of abuse of power or authority, and the effect this may have on undermining the position or status of professions. Also included is a review of some of the evidence used to conceptualise de-professionalisation as an economic signifier, defined by de-skilling, low productivity or output resulting from work activity. No claim is made for a direct relationship between these two meanings in terms of their internal attributes, apart from the fact that both would appear to have a corrosive impact. As regards the first, abuse of power is defined through incidents of physical or verbal abuse, or alternatively may involve an act of sexual abuse and invasion of personal privacy. There appears to be relatively little research done in this area relating to understanding the activities of professionals working in different sectors of public services. Available evidence seems to show that certain relationships rooted in social inequalities and power imbalances demonstrate how abuse can be projected from one individual onto another, by transferring or attributing an emotion or desire to another person, especially unconsciously. Specific studies discuss what it is about the nature of institutions that allowed abusive practices to take place within their confines. The term 'abjection' has been used to explain a process of discrediting others, and may apply in expressing attitudes towards vulnerable citizens, whom the state has a responsibility to protect, such that they become stigmatised and presented as discredited and discreditable. Different forms of power may corrupt or encourage dishonesty, and these may include turning a blind eye to corrupt practices.

The notion of a professional abuser is understood to refer to those individuals who prey on the weaknesses of others in the workplace: exploiting their vulnerability, taking advantage of their client's trust, not acting in their best interests and failing to keep professional boundaries. Professional sexual abuse as identified in some parts of mental health services is particularly relevant; however, challenging problems of preventing or responding to sex boundary violations has been ignored both in research and professional guidelines and is sometimes hidden by ineffective management responses. De-professionalisation as abuse of power may be associated with inadequate self-regulation and result in a diminution of service standards. This may be evidenced in the manner by which some professions have elected to deal with those individuals with 'performance problems', for example, wrongly prescribing drugs or sexual misconduct involving teachers, pointing towards a criminal standard of proof in fitness to practice – the Sexual Offences Act 2003 or Mental Health Act 1983/2007. In the current social climate there has been a focus on abuse of power in the workplace, particularly sexual abuse, involving activities of other types of public servant, examples being politicians holding public office or media celebrities with junior colleagues, usually women, and the need for appropriate procedures to be in place for organisations to respond to such incidents (or professional dilemmas).

De-professionalisation as a concept characterised by diminution of autonomy or status at work is contextualised perceptibly through the notion of low productivity, where, for example, a rise in low-skilled jobs has become blamed for static wages. Increases in productivity are as a result of deploying better raw materials, better trained or educated labour, or better machines. According to GDP figures, UK economic growth at the beginning of 2019 was as bad as in 2012. Instead of choosing public spending, the Conservative government has become consumed by ideological rows over Brexit; but perhaps ought to realise that the slow recovery from the 2008 crisis is about a deficiency of aggregate demand. Unemployment is low because involuntary part-time work is high, and at a level 42 per cent above what it was in 2008 – with a prevalence of low-paid, often part-time, insecure work throughout the economy (OECD, 2018; World Economic Forum, 2019).

Braverman's historical account of de-skilling is a leading and powerful version of the pessimistic position, which tends to use a definition of skill that emphasises the skill content of the job and the amount of task-specific training required to do it. This contrasts with the optimistic position, where exercising responsibility and obtaining increased educational qualifications would be seen as associated with up-skilling. The former evokes images of lacking an opportunity to demonstrate initiative, control or autonomy within the workplace. Despite an OBR assumption of growth, underpinned by a belief that labour productivity will grow briskly, there has been little evidence of an increase in productivity since the advent of the 2008 recession.

12

Conclusion: professionals as entrepreneurs in an age of austerity

De-professionalism, neo-liberalism and social inequalities

What is the future for professionalism and the public sector? There are several reasons why we should remain optimistic that professionalism as a trope concept should endure, not least because technological advances increase work productivity along with the demand for new skills. This is despite the fact that austerity policies in the United Kingdom (UK) embody a presence of continued uncertainty, lacking an evidential commitment to rebuilding public services. In past years a professional person with recognised expertise may have developed a life narrative, linear and cumulative, a narrative that made sense in a highly bureaucratic world. A different entrepreneurial world entailing 'creative destruction' (Reinert and Reinert, 2006: 55) requires people being at ease about not reckoning the consequences of change or not knowing what comes next. Neo-liberalism, involving a remaking of the state, reconfigured to serve the demands of capital, has meant that some professionals may have lost authority arguably because the state has lost its authority. Instead of celebrating the virtue of professional expertise, a system based on neo-liberal ideas tends to view professions as raw material within a general commodification process. This has given rise to a different rationale: it must ask what value the corporation has for the community, how it can serve civic interests rather than just its ledger of profit and loss. Whereas the state has a capacity to extend audit, intervention and knowledge transfer, an argument has been made that across areas of the public sector there has been a loss of autonomy in professional practice. De-professionalisation has become part of the neo-liberal lexicon defining a continuation of the marketisation agenda; hence it follows that if austerity finished tomorrow, it is likely that this de-professionalisation would continue.

De-professionalisation, defined by terms that circumscribe the reduced capacity of the public sector workforce, has become enmeshed in the wider debate around rising inequalities in the UK. Announced in May 2019, the Institute for Fiscal Studies (IFS) established an interdisciplinary research forum, chaired by Professor Angus Deaton, to examine disparities of income, wealth, health and political access. 'Amid fears Britain is on the cusp of sinking towards deep and ingrained inequalities following a decade of stagnant pay growth, there's a real question about whether democratic capitalism is working, when it's only working for part of the population' (IFS, 2019b: 26–7). A research puzzle to unravel needs to be based perhaps around the question of how far some professions have become fellow victims along with the rest of society, where widening inequalities in pay, health and opportunities are undermining trust in democracy.

Whereas belonging to a profession may have been celebrated in the past for admiring and rewarding expertise, a vast majority of the nation's wealth now accrues to shareholders, bosses, bondholders and those who don't earn it. The phenomenon of rent-seeking has been employed to describe what happens when a person or business uses their position or resources to get some additional benefit from the government. Rent-seeking results in reduced economic efficiency through misallocation of resources, reduced wealth creation, lost government revenue, heightened income inequality and potential national decline (Majaski, 2019). Making inequality reduction a central aim of government policy and wider society needs to be fully advanced, as it has been shown that the economic ideas adopted by the UK in the 1980s have led to vastly increased inequality. Globalisation and new technology have instilled an economy in which those with highly valued skills or talents can earn huge rewards. Attempting to reduce inequality via redistributive taxation is likely to fail because the global elite can easily hide their money in tax havens. 'The most entrenched, self-deluding and self-perpetuating justifications for inequality are about morality, not economy, and demand therefore a moral justification for selfishness' (Aldred, 2019: 20).

Economic productivity requires investment in human capital – training and development; and professionals continue to develop strategies to advance their own status. The opportunities for a professional entrepreneur are considerable, such as acquiring and consolidating new skills along with discovering and exploring new markets for channelling these skills. An entrepreneur has been defined as 'someone who creates and then organises and operates a new firm, as an innovator, and as someone who transforms interventions and ideas into economically viable entities' (Lowrey, 2003). This defined role of an entrepreneur as an economic agent is worthy insofar as their interventions are viewed as significant for the performance of the economy. One type of analysis of the role focuses broadly on the nature of the entrepreneur's influence; another on the management of survival, routine and the status quo. The notion of professionals as entrepreneurs lends itself to considering creation for advancement, for growth and dynamics, seeing the entrepreneur as an individual with a perpetual desire for achievement.

Investing in human capital embodies a constant factor as regards its impact on professionalisation processes, and part of its salvation is that it continues to be one of capitalism's failures not to properly value non-monetary work such as care, commitment or the depth of a personal work experience. Changes are required to address fundamental power imbalances that allow employers to shift risk onto their employees. Developments for example in artificial intelligence/robotics might reduce opportunities to display professionalism involving human interaction. A different type of political economy of work model is needed that values a range of work activities and places job quality centre-stage, restoring a firmer foundation for collectivist values.

In the UK, Brexit has become associated with reinforcing the neo-liberal model, now seen as somewhat ubiquitous, and as such acts as a kind of metaphor for retrenchment of professional autonomy because workers' rights may be diminished with the abandonment of European Union (EU) legislation and protection. Paradoxically, the term 'institutionalising the status quo' (Pridham 2008: 423) has become synonymous with remaining in the EU, referring to the fact that even more public sector contracts will likely go abroad. What explains both the governing class's lack of serious response to 2008's banking crash and the vast inequality that continues in its wake? A genre of financial elites has emerged as one solution to reducing social inequalities (Giridharadas, 2019). This author's study of the strategies used by members of the global financial elite to justify inertia shows how businesspeople have become elevated to 'leaders'. The findings reinforce the notion that this genre of elites believes and promotes the idea that social change should be pursued principally through the free market and voluntary action, not public life, the law and the reform of the systems that they have in common. Within neo-liberal ideology lies a suggestion that any solution to reducing inequalities should be supervised by the backers of capitalism and their allies, and not be antagonistic to meeting their needs. Members of the financial elite then make the argument that the biggest beneficiaries of the status quo should play a leading role in making progress towards shared opportunities. Their answer is to build an aggressive creative partnership that involves all levels of government, the private sector and non-government organisations to make it better.

De-professionalism and planning a workforce strategy

A mainstream view is that the Brexit project will ultimately advantage highly skilled people who elect to work in the UK. Many jobs that to date have been thought of as professional and lesser skilled, such as in social care, may require a reclassification in order that they become valued holistically and that their contribution is reappraised. In the present era of austerity, an argument has been made that the scientific status of competing models of social research has become seriously undermined through its deployment as a mechanism for rationing and controlling services. A recent public inquiry into an care home funded by the National Health Service (NHS) prompted one media commentator to ask whether it was the poor staff or the culture that led to an alleged abuse of vulnerable patients (Bodkin, 2019). It is a management choice whether or not to employ a professionalised workforce and, as with other types of market-led provision, it would appear that at least parts of the care sector will always go for the least expensive option (King's Fund, 2018a, 2018b). In England the workforce challenges, for example in the NHS, present a greater threat to health and social care than the funding challenges. A report by researchers from the Institute for Fiscal Studies found that overall spending on local services by English councils fell by 21 per cent between 2009/10 and 2017/18 (IFS, 2019a). A prediction was that the rising costs and demands of adult social care could require 60 per cent of local tax revenues within 15 years. One conclusion from this report was that either councils have to be provided with additional revenues, to enable them to continue providing existing services, let alone extend and improve them; or that government and society must accept that councils can afford to provide fewer or lower quality services than they currently do.

Key themes of a workforce strategy include supply and demand management, good employment practice, efficiency and productivity, and leadership and skills development; while an organisation needs to train, retain, recruit and skill its workforce to meet the needs of clients and customers. Publicly supported policies for entrepreneurship development may form a critical part of any workforce strategy involving professionally related activities and functions. This impacts on any future encouragement of socially and economically productive activities by individuals acting independently in business (Henrekson and Stenkula, 2009; NESTA, 2009; Ramlogan and Rigby, 2012). Policies may be implemented directly to address entrepreneurial needs, for example business advice programmes or through the broader macroeconomic policy frameworks, such as education policy. Focused on key actors, a central policy objective has been to seek to increase the competitiveness of an organisation. Is there a dissonance between working on behalf of the public sector and as a private sector entrepreneur? Although some fundamental organisational values may differ, a growing trend towards entrepreneurship has become evident across most domains driving public services.

Is higher education (HE)and further education (FE) –an example of a sector that would benefit from a workforce strategy? For instance, in higher education a close scrutiny has uncovered signs of internal disharmony as regards efforts to articulate this sector's dominant aims, allied to an argument that techniques of evidence-based practice in management have been misapplied (Sayer, 2014; Briner, 2015). Universities may act corporately as an entrepreneur for their locality or region; they may also choose to teach methodologies governing entrepreneurship through bespoke curricula. Most universities desire an international reputation for research, learning and teaching relevant to a fast-changing interconnected world. They realise this through enhancing their stature, reputation and influence; and by seeking to work in partnership with businesses to drive professionalism within a modern culture. Here, academic entrepreneurs act as traditional scientists and must also be like traditional entrepreneurs in their need to be focused, careful and critical in their thinking, while still being able to recognise business opportunities and create market value. If one of them discovers or invests something of commercial value, the university may help them create a start-up business to market it. The university views the individual as their employee and the inventions as the property of the university.

De-professionalism has become defined through measures to support a workforce strategy and stronger workforce unionisation. A major aim would be to reverse a decline in morale, professional autonomy or a readiness by employers to accept flexible or easily modified working arrangements, particularly as regards pay, qualifications and related entitlements. Entrepreneurship would be seen as a driving force crystallising the legitimate goals of the university sector in a space where subversivity or ambiguity might otherwise be attributed as challenging the sector's more traditional ethos. Professional teachers need to incorporate their entrepreneurial learnings into their curricula so that they can pass on knowledge to others. In the current environment those who teach entrepreneurship aim to strengthen links between education, research, entrepreneurship and innovation by leveraging their accommodating city or region as a unique asset on the international stage. This process of developing innovation projects into new ventures has been well circumscribed by the concept of the research active curriculum and encompasses knowledge application as well as knowledge discovery. It includes designing a research question, learning how to answer it and finding necessary sources, and is manifested through performance and evidence-based practice as well as through peer-reviewed journals and research council funding (The Russell Group, 2018).

The government-favoured terrain of resorting to evidence-based policy and practice has become pervasive and has 'to differing degrees influenced research activity and challenged professional identities in professions as diverse as medicine, social work, clinical psychology, nursing and education' (Trinder and Reynolds, 2008: 24). This methodology is here to stay and has been given a consistently high profile in both Conservative and Labour governments. There has been far less recognition of the extent to which such change comprises a new politically protected and closed knowledge system – a professional knowledge industry – that operates in line with the still dominant neo-liberal political ideology of government. One effect is that this has considerable implications for the role of HE, the nature of research and the accreditation of professional competence (Tunstill and Blewett, 2019).

There have been various demands expressed for a workforce strategy to consolidate the benefits of public services and to halt fragmentation along with the national staffing crisis (CIPD, 2018b). It has been reported by the government's Migration Advisory Committee that psychologists, occupational therapists, midwives and vets were among the professions that should be added to the official shortage list (MAC, 2019b; Siddique, 2019). A strategy would include identifying skills gaps, targeting specific and identified efficiencies, starting employee retention initiatives and improving the quality of outputs. A programme based on progressive taxation, investment in education, a cradle-to-grave welfare state and collective bargaining would help to rebuild parts of society where austerity measures in particular have had profoundly damaging effects on much of the population.

The provision (or lack) of further education opportunities across the UK represents a critical area where there has been a reported major under-investment and a 25 per cent fall in student funding since 2010 (Adams, 2019). An attempt to forearm any future bid for a workforce strategy arrived with the Augar Review of post-18 education and funding (DfE, 2019b). This report painted a picture of a bloated HE sector and recommended a shift in funding away from universities towards FE and vocational training. It critiqued the ethos of universities for offering too many 'low value' courses. One purpose of the review was to make degrees less attractive by increasing student loan repayments by low- and middle-income graduates, including some professional groups. It recommended loan repayments starting at a lower salary level and their timeframe being extended from 30 years to 40 years. Main proposals included cutting undergraduate tuition fees from £9,250 to £7,500 and to use 'replacement funding' to target those students who go on to high-paying graduate jobs and also to transfer more funding to FE with a provision of student loans similar to that of universities. The funding of FE and HE should not be perceived as 'a zero-sum game' in so far as any utility gain in one sector (FE) would not be balanced by a loss in another sector (HE). Nevertheless, this policy proposes challenges to planning any workforce strategy involving FE and HE teachers; and would consider ways of calculating the transferable skills and features distinctive to each of the two separate sectors.

One characterisation of the Augar proposals is that of extending de-professionalism within the HE sector. This will be appreciated by highlighting their likely impact on those who teach in HE and on those professionals in training, for example in relation to graduates in nursing or teaching, who would pay more in loan repayments overall. A possible prejudice of the report would be in its feigned attack on those HE teachers, who by dint of their professional qualifications remain essential as pedagogues and mentors. Augar was requested to adjust support for different subjects to reflect the economic and social value of degrees, and how much they cost to teach. Some of its recommendations, however, appeared to neglect the fact that many degree courses are designed as feeders for particular forms of employment and therefore focus on producing graduates with higher level transferable skills. There is an acknowledged prejudice against those who teach on arts and humanities degrees where most graduates receive poorer wages, at least in the early stages of their career; the university would receive lowered fees, which would cut jobs and inherently damage professional development (Fazackerley, 2019). To receive the same income from student fees, classes might then need to become larger, prohibiting a focus on one-to-one tuition, often regarded as an essential feature for the healthy survival of professional training.

There are a number of perspectives and frameworks that underpin a workforce strategy. Professionalism involves qualities such as a high level of competence, efficiency and willingness to innovate, together with altruism and integrity and an expectation that individuals are keen to widen their educational qualifications and skills profile. These virtuous qualities, which include being given the opportunity or authority to take charge, may be less visible to some outsiders – who instead question the value of professionals to the national economy, in contrast to other groups who are seen to create wealth. This argument has been taken up by managerialist ideology, which has become an all-pervasive force in shaping organisations that employ large numbers of the public sector workforce. This model is embedded ubiquitously throughout professional practices to scope demands for increased efficiency, accountability and achieving greater responsiveness to clients and service users. It complements a neo-liberal approach that propagates those actions that increase flexibility, mobility and individualisation. However, the model reduces the likelihood of some professionals, for example social workers, being able or willing to take a socially critical position in their day-to-day work, to the detriment of the integrity of the profession (Garrett, 2018).

An alternative approach, underpinned by an ideology combining democratic and collaborative professionalism, has been distinguished by a sensitivity to the interests of a range of external stakeholders and representatives, and a dedication to finding ways of deepening accountability towards more collectivist values. Democratic professionalism is as much a practice as it is a constellation of values, a practice that is built around models of active and collaborative democratic change. A problem inherent in this model is that professionals may engage only in technocratic professionalism (concerned with technical and self-interested practices and motivations driven by commercial profit) instead of civic professionalism, which invests professional practice with moral meaning and with democratic value (Maharg, 2012). Collaborative professionalism in contrast is perhaps more prescriptive. This approach is about how to collaborate more deeply in ways that achieve greater impact. In an educational setting, collaborative professionalism is about how teachers and other educators transform teaching and learning together to work with all students to develop fulfilling lives of meaning, purpose and success. It is evidence-informed and based on a high level of trust and precision, where teachers have strong relationships, trust each other and feel free to take risks and make mistakes (Hargreaves and O'Connor, 2018).

Throughout this discourse, an analytical framework has evolved as a way of conceptualising the professionalism/de-professionalism nexus. This framework is presented as transgressive in so far as it acknowledges perspectives drawn from different disciplines, involves a limited violation of accepted or imposed boundaries and includes references to measures aimed at reversing de-professionalisation. One effect has been to draw attention to visceral human factors such as loss of autonomy, vulnerability of identity and the impact of external control on personal motivation, along with obviating any requirement for specialist knowledge. An argument has been made that the process of de-professionalisation needs to be evaluated through objective indicators such as staff shortages or reduced work output, but may also be expressed experientially, for example through feelings of low morale and motivation. Professional organisations have suggested, for example, that the price for a badly underfunded NHS is being paid for by the nation's doctors, along with all the other overworked and demoralised health professionals (BMA, 2018; Nuffield Trust, 2019).

A commitment towards professionalised public services?

It must be encouraging to see policies change in response to outsourcing failures as some NHS bosses have begun to make the case against competition in the health service. The NHS Long Term Plan sought to redress the chronic staff shortage by a financial injection of £20.5 billion for annual improvements between 2019/20 and 2023/4 – it was short of around 103,000 doctors, nurses and other personnel, making it hard to drive the measurable progress they are seeking. Additionally, the number of full-time general practitioners (GPs) in England fell from 29,138 in March 2018 to 28,697 in June 2019 – a loss of 441 family doctors. That is despite the Conservative government's pledge in 2015 to increase the number of GPs by 5,000 by 2020. The long-delayed NHS Plan (DHSC, 2019) was published in January 2019, promising 'a new service model for the 21st Century', which would entail 'major practical changes' (pp 1–2). These included boosting out-of-hospital care, dissolving the historic divide between primary and community health services, and embedding local partnerships with local authority-funded services through new integrated care systems.

Social care represents possibly the most unaddressed social policy of our age, with councils unable to meet obligations to a rapidly ageing population. The deteriorating prospects for local government mean that nearly one in five councils in England may be forced to impose drastic spending controls to stave off bankruptcy; this was a warning issued by the Local Government Association (Butler, 2019a). Around 400 care homes have closed between 2014 and 2019, with low pay cited as the main reason for difficulties recruiting staff. Retaining the sector's 1.4 million workers has become a bigger challenge than recruitment, according to experts, particularly as an estimated 100,000 of them are non–British EU nationals who may be affected adversely by Brexit (Brindle, 2019).

The de-professionalism argument arises from an urgent need to restore the funding to providing a basic standard of care and to achieve a firmer integration of the two – health and social care – providers. In 2017 the Conservative government promised to publish a consultative Green Paper on Social Care, but over two years later this has still not yet surfaced. In July 2019 the government was urged to spend £8 billion immediately to address the 'national scandal' of the UK's social care system by introducing free personal care, according to a Report from the House of Lords (Payne, 2019). An inquiry by the Lords' Economic Affairs Committee warned that the present system was 'severely unfunded', with 1.4 million adults unable to access adequate care. This report also highlighted the disparity in prices paid by local authorities versus those who are self-funded. The chair of the Lords' Committee, Michael Forsyth, said in an interview that 'it was necessary to do something about care workers who are paid next to nothing, and then would leave to work in a supermarket' (Economic Affairs Committee, 2019). Political failure and Treasury reluctance appear to be at the heart of this matter, along with a need to value care-giving as a professional activity.

Targets for mental health care remain opaque, and it has become evident that further training and education are required for staff to obtain knowledge/skills to carry out complex technical and behavioural assessments and interventions. For instance, in this specialty, where there is a dire staff shortage and retention problem and where stigma exists, new roles have emerged – well-being coordinator, physician associate – to fill a skills gap (Andalo, 2019). Most professions now recognise that learning and professional development are lifelong through continuing professional development methods. Having suffered a succession of austerity measures, new strategies will be needed to reverse the effects of such processes. These include bolstering government ownership of public services, rewarding specialist expertise and fully implementing human rights and related social legislation.

Reversing de-professionalisation will require a re-ownership of the 'Whig narrative' of the welfare state, or a social citizenship-based progressive agenda. This term is often used pejoratively to present the past in the context of the inexorable march of progress, but if only accepted as a figurative expression it portrays a need to re-examine some of the values pre-empted by the welfare state consensus. Rights to legal protection, to housing, social services and to employment protection are examples where professional advocacy will become salient. In the case of legal protection, legal aid was partly abolished in 2013, means-tested and severely curtailed. Whereas the numbers in need have increased greatly, owing to housing, divorce and family breakdown, with the decline in legal aid there has been a large increase in the numbers of people representing themselves. Legal aid reforms were set out in the Legal Aid, Sentencing, Punishment of Offenders Act 2012, targeting only the highest priority cases and instead offering more encouragement of the use of mediation to resolve disputes. Everyone has been affected: parents going through the family courts, tenants fighting landlords, patients fighting hospitals and so on; defendant's costs orders have meant that even if proved innocent a person is now required to pay their costs (Hill and Bowcott, 2018). More than half of all magistrates courts in England and Wales have closed between 2010 and 2018, reducing access to social rights protection (Bowcott and Duncan, 2019). Legal aid fees for solicitors have been cut, and expenditure on legal aid has fallen by over a third in real terms. Accessing the legal aid system without expert help and removing people's right to have expert legal representation implies that justice is now denied to the majority (Home Office 2016; Croft, 2018).

In the context of debating a person's right to housing and shelter, it has been well-publicised that there was an estimated 98 per cent rise in the number of rough sleepers in the UK between 2010 and 2018 (Heriot Watt University, 2018). According to research by the charity Crisis, nearly 600 homeless people died on the streets or in temporary accommodation in England and Wales in 2017, up 24 per cent in five years (Butler, 2018c). Deaths due to homelessness have risen every year – from 475 in 2014 to 597 in 2017. This research has suggested that 12,300 people are currently sleeping rough on the street, well over double the official figure, and that formal estimates for rough sleeping have failed to capture the true scale of the crisis facing tens of thousands of people who have no permanent home but do not show up in council records (Heriot Watt University, 2018). In a report, the Commission on the Future of Social Housing has estimated that more than 3 million new social homes will be needed by 2040, concluding that there needs to be a profound shift to see social housing as a national asset like any other infrastructure (Shelter, 2019). This would effectively become an overriding government responsibility and enshrine an individual's right to a home, and, at the very least, bring about a halt to too much public money going to private landlords, in other words rent-seeking (Greenfield, 2018).

Can we reverse a process whereby services have been taken over by high-performing local authorities and teams of experts, and unalloyed freedoms being granted to any approved organisation that may choose to respond to a particular policy agenda? An organisation may then have a right to take over aspects of service delivery for a given local area and proceed to run it as it sees fit, perhaps relying less on the expertise – or otherwise – of trained professionals and instead preferring to train its own staff. A topical example that illustrates this important argument concerns home schooling, as this currently operates outside any national or local jurisdiction, and therefore implicitly questions the virtue of deploying professionals as educators. Parents are now facing an obligation to register children being educated at home under government proposals intended to prevent young people from disappearing under the radar. An estimated 60,000 children are currently thought to be educated at home – a figure that is rising annually. The register will, for the first time, enable authorities to see where children are if they are not in school and intervene more effectively if required (Weale, 2019b). Outside regulators would not place any specific requirements on professional support and access, so although parents in the future may have a responsibility to register their child, there is still no guarantee that the child will receive an education to any acceptable or approved standard – and in this sense s/he might remain vulnerable. The training gap within the public sector workforce has resulted in a failure to equip staff with the right skills (upskilling), and in the education sector, to employ an adequate number of specialist teachers in schools and colleges, resulting in a lack of commonality of service standards (Moorhead, 2016b).

De-professionalism, regulation and valuing expertise

Austerity was a political choice made by the Conservative government that has recycled savings from austerity into tax breaks for the better-off. Unnecessary, uncaring cuts to public services testify to the fact that both the present Conservative and previous Coalition government in the UK have chosen private profit over civic service. Austerity has become foregrounded as a weasel word used to promote rhetoric that there is no alternative, that anaesthetises public anger as we are led to believe that there is no choice. 'We have to build in our communities and in our daily conversations a challenge to the dialogue of cuts as economic necessity. Government politicians have ignored the impact of austerity and refused to measure it. Instead they have chosen to put blame on to the victims and the responsibility on to charities that buckle under the strain' (Clough, 2018: 6). If our 'decade of shame' is not to become permanent, recognition is required that a strong society is one in which everyone is strong (CPAG, 2017; Chakrabortty, 2018b).

These policy failures are significant in the context of developing an overall strategy for delivering public services, for encouraging innovation and productivity, and for benchmarking the values of professionalism to the economy as a whole. Evidence staking out a commitment towards a professionalised public service model would be enlivened through an ongoing debate around standards and regulation. Reports from bodies such as NHS England (2018b), Monitor (2018), the NHS Trust Development Authority (2018) and the National Audit Office (2018) have described challenging times in the health and social care sector in particular, pointing out frequently that the adult social care system has been on the brink of collapse. With the forthcoming expectation of a more integrated National Health and Social Care Service, a formal framework governing the pay, skills and qualifications of social care staff might then become recognised. An intention would be to remove piecemeal workforce planning and to subsume the workforce under the Agenda For Change regulations, which honour agreements on the national living wage, pay restraint and incremental scales (NHS Employers, 2019).

The state of care Care Quality Commission (CQC) report for 2017/18 (CQC, 2018e) referred to examples of poor treatment standards with more progress required as regards quality and regulation. This would include encapsulating how far a government and the public may put a premium on the kind of specialist knowledge, skills and experience of those who provide services to people. To buttress the authority of professionalism from within an agenda of austerity, bank bailouts and globalisation, individuals need to be valued for those particular qualities endemic to the services that they provide, such as empathy, communication, problem-solving. With an increasing need for long-term care, the reconciliation of employment and caring has become a salient social issue. For instance, a recent study has demonstrated that provision of paid services to people cared for by working carers, sometimes known as replacement care, would result in an increased demand for and expansion of paid home care work in England (Pickard, 2019). This is a sector characterised by poor wages and conditions (Hussein et al, 2011; House of Commons, 2017) and, by implication, a replacement care policy could lead to an expansion of poorly paid work together with its onerous characteristics, which include carer demoralisation and stress. A majority of home care providers have argued for higher hourly rates if these conditions are to change (United Kingdom Home Care Association, 2015); and it has been claimed that the average hourly rates for home care since 2015/16 have been compatible with the introduction of an Ethical Care Charter by a number of councils in England (House of Commons, 2017). The Ethical Care Charter was created in 2012 by UNISON, one of the largest trade unions in the UK, and includes the national living wage, payment for travel time, paid sick leave, no zero-hours contracts and provision for training (UNISON, 2012, 2013).

Valuing expertise means placing a social and economic value on the skills, knowledge and technical expertise acquired over time by a professional group engaged in a specified activity. In the context of current demographic changes, empirical researchers have presented a strengthened economic case for public investment in social care services for older and disabled people cared for by working carers (Kroger and Yeandle, 2013; Burchardt et al, 2015; Edmiston et al, 2017; Brimblecombe et al, 2017, 2018; Pickard, 2019). There would appear to be little appreciation of the economic cost to societies of over-reliance on informal care givers. Governments, statutory agencies and executives should not only privilege those individuals who 'create wealth' through whatever means in order to benefit a small number of people, but also those who, as part of a larger human services workforce, help to build a more civilised society. As many professionals adapt to taking on more entrepreneurial roles, they continue to engage with the demands of a fluctuating social policy agenda by transferring their skills to other areas, influenced by opportunities created from new technologies.

Professions do not exist in monolithic form; they are not uniform and there are disparities dividing them, for example in terms of their social status, power and command over resources. Such differences that exist among professions have throughout this discussion only been touched upon, specifically the extent to which the neo-liberalist ideology and austerity may have impacted and widened these differences, for example by enabling entrepreneurship and by foreshadowing a greater or lesser professionalisation. Professionals and non-professionals assign different status to the sub-specialties of the various professions. This follows from their different bases for prestige assignment. Intra-professional status rests on the exclusion of non-professional issues or of professional issues irrelevant in a particular case (Abbott, 1988). For example, a recent research study has shown that privately educated graduates are a third more likely to enter into high-status occupations than state-educated graduates from similarly affluent families and neighbourhoods, largely owing to differences in educational attainment and university selection (Macmillan et al, 2015). A perspective for analysing differences among professions was presented by Klegon (1978), where the argument was that 'the ability to obtain and maintain professional status is closely related to concrete occupational strategies and to wider social forces and arrangements of power' (pp 371–2). Such a perspective leads to a consideration of the social meaning of occupational tasks, the resources behind the emergence and continuation of professionalism, and the social consequences of professionalism. For example, the UK may employ a huge social care workforce but the status of workers as a group is fragmented and they have limited resources to organise and obtain proper employment rights.

The UK political establishment remains entrenched in its willingness to protect and grant, and occasionally abuse, unlimited funds for diverse parliamentary activities as a price for sustaining the workings of its constitutional framework. A more expensive concept of government as provider is the social welfare state: government can cushion the inability of citizens to provide for themselves, particularly in the vulnerable conditions of youth, old age, sickness, disability and unemployment due to economic forces beyond their control. At its best, however, it is providing an infrastructure of care to enable citizens to flourish socially and economically in the same way that an infrastructure of competition does (Slaughter, 2017). The argument becomes one of prioritising protection of the workings of sacrosanct agencies over valuing more contentious human rights legislation. According to Hannum (2016), this tendency has been evidenced by the conflation of human rights with individual criminal responsibility, by a marginalisation of the role of government and by failure to appreciate the inherent flexibility of human rights norms. An outcome is that social progress can only be achieved by appealing to law, politics and morality, not by promoting human rights as a panacea that can remedy all wrongs (Hannum, 2016).

A virtue of professionalism, which embodies a public interest legitimacy, is that of adaptation, a demonstration of a learned ability to displace and transfer one's skills within a changing work environment. Has de-professionalism negatively affected the quality of a service's 'outputs'? Returning to the previous example of university teaching, this may involve a preoccupation with doing things that will increase the exchange value of academic labour in terms of the resources that flow, directly or indirectly, from a strong performance on the measures of research output and teaching quality. Included here is the idea of paying deference to the notion that universities with the best qualified staff will have more to offer to their students. Professions have needed to offer an implicit approval, within the managerialist model, that the services they deliver might be measured and evaluated in terms of the potential outcomes that they have been designed to achieve, taking student performance rates as one contributor to this profile. Professional regulation in the public interest has undoubtedly become a high-profile topic in the social sciences internationally and been an increasing priority for governments across the globe, in the developed and developing world (Chamberlain, 2018).

How do professions deal with performance problems, for example wrongly prescribing drugs, sexual misconduct, failure to teach or lead effectively, or maintaining correct boundaries? Challenging the abuse of power by professionals has become an issue of erosion of trust, closely tied to the failure of both the regulatory agencies and the professional associations to uphold their mandates. These regulatory failures have been clearly exemplified by the expansion of the for-profit private provision of health, education, social care and criminal justice services; and the general failures in implementing and enforcing existing regulations. Hidden by ineffective management response and inadequate self-regulation, such failings have often become a serious governance issue. The extensive evidence taken from an increase in the number of CQC or Ofsted inquiries over recent years serves as a reminder.

Bringing service users into the matrix contributes to an extension of knowledge and, for example, confronts biomedical knowledge with new perspectives of lay knowledge. Titles and qualifications, which formerly gave access to market power and state protection, no longer guarantee these privileges. Against the backdrop of marketisation, there is an increasing need for reliable data to allow for informed decisions and to improve the safety of consumers, patients, students and the public at large. This offers opportunities and challenges as it creates an arena of competition where there are winners and losers. Changes in the building of trust confirm that nowadays the effectiveness and efficiency of the formalised expert system have to be justified using tools borrowed from management, and the knowledge of practitioners needs the proof of a scientific community emboldened by its own bureaucracy.

De-professionalism and identity – a research agenda?

There is a pressing need for an empirical research agenda to deliver evidence in the field of professionalism and public services. The aim would be to offer insights into professional identity, where subjects would be asked to define the distinctive characteristics of their work, and what they think makes them a professional and their field a profession. Whether they choose to focus on autonomy, subject specialisation or leadership, participants would be asked what frustrates them about their work when they feel that their professionalism is being undermined. The results would be constructive in building a picture of what drives professionals and helps sustain their goals in the current era. Subjects might also be asked about the changes they have seen in their profession over recent years and how they describe the outputs or outcomes of their work. Probing may help to clarify their meanings, so it becomes possible to translate their responses into theoretical concepts.

Professional identity is an aspect of social identity that develops in professional personnel as a result of their work activities. Factors such as professional competence, professional development, professional ethics and professional specialisation can contribute to this identity, along with role perception and self-concept. Webb and colleagues have drawn attention to 'emergent areas for research and possible future directions for a concentrated study of professional identity' (Webb 2017: 236) particularly as this relates to the social work profession. The contention here is that professional identity is 'interiorized and structured for practitioners by wider contexts' (Webb, 2017: 236), with recognition made of the influence of workplace values, professional associations and government austerity measures. The impact of multidisciplinary working on professional identity comprises an understanding of intra-professional group differences, especially as this relates to topical issues, mapping out discourses or discursive practices. In the light of cumulative evidence presented in preceding chapters, it may be helpful to couch research aims in terms of formal hypotheses:

1. That reversing the culture of neo-liberalism, austerity and managerialism will lead to improvements in recruitment and retention.
2. That changes to the work environment – reducing individual workload, addressing low pay, improving safeguarding and providing mentoring/supervision – will lead to improvements in workforce morale.
3. That incentivising public sector workers to enhance their specialist knowledge will contribute to an improvement in service outputs, as defined within each sector.

4. That deepening the multidisciplinary work experience of individual staff members will act as a progressive force in enhancing their professional identity.

Research questions include:

- How does one develop a professional identity, for example through group experiential learning (Falgares et al, 2017) or by working with para-professionals with short-term goal-directed counselling (Gazzola et al, 2011)?
- How have perceptions of professional practice changed and how has multidisciplinary work helped reshape a profession's role (Baldwin, 2012; Machin et al, 2012; Department of Health and Social Care, 2018)?
- Transitioning from student to professional – how far has a Higher Education Institution 'owned' the notion of professional identity and carried this forward from an educational setting into practice by creating authentic learning experiences (Mylrea et al, 2019)?
- How far has work experience, based on acquired values, helped to develop professional identity (Wood et al, 2015; Metz, 2017)?
- How has increased workload and uncompetitive pay impacted on identity, and how has identity been challenged by technology, limiting parts of a professional's role (Larsson et al, 2009; RCM, 2017)?
- Has professional identity thrived through creation of one's own culture through self-development (Einion, 2016)?
- Has having an ethical code helped shape a profession's identity by deriving values and methods to cultivate such values (Madison, 2017)?
- How has professionalisation altered not only professionals in training but also the 'fundamental machinery of identity construction – constitutive roles, narratives, normative commitment' (Bliss, 2016: 6)?
- Has professional identity been shaped by translating and unpacking the goals of a service, for example security or rehabilitation (Bruhn et al, 2010; Pidd, 2019)?
- Has professionalisation and acquiring identity become confused and conflicted through a perceived dissonance in values and through extreme work pressures (Schaible, 2018)?

Finally, research might usefully gather evidence about trust relations among different parties. There is a clear argument for a comprehensive study that explores the salience and nature of trust relations in the organisation and practice of running a public service, and what shapes these relationships. It would include investigation of the relationship between the state regulatory institutions (examples being Ofsted, Care Quality Commission, Monitor, NHS Improvement) and those regulated; between financing agencies, provider organisations in the public and private sectors, and professionals; and between provider organisations in the public and private sectors, and professionals.

References

5RB (2018) 'Foster carer settles anonymous letter claim', 21 June, www.5rb.com/news/foster-carer-settles-anonymous-letter-claim/

Abbott, A. (1988) *The System of the Professions: An Essay on the Division of Expert Behaviour*, London: University of Chicago Press.

Abbott, A. (1991) 'The order of professionalisation: an empirical analysis', *Work and Occupations*, 18: 355–84.

Abbott, P. and Sapsford, R. (1990) 'Health visiting: policing the family', in P. Abbott and C. Wallace (eds) *The Sociology of the Caring Professions*, London: Falmer Press, pp. 50–66.

Academy of Medical Royal Colleges (2019) 'Policies and activities statement of purpose: education, training, Brexit'. Available at: www. aomrc.org.uk (accessed 4 October 2019).

Adams, R. (2017) 'Thousands of schools in England face big budget cuts, unions warn', *The Guardian*, 4 January.

Adams, R. (2018a) 'Grammar schools given £50million to admit disadvantaged pupils', *The Guardian*, 11 May.

Adams, R. (2018b) 'Ministers accused of using inaccurate data to defend schools funding', *The Guardian*, 5 October.

Adams, R. (2018c) 'Struggling UK universities warn staff of possible job cuts', *The Guardian*, 11 December.

Adams, R. (2019) 'Universities hit back after report proposing funding cuts', *The Guardian*, 30 May.

ADASS (2016) 'Making safeguarding personal: temperature check 2016', Association of Directors of Adult Social Services. Available at: https://www.adass.org.uk/making-safeguarding-personal-temperature-check-2016 (accessed 4 October 2019).

Adcroft, A. and Willis, R. (2006) 'Postmodernism, de-professionalisation and commodification (the outcomes of performance measurement in higher education)', *Journal of Finance and Management in Public Services*, 6(1): 43–60.

Adu, A. (2018) 'Sick and pay: Care company branded "obscene" after fining staff £50 for calling in ill', *The Sun*, 23 December.

Age UK (Ben Franklin) (2016) *The End of Formal Adult Social Care?* London: Age UK.

Aldred, J. (2019) *Licence to Be Bad: How Economics Corrupted Us*, London: Penguin Books/Allen Lane.

Allan, C. (2017) 'We need to address the mental health crisis, not more empty words', Opinion Mental Health, *The Guardian*, 30 August.

Allen, K. (2017) 'In just 28 hours, top bosses are paid more than a typical salary', *The Guardian*, 4 January.

Alvesson, M. (2013) *Understanding Organisational Culture* (2nd edn), London: Sage.

Anandaciva, S., Jabbal, J., Maguire, D., Wood, D. and Gilburt, H. (2018) 'How is the NHS performing?' The King's Fund Centre, Quarterly Monitoring Report, 21 December.

Andalo, D. (2019) 'New to the game: changing roles in mental health', The Guardian [online] 15 May, Available at: www.theguardian.com/society/mental-health (accessed May 2019).

Anderson, E. (2014) 'John Lewis wrong on workforce comments, government says', *Daily Telegraph*, 12 November.

Anderson, S. (2019) 'Employment rights for foster carers are essential to give children stability', *The Guardian*, 13 February.

Anning, A. and Edwards, A. (1999) *Promoting Children's Learning from Birth to Five: Developing the New Early Years Professional*, Buckingham: Open University Press.

Antonakis, J. (2011) 'Predictors of leadership: the usual suspects and the suspect traits', in A. Bryman, D. Collinson, K. Grint, B. Jackson and M. Uhl-Bien (eds) *The Sage Handbook of Leadership*, London: Sage, pp. 269–85.

Arblaster, A. (1985) *The Rise and Decline of Western Liberalism*, Oxford: Blackwell.

Asthana, A. (2016) 'More grammar schools would be a disaster, says social mobility tsar', *The Guardian*, 8 September.

Asthana, A. (2017) 'Maternity wards closed 400 times as shortage of beds and staff grows', *The Guardian*, 8 August.

Bagot, M. (2019) 'Tory NHS "revolution": wrong medicine', *Daily Mirror*, 8 January.

Baker, A., Epstein, G. and Montecino, J. (2018) 'The UK's finance curse? Costs and processes', Research Report, 5 October. PERI (Political Economy Research Institute), Gordon Hall, 418 North Pleasant St, Suite A, Amherst, MA, 01002.

Baldwin, S. (2012) 'Exploring the professional identity of health visitors', *Nursing Times*, 108(25): 12–15.

Ball, S. (2008) *The Education Debate*, Bristol: Policy Press.

Ball, S. and Olmedo, A. (2011) 'Global social capitalism: using enterprise to solve the problems of the world', *Citizenship, Social & Economics Education*, January.

Barber, B. (1963) 'Some problems in the sociology of the professions', *Daedalus* 92(4): 669–88.

Barham, P. (1992) *Closing the Asylum: The Mental Patient in Modern Society*, London: Penguin.

Baron-Cohen, S. (2019) 'If anything can bring healing to Israel-Palestine, it's empathy', *The Guardian*, 22 January.

Barr, H. and Ross, F. (2006) 'Mainstreaming Interprofessional Education in the UK: a position paper', *Journal of Interprofessional Care*, 20(2): 96–104.

Barry, A. and Yuill, C. (2016) *Understanding the Sociology of Health* (4th edn), London: Sage.

Barth, T. (2010) 'Crisis management in the Catholic Church: lessons for public administration', *Public Administration Review*, 70(5): 780–91.

Barton, R. (1959) *Institutional Neurosis*, Bristol: John Wright & Sons.

Batty, E., Beatty, C., Foden, M., Lawless, P., Pearson, S. and Wilson, I. (2010) *The New Deal for Communities Experience: A Final Assessment*, London: Department for Communities and Local Government.

Bauman, Z. (1998) *Work, Consumerism and the New Poor*, Milton Keynes: Open University Press.

Bawden, A. (2016) 'Foster carers vote to unionise over pay', *The Guardian*, 21 September.

BBC News (2012) 'Academies told they can hire unqualified teachers', Angela Harrison, education correspondent, 27 July.

BBC News (2014) 'John Lewis chairman: UK workforce needs a step change', 12 November. Available at: https://www.bbc.co.uk/news/uk-30019547 (accessed 4 October 2019).

BBC News (2017a) 'Public sector morale at "critical levels"', 4 July. Available at: https://www.bbc.co.uk/news/uk-40489256 (accessed 4 October 2019).

BBC News (2017b) 'Secondary school pupil numbers set for 19% rise by 2026', 14 July. Available at: https://www.bbc.co.uk/news/education-40608795 (accessed 4 October 2019).

BBC News (2018a) 'Brexit: Theresa May says it's Chequers or no deal', Panorama interview, 17 September.

BBC News (2018b) 'Budget 2018: Chancellor abolishes PFI for future projects', 29 October. Available at: https://www.bbc.co.uk/news/av/uk-politics-46023089/budget-2018-chancellor-abolishes-pfi-for-future-projects (accessed 4 October 2019).

BBC News (2018c) 'Police look at bishops' "failure to act" over sex abuse claims', 5 March. Available at: https://www.bbc.co.uk/news/uk-england-43228491 (accessed 4 October 2019).

BBC News (2018d) 'Child abuse inquiry says orphanages were places of "threat" and "abuse"', 11 October. Available at: https://www.bbc.co.uk/news/uk-scotland-45812269 (accessed 4 October 2019).

BBC News (2019) 'Poverty in the UK is "systemic" and "tragic"', says UN special rapporteur', 22 May. Available at: https://www.bbc.co.uk/news/uk-48354692 (accessed 4 October 2019).

BBC News Interview (2019) 'GPs out of hours: "Money and begging emails not filling gaps"', 24 July. Available at: https://www.bbc.co.uk/news/uk-wales-politics-49088735 (accessed 4 October 2019).

BBC Radio 4 (2016) *Today Programme*, 26 April.

BBC Radio 4 (2018) 'Inside public services. Working with dignity and respect: improving mental health services with digital stories'.

Beatty, C. and Fothergill, S. (2013) 'Hitting the poorest places hardest: the local and regional impact of welfare reform', Sheffield: SHU Centre for Regional Economics and Social Research. Available at: www.shu.ac.uk/research/crest/sites/shu.ac.uk/files/hitting-poorest-placeshardest O.pdf (accessed 4 October 2019).

Beder, S. (2000) *Selling the Work Ethic: From Puritan Pulpit to Corporate PR*, London: Zen Books.

Behr, R. (2018) 'Britain's magical thinking won't make the EU accept the impossible', Opinion Brexit, *The Guardian*, 16 October.

Béland, D. (2007) 'The social exclusion discourse: ideas and policy change', *Policy and Politics*, 35(1): 123–39.

Benbow, D. (2013) 'Professional boundaries: when does the nurse-patient relationship end?', *Journal of Nursing Regulation*, 4(2): 30–3.

Berlin, I. (1954) *Historical Inevitability*, New York: Oxford University Press.

Berlyne, J. (2016) 'The problems in Britain's education system are political in origin – and they require a political solution', Student Opinion, *The Independent*, 18 August.

Bertilsson, M. (1990) 'The welfare state, the professions and citizens', in R. Torstendahl and M. Burrage (eds) *The Formation of Professions, Knowledge, State and Strategy*, London: Sage, pp. 114–33.

Blakemore, K. and Warwick-Booth, L. (2013) *Social Policy: An Introduction* (4th edn), Maidenhead: Open University Press.

Bliss, J. (2016) 'The professional identity of lawyers', *The Practice* (Center on the Legal Profession, Harvard Law School), 2(3), March/April. Available at: https://thepractice.law.harvard.edu/article/the-professional-identity-formation-of-lawyers/ (accessed April 2019).

Blomberg, T., Brancale, J., Beaver, K. and Bales, W. (eds) (2016) *Advancing Criminology and Criminal Justice Policy*, London: Routledge.

Blyth, M. (2013) *Austerity: The History of a Dangerous Idea*, Oxford: Oxford University Press.

BMA (British Medical Association) (2016) 'End of life care and physician-assisted dying', London: BMA. Available at: www.bma. org.uk/collective-voice/policy-and-research/ethics/end-of-life-care (accessed 4 October 2019).

BMA (British Medical Association) (2018) 'Feeling the squeeze: the local impact of cuts to public health budgets in England', London: BMA. Available at: https://www.bma.org.uk/-/media/files/pdfs/ collective voice/policy (accessed 4 October 2019).

BMA (British Medical Association) (2018) 'Working in a system that is under pressure', March, London: BMA. Available at: https:// www.bma.org.uk/collective-voice/influence/key-negotiations/nhs-pressures/working-in-a-system-under-pressure (accessed 4 October 2019).

Boas, T. and Gans-Morse, J. (2009) 'Neo-liberalism: from new liberal philosophy to anti-liberal slogan', *Studies in Comparative International Development*, 44(2): 137–61.

Bodkin, H. (2019) 'Ten Whorlton Hall staff arrested on suspicion of physical and psychological abuse', *Daily Telegraph*, 24 May.

Boffey, D. (2011) 'Public sector workers need discipline and fear, says Oliver Letwin', *The Observer*, 30 July.

Boffey, D. (2014) 'The care workers left behind as private equity targets NHS', *The Observer*, 10 August.

Boffey, D. (2015) 'Schools must share teaching staff if they are to survive, head teachers' leader calls for a united solution to recruitment crisis', *The Observer*, 3 May.

Bonoli, G. and Natali, D. (eds) (2012) *The Politics of the New Welfare State*, Oxford: Oxford University Press.

Booth, R. (2018a) 'UK must act on poverty now, expert tells Rudd', *The Guardian*, 21 November.

Booth, R. (2018b) 'UN expert considers branding benefits regime "inhuman"', *The Guardian*, 16 November.

Borland, S. (2019) 'NHS goes to war on cigarettes and alcohol', *Daily Mail*, 5 January.

Borland, S., Payne, T. and Dilworth, M. (2018) 'Midwives in baby deaths probe were praised by experts', *Daily Mail*, 1 September.

Boseley, S. (2018) 'Gosport doctor breaks silence over hospital deaths blaming NHS resources', *The Guardian*, 28 June.

Boseley, S. and Weaver, M. (2016) 'Junior doctors' row: BMA announces three more five-day strikes', *The Guardian*, 1 September.

Bottery, S., Ward, D. and Fenney, D. (2018) 'Adult social care – our work on social care policy, services and reform', Social Care 360, 16 May, London: King's Fund Centre.

Bounds, A. (2019) 'How struggling towns are starting to shape UK politics', *Financial Times*, 18 April.

Bourdieu, P. (1984) *Distinction: A Critique of the Social Judgement of Taste*, London: Routledge.

Bourne, T., Wynants, L., Peters, M., Van Audenhove, C., Timmerman, D., Van Calster, B. and Jalmbrant, M. (2015) 'The impact of complaints procedures on the welfare, health and clinical practice of 7926 doctors in the UK: a cross-sectional survey', *British Medical Journal/Journal of Neuro Interventional Surgery*, 5(1): 1–12.

Bowcott, O. and Duncan, P. (2019) 'Half of all magistrates courts axed since 2010', *The Guardian*, 28 January.

Bowling, A. (1995) *Measuring Disease*, Buckingham: Open University Press.

Boyle, D., Coote, A., Sherwood, C. and Slay, J. (2010) *Right Here, Right Now: Taking Co-Production into the Mainstream*, discussion paper, London: NESTA. Available at: https://www.nesta.org.uk/report/co-production-right-here-right-now (accessed 4 October 2019).

Bradley, K. (2009) 'The Bradley Report: Lord Bradley's review of people with mental health problems or learning disabilities in the criminal justice system', London: Department of Health.

Braverman, H. (1974) *Labour and Monopoly Capital: The Degradation of Work in the 20th Century*, New York: Monthly Review Press.

Brennan, J. (2016) *Against Democracy*, Princeton, NJ: Princeton University Press

Brignall, M. (2016) 'Huge differences in youth unemployment across UK', *The Guardian*, 15 May.

Brimblecombe, N., Pickard, L., King, D. and Knapp, M. (2017) 'Perceptions of unmet needs for services in England: a comparison of working carers and the people they care for', *Health and Social Care in the Community*, 25(2): 435–46.

Brimblecombe, N., Pickard, L., King, D. and Knapp, M. (2018) 'Barriers to receipt of social care services for working carers and the people they care for in times of austerity', *Journal of Social Policy*, 47(2): 215–33.

Brind, R., McGinigal, S., Lewis, J., and Ghezelayagh, S. (2014) 'Childcare and early years providers survey 2013', TNS BMRB Report JN 117328, London: DfE.

Brind, R., Norden, O. and Oseman, D. (2012) 'Childcare provider finances survey', DfE-RR213, London: DfE.

Brindle, D. (2015) 'Fears of benefit cap for older people if councils take charge', *The Guardian*, 17 December.

Brindle, D. (2019) 'Interview: Julie Ogley "we need a proper, meaty dialogue about funding"', *The Guardian*, 3 July.

Briner, R. (2015) 'Universities are mismanaging performance', *Times Higher Education Supplement*, 7 May.

Bröckling, U. (2016) *The Entrepreneurial Self: Fabricating a New Type of Subject*, London: Sage.

Brown, R., Barber, P. and Martin, D. (2015) *The Mental Capacity Act 2005: A Guide for Practice* (3rd edn), London: Sage.

Bruhn, A., Nylander, P. and Lindberg, O. (2010) 'The prison officer's dilemma: professional representations among Swedish prison officers', *Les Dossiers des Sciences de L'Education*, 23(1): 77–93.

Bryman, A. (1992) *Charisma and Leadership in Organisations*, London: Sage.

Buchan, I., Kontopantelis, E., Sperrin, M., Chandola, T. and Doran, T. (2017) 'North–south disparities in English mortality 1965–2015: longitudinal population study', *Journal of Epidemiology & Community Health*, 71(9): 928–36.

Bullogh, O. (2018) 'The finance curse: how global finance is making us all poorer – review', Economics Book Reviews, *The Guardian*, 23 October.

Burchardt, T., Obolenskaya, P. and Vizard, P. (2015) *The Coalition's Record on Adult Social Care: Policy, Spending and Outcomes 2010–2015*, London: CASE.

Burrows, R. and Loader, B. (eds) (1994) *Towards a Post-Fordist Welfare State?*, London: Routledge.

Burton, M. (2016) *The Politics of Austerity: A Recent History*, London: Palgrave Macmillan.

Buse, K., Mays, N. and Walt, G. (2005) *Making Health Policy* (2nd edn), Maidenhead: Open University Press.

Butler, I. and Drakeford, M. (2005) *Scandal, Social Policy and Social Welfare*, Bristol: Policy Press.

Butler, P. (2016) 'Ministers ignored repeated warnings on Kids Company', *The Guardian*, 21 February.

Butler, P. (2018a) 'Bankrupt council "should be scrapped"', *The Guardian*, 10 March.

Butler, P. (2018b) 'Cuts plunge children's services in England into crisis, charities warn', *The Guardian*, 10 November.

Butler, P (2018c) 'Homelessness rates "more than double the official estimate"', *The Guardian*, 14 December.

Butler, P. (2019a) 'Councils warn of fresh cuts in fight to avoid bankruptcy', *The Guardian* 2 July.

Butler, P. (2019b) 'Poorest hit hardest as councils forced to close Sure Start children's centres', *The Guardian*, 17 June.

Butler, P. (2019c) Social services accused of failing toddlers murdered in their homes', *The Guardian*, 6 June.

Butler, P (2019d) 'The care crisis: cuts, chaos and children', *The Guardian*, 6 June.

Butler, P. (2019e) 'Sure Start numbers plummet as cuts hit children's services', *The Guardian*, 16 June.

Butterfield, H. (1931) *The Whig Interpretation of History*, London: G. Bell & Sons.

Butterfield, H. (1944) *The Englishman and His History*, London: G. Bell & Sons.

Cahill, D. and Wilkinson, P. (2017) 'Child sexual abuse in the Catholic Church: an interpretative review of the literature and public inquiry reports', August, Centre for Global Research, RMIT University, Melbourne.

Callender, C. (2012) 'Lifelong learning and training', in P. Alcock, M. May and S. Wright (eds) *The Student's Companion to Social Policy* (4th edn), Oxford: Wiley-Blackwell, pp. 345–51.

Cambridge, P. (1999) 'The first hit: a case-study of the physical abuse of people with learning disabilities and challenging behaviour in a residential setting', *Disability and Society*, 14(3): 285–308.

Cameron, H. (2000) 'Colleagues or clients? The relationship between clergy and church members', in N. Malin (ed.) *Professionalism, Boundaries and the Workplace*, London: Routledge, pp. 106–20.

Campbell, D. (2015a) 'Prestigious Hospital in Special Measures Over Staff Shortage: CQC Says Safety Being Put at Risk at Addenbrooke's', *The Guardian*, 22 September.

Campbell, D. (2015b) 'Rationing in NHS hitting patient care, say doctors', *The Guardian*, 9 December.

Campbell, D. (2015c) 'Seven day NHS pledge doomed to fail, warns doctors' chief', *The Guardian*, 14 October.

Campbell, D. (2015d) 'Social care cuts leave 1 million pensioners struggling', *The Guardian*, 21 October.

Campbell, D. (2016a) 'Number of mental health nurses falls 10%', *The Guardian*, 25 January.

Campbell, D. (2016b) 'Junior doctors may follow April strikes with indefinite walkout', *The Guardian*, 21 April.

Campbell, D. (2016c) 'NHS chief says junior doctors walkouts may put seriously ill at risk', *The Guardian*, 8 September.

Campbell, D. (2017a) 'Biggest headache for NHS boss is own plan', *The Guardian*, 1 February.

Campbell, D. (2017b) 'Head Of top NHS trust quits over cash squeeze', *The Guardian*, 11 December.

Campbell, D. (2017c) 'Junior doctor Nadia Masood: Hunt's driven a lot of us out of the NHS', *The Guardian*, 2 January.

Campbell, D. (2017d) '"Lack of staff" causes 80% of full-term stillbirths', *The Guardian*, 28 November.

Campbell, D. (2017e) 'Patients put at risk from drugs and tests "they do not need"', *The Guardian*, 22 October.

Campbell, D. (2017f) 'Rogue doctors use superhero status to abuse patients', *The Observer*, 26 August.

Campbell, D. (2017g) 'Soaring NHS vacancies prompt warnings of "desperate" understaffing', *The Guardian*, 25 July.

Campbell, D. (2017h) 'Waiting list for NHS hospital care hits a 10-year high of four million', *The Guardian*, 11 August.

Campbell, D. (2018a) 'Fears over standards of care as more patients re-admitted to hospital', *The Guardian*, 1 June.

Campbell, D. (2018b) 'Figures reveal rise in sexual assaults on ambulance staff', *The Guardian*, 23 April.

Campbell, D. (2018c) 'Limits on non-EU doctors to be relaxed to plug NHS gaps', *The Guardian*, 30 November.

Campbell, D. (2018d) 'May must be bold to fix social care, says regulator', *The Guardian*, 3 July.

Campbell, D. (2018e) 'More than 200 suicides recorded at mental health units over seven years', *The Guardian*, 14 August.

Campbell, D. (2018f) 'More women than men take their own lives in mental health units', *The Guardian*, 14 August.

Campbell, D. (2018g) 'NHS trust at centre of baby deaths inquiry deemed unsafe – Shrewsbury and Telford Hospitals A&E and maternity care is inadequate – Regulator', *The Guardian*, 29 November.

Campbell, D. (2018h) 'Scores of "ghost wards" in hospitals due to NHS crisis', *The Guardian*, 13 April.

Campbell, D. (2019a) 'NHS care failures leave children with autism in danger of suicide', *The Guardian*, 17 June.

Campbell, D. (2019b) 'NHS chiefs accused of breaking law over scanner contract', *The Guardian*, 27 May.

Campbell, D. (2019c) 'Operations cancelled in standoff with consultants', *The Guardian*, 8 July.

Campbell, D. (2019d) 'Time to curb privatisation of care, NHS chiefs tell PM', *The Guardian*, 8 January.

Campbell, D. and Johnson, S. (2016) 'Hunt's cuts force NHS watchdog to reduce inspections: hospitals and care homes to undergo less scrutiny', *The Guardian*, 24 May.

Campbell, D. and Siddique, H. (2016) 'Junior doctors strike for first time in 40 years as last-ditch talks end in deadlock: poll findings reveal 66% public support for action', *The Guardian*, 12 January.

Campbell, D. and Stewart, H. (2018) 'Labour: calls to relax visa rules for NHS staff', *The Guardian*, 10 September.

Campbell, D., Walker, P., Mason, R. and Weaver, M (2018) 'Hospital bosses tell Jeremy Hunt to spend now to rescue NHS', *The Guardian*, 11 January.

Campling, J. and Payne, M. (2000) *Teamwork in Multi-Professional Care*, Basingstoke: Macmillan International Higher Education, Red Globe Press.

Carchedi, G. (1975) 'On the economic identification of the new middle class', *Economy and Society*, 4(1): 1–86.

Care Act (2014) London: The Stationery Office.

Care Home Professional (2019) 'Former CQC head, Sir David Behan, joins HC-One', Lee Peart, 18 January. Available at: https://www.carehomeprofessional.com/former-cqc-head-sir-david-behan-joins-hc-one/ (accessed 4 October 2019).

Care Standards Act (2000) London: The Stationery Office.

Carers UK (2017) *Overview of the UK Population*, Office for National Statistics. Available at: https://www.ons.gov.uk/peoplepopulation andcommunity/populationandmigration/populationestimates/articles/overviewoftheukpopulation/november2018 (accessed 4 October 2019).

Carpenter, J. and Dickinson, H. (2008) *Interprofessional Education and Training*, Bristol: Policy Press.

Carr, E.H. (1964) *What is History?*, Harmondsworth: Penguin.

Carrell, S. and McEnaney, J. (2018) 'Teach First briefed heads at Prince Charles event in Scotland', *The Guardian*, 27 March.

Casey, L. (2014) 'The National Troubled Families Programme', *Social Work & Social Sciences Review*, 17(2): 57–62.

Center for Constitutional Rights on Behalf of the Survivors Network of Those Abused by Priests (2013) *Fighting for the Future: Adult Survivors Work to Protect Children and End the Culture of Clergy Sexual Abuse: An NGO Report*, New York: Center for Constitutional Rights.

Cerny, P. (1997) 'Paradoxes of the competition state: dynamics of political globalisation', *Government and Opposition*, 32(2): 251–74.

Cervero-Liceras, F., McKee, M. and Legido-Quigley, H. (2015) 'The effects of the financial crisis and austerity measures on the Spanish health care system: a qualitative analysis of health professionals' perspectives in the region of Valencia', *Health Policy*, 119(1), January, 100–6 (https//doi.org/10.1016/j.healthpol.2014.11.003).

Chakelian, A. (2019) '14 damning findings by the UN inspector who investigated UK poverty', *New Statesman*, 22 May.

Chakrabortty, A. (2016) 'We're watching the death of neoliberalism – from within', *The Guardian*, 14 March.

Chakrabortty, A. (2017) 'Haringey taken over by Momentum? It's just locals taking back control', *The Guardian*, 12 December.

Chakrabortty, A. (2018a) 'In boardrooms, Brexit is already here. And the warning is stark', *The Guardian*, 10 October.

Chakrabortty, A. (2018b) 'It took a UN envoy to hear how austerity is destroying lives', *The Guardian*, 14 November.

Chamberlain, J. (2018) Introduction: 'Professional health regulation in the public interest', in J. Chamberlain, M. Dent and M. Saks (eds) *Professional Health Regulation in the Public Interest: International Perspectives*, Bristol: Policy Press, pp. 1–16.

Charlesworth, A. (2018) 'Response to the Autumn Budget 2018 – day to day spending on the wider health budget will fall by £1bn in real terms next year', 30 October, the Health Foundation.

Charlesworth, A. and Thorlby, R. (2012) *Reforming Social Care: Options for Funding*, London: Nuffield Foundation.

CIPD (Chartered Institute for Personnel Development) (2018a) 'Why is no one exposing our failing firms in advance? Hidden figures: research shows important people data is missing from corporate reports', 22 February.

CIPD (Chartered Institute of Personnel Development) (2018b) 'Workforce planning practice. Guide', May. Available at: https://www.employment-studies.co.uk/resource/workforce-planning-practice (accessed 4 October 2019).

CPAG (Child Poverty Action Group) (2017) *The Austerity Generation: The Impact of a Decade of Cuts on Family Incomes and Child Poverty*, London: CPAG. Available at: https://cpag.org.uk/policy-and-campaigns/report/austerity-generation-impact-decade-cuts-family-incomes-and-child-poverty (accessed 4 October 2019).

Children's Commissioner (2019) Report: 'Who Are They? Where Are They? Children Locked Up', 16 May. Available at: https://www.childrenscommissioner.gov.uk/publication/who-are-they-where-are-they/ (accessed 4 October 2019).

Church of England (2017) 'Elliott Review: one year progress report', 31 March. Available at: www.churchofengland.org/media-centre/news/2016/03/elliott-review-findings.aspx.

Clarke, J. and Newman, J. (1997) *The Managerial State: Power, Politics and Ideology in the Remaking of Social Welfare*, London: Sage.

Clarke, R. (2016) 'These leaks show Hunt's deception on the seven-day NHS', *The Guardian*, 23 August.

Clay, F. (2016) 'We have to convert the pressure and frustration to a sense of possibility: NHS boss calls for new deal to care for the old', *The Guardian*, 19 January.

Clough, R. (2018) 'Rage against the cruelty of so-called austerity and public sector cuts', *The Guardian* [online] 15 November. Available at: gu.com/letters.

Cole, W. (2019) 'More than 300 "overworked" NHS nurses have taken their own lives in last 7 years, sparking calls for government inquiry into shocking toll', *Mail Online*, 28 April. Available at: https://www.dailymail.co.uk/news/article-6969149/More-300-overworked-NHS-nurses-taken-lives-seven-years.html (accessed 4 October 2019).

Colton, M. (2002) 'Factors associated with abuse in residential child care institutions', *Children & Society*, 16(1): 33–44.

Commission on Growth and Development (2008) The Growth Report: Strategies for Sustained Growth and Inclusive Development. The International Bank for Reconstruction and Development/the World Bank. Available at: http://documents.worldbank.org/curated/en/120981468138262912/The-growth-report-strategies-for-sustained-growth-and-inclusive-development (accessed 4 October 2019).

Committee on Standards in Public Life (1995) First Report of the Committee on Standards in Public Life: guidance on the seven principles of public life. Available at: https://www.gov.uk/government/publications/the-7-principles-of-public-lifem (accessed 4 October 2019).

Commons Select Committee (2018) 'Sexual harassment at work: government responds to committee report', 18 December. Available at: https://www.parliament.uk/business/committees/committees-a-z/commons-select/women-and-equalities-committee/news-parliament-2017/sexual-harassment-workplace-government-response-17-19/m (accessed 4 October 2019).

Commons Select Committee (2018a) 'Five-point plan to tackle sexual harassment in the workplace', 25 July. Available at: https://www.parliament.uk/business/committees/committees-a-z/commons-select/women-and-equalities-committee/news-parliament-2017/sexual-harassment-workplace-report-published-17-19/ (accessed 4 October 2019).

Connolly, K. and Boffey, D. (2018) 'Merkel says Germany making contingency plans for no-deal Brexit', *The Guardian*, 17 October.

Cooper, R. and Law, J. (1995) 'Organisation: distal and proximal views', in Bacarach, S., Gagliardi, P. and Mundell, B. (eds), *Studies of Organizations in the European Tradition*, London: JAI Press, pp. 237–74.

Cooper, V. and Whyte, D. (eds) (2017) *The Violence of Austerity*, London: Pluto Press.

Coram Voice (2019) 'Coram Voice responds to the Children's Commissioner's report on "Children Locked Up by the State"', 16 May.

Corbett, D. (1991) *Public Sector Management*, Sydney: Allen and Unwin.

Corbett, S. and Walker, A. (2019) 'Between neoliberalism and nationalist populism: what role for the 'European social model' and social quality in post-Brexit Europe?', *Social Policy and Society*, 18(1): 93–106.

Coughlan, S. (2016) 'Academy rejects call for parent governors', BBC News Education Correspondent, 15 September.

Coward, R. (2011) 'Southern Cross wakes us up to the business of caring', *The Guardian*, 11 July.

CQC (Care Quality Commission) (2015a) 'Addenbrookes and the Rosie hospitals quality report', 21 April. Available at: https://www.cqc.org.uk/sites/default/files/new_reports/AAADO111.pdf (accessed 4 October 2019).

CQC (Care Quality Commission) (2015b) 'Annual report 2014/15', 21 July. Available at: www.cqc.org.uk/content/annual-report-201415.pdf (accessed 4 October 2019).

CQC (Care Quality Commission) (2016a) 'Brighton and Sussex University Hospitals NHS Trust. CQC', 17 August. Available at: www.cqc.org.uk/provider/RXH (accessed 4 October 2019).

CQC (Care Quality Commission) (2016b) 'CQC tells Brighton and Sussex University Hospitals NHS Trust to improve services', 14 July. Available at: www.cqc.org.uk/cqc-tells-brighton-and-sussex-universityhospitals-nhs-trust-improve-services (accessed 4 October 2019).

CQC (Care Quality Commission) (2016c) 'Shaping the future: consultation document', 1 January, (www.cqc.org.uk/files/20160119/strategyconsultation/final_web.pdf).

CQC (Care Quality Commission) (2017) 'The state of care in mental health services 2014 to 2017', CQC-380-072017.

CQC (Care Quality Commission) (2018a) 'Chief Inspector of Hospitals recommends Norfolk and Suffolk NHS Foundation Trust remains in special measures', press release,28 November.

CQC (Care Quality Commission) (2018b) 'Norfolk and Suffolk NHS Foundation Trust: Hellesdon Hospital, Norwich, Norfolk NR65BE, PDf inspection report', 28 November.

CQC (Care Quality Commission) (2018c) 'Opening the door to change. NHS safety culture and the need for transformation', December.

CQC (Care Quality Commission) (2018d) 'Sexual safety on mental health wards', September.

CQC (Care Quality Commission) (2018e) *The State of Health Care and Adult Social Care in England 2017/18*, House of Commons, 10 October, Newcastle: CQC.

CQC (Care Quality Commission) (2019) *The State of Health Care and Adult Social Care in England 2018/19*, Newcastle: CQC.

Croft, J. (2018) 'One million fewer legal aid claims per annum: cost burden has shifted to social services', *Financial Times*, 3 August.

Croisdale-Appleby, D. (2014) *Re-visioning Social Work Education: An Independent Review*, London: DfE.

Cronquist, R. (2011) 'Nurses and social media: regulatory concerns and guidelines', *Journal of Nursing Regulation*, 2(3), October: 37–40.

Crossley, S. and Lambert, M. (2017) Introduction: '"Looking for trouble?" Critically examining the UK government's Troubled Families Programme', *Social Policy and Society*, 16(1): 81–5.

Culverhouse, B. (2016) 'Teachers are deserting the UK in droves. Excellent work, Michael Wilshaw', *The Guardian*, 29 February.

Dale-Davidson, D. and Rees-Mogg, W. (updated edition, 2012) *The Sovereign Individual: Mastering the Transition to the Information Age*, London: Simon & Schuster.

Daly, M. (2015) 'Parenting support as policy field: an analytic framework', *Social Policy and Society*, 14(4): 597–608.

Daly, M. (2019) 'The implications of the departure of the UK For EU social policy', *Social Policy and Society*, 18(1): 107–17.

Daly, M. and Bray, R. (2015) 'Parenting support in England: the bedding down of a new policy', *Social Policy and Society*, 14(4): 633–64.

Dasgupta, P. (1990) 'Trust as a Commodity', in D. Gambetta (ed.), *Trust: Making and Breaking Cooperative Relations* (revised edn), Oxford: Blackwell, pp. 49–72.

Dasgupta, R. (2018) 'The demise of the nation state', *The Guardian*, 5 April.

Davies, R. (2018) 'Four Seasons Health Care rescue talks suffer setback', *The Guardian*, 11 January, p. 23.

Davies, W. (2017) *The Limits of Neo-Liberalism: Authority, Sovereignty and The Logic of Competition* (revised edn), London: Sage.

Davis, M. (1980) 'A multidimensional approach to individual differences in empathy', *JSAS Catalog of Selected Documents in Psychology*, 10: 85.

DCLG (Department of Communities and Local Government) (2012) *Working with Troubled Families*, London: DCLG.

DCLG (Department of Communities and Local Government) (2013) 'Troubled families programme', Available at: www.gov.uk/government/uploads/system/uploads/attachment_data/file/336430/understanding-Troubled-Families-web_format.pdf

Deacon, B. (2007) *Global Social Policy and Governance*, London: Sage.

Dearing Report (1997) *The National Committee of Inquiry into Higher Education: Report of the Committee*, London: HMSO.

Delamotte, E. (2016) 'De La Professionalisation a L'industrialisation' [From Professionalisation to Industrialisation], in Pierre Moeglin (ed.), *L'industrialisation de la formation. État de la question*, Centre de National de Documentation Pedagogique, pp. 75–92. Actes et Rapports pour L'education 2-240-0060-4. Available at: http://hal.archives-ouvertes.fr/hal-01387562 (accessed 7 October 2019).

Demailly, L. (2003) 'L'evaluation de l'action educative comme apprentissage et negociation', *Revue Francoise de Pedagogie*, 142(1): 115–29.

Demailly, L. and De La Broise, P. (2009) 'Les enjeux de la de-professionalisation: Etudes de cas et pistes de travail', *Socio-Logos, Revue de L'association francaise de Sociologie*, 4, 7 May, Available at: http://socio-logos.revues-org/2305 (accessed 7 October 2019).

Demello, S. and Furseth, P. (2016) *Innovation and Culture in Public Services: The Case of Independent Living*, Cheltenham: Edward Elgar.

Department for Communities and Local Government (2012) 'Regeneration to Enable Growth: A Toolkit Supporting Community-led Regeneration', January. Available at: https://assets.publishing.service.gov.uk/government/uploads/system/uploads/attachment_data/file/5983/2064899.pdf (accessed 4 October 2019).

DEFRA (Department for Environment, Food and Rural Affairs) (2013) 'Rural proofing guidance. UK government', 16 May.

Derrida, J. (1978) *Writing and Difference*. Chicago: University of Chicago Press.

Deverell, K. and Sharma, U. (2000) 'Professionalism in everyday practice: issues of trust, experience and boundaries', in N. Malin (ed.) *Professionalism, Boundaries and the Workplace*, London: Routledge, pp. 25–46.

DfE (Department for Education) (2013a) *More Affordable Childcare*, London: DfE.

DfE (Department for Education) (2013b) *Evidence to Inform the Childcare Commission: Part 1 – International Evidence on Childcare Policies and Practices*, London: DfE.

DfE (Department for Education) (2013c) *Sure Start Children's Centres Statutory Guidance for Local Authorities, Commissioners of Local Health Services and Jobcentre Plus*, London: DfE.

DfE (Department for Education) (2015) Review of Childcare Costs: The Analytical Report, DfE -00295-2015, London: DfE.

DfE (Department for Education) and DH (2011) *Supporting Families in the Foundation Years*, London: DfE.

DfE (Department for Education) (2019a) 'Edward Timpson publishes landmark exclusions review', 7 May.

DfE (Department for Education) (2019b) *Independent Panel Report: Review of Post-18 Education and Funding (The Augar Review)*, 30 May.

DHSC (Department of Health and Social Care) (2012) *Policy Paper: Caring for Our Future- Reforming Care and Support*, London: The Stationery Office.

DHSC (Department of Health and Social Care) (2017) 'Department of Health annual report and accounts 2016–2017', 18 July.

DHSC (Department of Health and Social Care) (2018) 'Guidance – public health grants to local authorities: 2018 to 2019. The public health allocations and monetary conditions for local authorities to improve health in local populations'. Available at: https://www.gov.uk/government/publications/public-health-grants-to-local-authorities-2018-to-2019 (accessed 4 October 2019).

DHSC (Department of Health and Social Care) (2019) *The NHS Long Term Plan*, London: DHSC.

DHSS (Department of Health and Social Security) (1972) *Report of the Committee on Nursing. The Briggs Report*, London: HMSO.

DHSS (Department of Health and Social Security) (1986) *Neighbourhood Nursing: A Focus for Care (Report of the Community Nursing Review)*, London: HMSO.

Dingwall, R. (2016) 'Graduate Jobs Must Move with the Times', *The Guardian* letters, 9 May, response to Editorial, 'The University Industry Churns Out Degrees, but not Destinations', 4 May.

Dingwall, R. and Lewis, P. (eds) (1983) *The Sociology of the Professions*, London: Macmillan.

Dobbins, T. and Dundon, T. (2017) 'The chimera of sustainable labour-management partnership', *British Journal of Management*, 28(3): 519–33.

Dobbins, T. and Plows, A. (2017) 'Labour market intermediaries: a corrective to the human capital paradigm (mis)matching skills and jobs?', *Journal of Education and Work*, 30(6): 571–84.

Dodd, V. (2019) 'Public being misled over school funding – former Ofsted head', *The Guardian*, 27 May.

Doel, M., Allmark, P., Conway, P., Flynn, M., Nelson, P. and Tod, A. (2009) *Professional Boundaries*, London: General Social Care Council.

DoH (Department of Health) (1988) *Working for Patients*, Cm 555, London: HMSO.

DoH (Department of Health) (2010) *Building the National Care Service. HM Government White Paper,* Cm 7854, London: The Stationery Office.

DoH (2015) *Winterbourne View: transforming care two years on*, London: The Stationery Office.DoH & LGA (Department of Health & Local Government Association), Directors ADASS -adult social services, The Children's Society (2014) The Care Act and Whole Family Approaches. Final Draft 14 January 2015. http://professionals.carers.org/whole-family-approach-practice-examples.

Donaldson, Sir L. (2006) *Good Doctors, Safer Patients: A Report by the Chief Medical Officer*, London: Department of Health.

Donnelly, K., Ainley, D., Glatter, R. and Shaw, P. (2017) 'UK education is eroded by the Ebacc, academies and tuition fees', *The Guardian* letters, 14 August.

Dorling, D. (2014) *Inequality and the 1%*, London: Verso.

Doward, J. (2017) 'Austerity puts public sector workers' wages below private sector', *The Observer*, 21 October.

Doyle, T., Sipe, A. and Wall, P. (2006) *Sex, Priests and Secret Codes: The Catholic Church's 2000-Year Paper Trail of Sexual Abuse*, Los Angeles: Volt Press.

Du Gay, P. (2000) *In Praise of Bureaucracy: Weber, Organisation and Ethics*, London: Sage.

Dumas, C. (2018) *Populism and Economics – Examines How Populism Has Affected Economics. OECD Region Social Mobility*, London: Profile Books.

Durkheim, E. (1966, trans. G. Simpson) *The Division of Labour in Society*, New York: The Free Press.

Dwyer, P. and Wright, S. (2014) 'Universal credit, ubiquitous conditionality and its implications for social citizenship', *Journal of Poverty and Social Justice*, 22: 27–35.

Eaton, G. (2018) 'Budget 2018: the OBR shows how Brexit has hurt the UK economy', *New Statesman*, 29 October.

EC/EACEA/Eurydice/Eurostat (2014) *Key Data on Early Childhood Education and Care in Europe. 2014 edition. Eurydice and Eurostat Report*, Brussels: EACEA.

Economic Affairs Committee (2019) 'Social care funding: time to end a national scandal'. Available at: https://publications.parliament.uk/pa/ld201719/ldselect/ldeconaf/392/392.pdf (accessed 7 October 2019).

Edgell, S. (2012) *The Sociology of Work: Continuity and Change in Paid and Unpaid Work* (2nd edn), London: Sage.

Edgley, A. and Avis, M. (2006) 'Interprofessional collaboration: sure start, uncertain futures', *Journal of Interprofessional Care*, 20(4): 433–5.

Edmiston, D. (2017) 'Welfare, austerity and social citizenship in the UK', *Social Policy and Society*, 16(2): 261–70.

Edmiston, D., Patrick, R. and Garthwaite, K. (2017) 'Introduction: austerity, welfare and social citizenship', *Social Policy and Society*, 16(2): 253–9.

Edmond, N. and Price, M. (2012) 'Professionalism in the children and young people's workforce', in N. Edmond and M. Price (eds) *Integrated Working with Children and Young People: Supporting Development from Birth to Nineteen*, London: Sage, pp 29–45.

Education Endowment Foundation (EEF) (J. Sharples, R. Webster and P. Blatchford) (2016) *Making Best Use of Teaching Assistants. Guidance Report*, 14 November, London: Education Endowment Foundation.

Einion, A. (2016) 'Resilience, midwifery and professional identity: changing the script of midwifery culture through narrative, pt 1', *The Practising Midwife TPM Journal all4maternity*, 19(6) (June): 30–2.

Eldridge, J. (1971) *Max Weber: The Interpretation of Social Reality*, London: Michael Joseph.

Elgot, J. (2019) 'We won't be bribed, Labour MPs warn May as £1.6bn goes to struggling towns', *The Guardian*, 4 March.

Elgot, J. and Campbell, D. (2016) 'Seven-day NHS "might not cut deaths". Report casts doubt on key point in dispute', *The Guardian*, 16 February.

Elgot, J., Stewart, H. and Walker, P. (2018) 'Hard Brexit would cost public finances £80bn, says secret analysis', *The Guardian*, 7 February.

Elliott, L. (2015a) 'Corbyn has the vision, but his numbers don't yet add up', *The Guardian*, 21 August.

Elliott, L. (2015b) 'Poorest parts of Britain face 40% public sector job cuts', *The Guardian*, 12 June.

Elliott, L. (2015c) 'Rise in low-skilled jobs blamed for static wages', *The Guardian*, 24 September.

Elliott, L. (2017) 'Employers call for productivity watchdog', *The Guardian*, 28 November.

Elliott, L. (2018a) 'A new world of technology is heading our way, and we'll need state help to navigate it', *The Guardian*, 18 June.

Elliott, L. (2018b) 'The rise in zero-hours can only be halted by strong unions', *The Guardian*, 14 September.

Elliott, L. (2018c) 'The Left case for leave is gaining strength as it becomes clear that this Europe is not for turning', The Guardian, 1 October.

Elliott, P. (1972) *The Sociology of Professions*, London: Macmillan.

Ellison, N. (2009) 'The socio-economic context of social policy', in H. Bochel and G. Daly (eds) Social Policy, 3rd edn, London: Routledge, pp. 13–38.

Esping-Andersen, G. (2002) 'A child-centred social investment strategy', in G. Esping-Andersen, D. Gallie, A. Hemerijck and J. Myles (eds) *Why We Need a New Welfare State*, Oxford: Oxford University Press, pp. 26–67.

Etzioni, A. (1969) 'The semi-professions and their organisation: teachers, nurses, social workers', in A. Etzioni (ed.) *Modern Organisations*, New York: The Free Press.

Evans, J. (2003) 'Independent living movement in the UK', European Network on Independent Living, Cornell University ILR School DigitalCommons@ ILR. Available at: https://www.independentliving.org/docs6/evans2003.html (accessed 7 October 2019).

Evans, R. (2018) 'Activist seeks prosecution of police spy over sexual relationship', *The Guardian*, 1 May.

Evans, T. (2013) 'Organisational rules and discretion in adult social work', *British Journal of Social Work*, 43(4): 739–58.

Evans, T. (2015) 'Professionals and discretion in street-level bureaucracy', in P. Hupe, M. Hill and A. Buffat (eds) *Understanding Street-Level Bureaucracy*, Bristol: Policy Press, pp. 279–94.

Evetts, J. (2009) 'New professionalism and new public management: changes, continuities and consequences', *Comparative Sociology*, 8(2): 247–66.

Fairclough, N. and Graham, P. (2002) 'Marx as a critical discourse analyst', *Estudios de Sociolinguistica*, 3(1): 185–229.

Falgares, G., Venza, G. and Guarnaccia, C. (2017) 'Learning psychology and becoming psychologists: developing professional identity through group experiential learning', *Psychology Learning and Teaching*, March. Available at: https://doi.org/10.1177/1475725717695148.

Farnsworth, K. and Irving, Z. (eds) (2015) *Social Policy in Times of Austerity*, Bristol: Policy Press.

Faulkner, A. (2008) '"Strange bedfellows" in the laboratory of the NHS? An analysis of the new science of health technology assessment in the United Kingdom', *Sociology of Health and Illness*, 19(19B): 183–208.

Fazackerley, A. (2018) 'We haven't got a Plan B – academics race to safeguard research amid Brexit fears', *The Guardian*, 16 October.

Fazackerley, A. (2019) 'Arts under fire: universities rail at "catastrophic" plan to link fees to graduate pay', *The Guardian*, 11 June.

Featherstone, B., Gupta, A., Morris, K. and Warner, J. (2018) 'Let's stop feeding the risk monster: towards a social model of child protection', *Families, Relationships and Societies*, 7(1): 7–22.

Ferguson, D. (2018) 'Teachers on charity: "It was humbling. I never thought it would happen to me"', The Guardian, 26 June.

Ferguson, I., Ioakimidis, V., and Lavalette, M. (2018) *Global Social Work in a Political Context: Radical Perspectives*, Bristol: Policy Press.

Fielding, M. (2004) '"New wave" student voice and the renewal of civic society', *London Review of Education*, 2(3): 197–216.

Fischer, H., Houchen, B. and Ferguson-Ramos, L. (2008) 'Professional boundaries violations: case studies from a regulatory perspective', *Nursing Administration Quarterly*, 32(4), 317–23.

Fleming, P. (2015) *The Mythology of Work*, London: Pluto.

Flynn, M. (2012) 'Winterbourne View Hospital: a serious case review. Gloucester: South Gloucestershire Safeguarding Adults Board' (www. south-glos.gov.uk/news/serious-case-review-winterbourne-view/).

Foley, M. and Cummins, I. (2018) 'Reporting sexual violence on mental health wards', University of Salford. Available at: https://usir. salford.ac.uk/46498 (accessed 7 October 2019).

Foucault, M. (1965) *Madness and Civilization*, New York: Random House.

Foucault, M. (1973) *The Order of Things*, New York: Vintage Books.

Foucault, M. (1977a) *Discipline and Punish: The Birth of the Prison*, Harmondsworth: Penguin.

Foucault, M. (1977b) *The Birth of the Clinic: An Archeology of Medical Perception*, New York: Vintage.

Foucault, M. (1980) *Power/Knowledge*, Brighton: The Harvester Press.

Fournier, V. (2000) 'Boundary work and the (un)making of the professions', in N. Malin (ed.) *Professionalism, Boundaries and the Workplace*, London: Routledge, pp. 67–86.

Fouzder, M. (2018) 'Justice centre stage in week of events', 29 October, https://www.lawgazette.co.uk/news/5068112/article.

Foy, M. (2018) 'Clinical negligence: can we afford it?', *Bone & Joint 360*, 7(1): 41–2.

Francis, R. (2013) *Report of the Mid-Staffordshire NHS Foundation Trust Public Inquiry*, London: The Stationery Office.

Francis Inquiry Report (Report of the Mid-Staffordshire NHS Foundation Trust public inquiry and the Government's response, 2 December 2013) SN/SP/6690 House of Commons Library.

Fraser, D. (1973) *The Evolution of the British Welfare State*, London: Macmillan.

Freeman, M., Miller, C. and Ross, N. (2000) 'The impact of individual philosophies of teamwork on multi-professional practice & the implications for education', *Journal of Interprofessional Care*, 14: 237–47.

Freidson, E. (1970) *Profession of Medicine: A Study in the Sociology of Applied Knowledge*, New York: Dodd, Mead & Co.

Freidson, E. (2001) *Professionalism: The 3rd Logic*, Cambridge: The Polity Press.

Friedman, T. (2000) *The Lexus and the Olive Tree*, London: Harper Collins.

Frost, N. and Robinson, M. (eds) (2016) *Developing Multi-Professional Teamwork for Integrated Children's Services* (3rd edn), London: Open University Press.

Frostenson, M. (2015) 'Three forms of professional autonomy: de-professionalisation of teachers in a new light, in Autonomy in Education', *NordSTEP, Nordic Journal of Studies in Educational Policy*, 1(2), 3 July: 20–9.

Fukuyama, F. (1989) *The End of History?*, Harmondsworth: Penguin.

Furedi, F. (2004a) *Therapy Culture: Cultivating Vulnerability in an Uncertain Age*, New York: Routledge.

Furedi, F. (2004b) 'Plagiarism stems for a loss of scholarly ideals', *Times Higher Education Supplement*, 6 August.

Gallagher, A (2014) 'The "caring entrepreneur": childcare policy and private provision in an enterprising age', *Environment and Planning*, 46: 1108–23.

Gambaro, L. (2012) 'Why are childcare workers low paid? An analysis of pay in the UK childcare sector, 1994–2008', unpublished PhD thesis, the London School of Economics and Political Science.

Gambetta, D. (1988) 'Can we trust trust?' in D. Gambetta (ed.) *Trust: Making and Breaking Cooperative Relations*, Oxford: Blackwell, pp. 213–38.

Gani, A. (2015) 'It's not just about pay, it's about the future of the NHS', *The Guardian*, 17 October.

Garrett, P.M. (2009) *'Transforming' Children's Services: Social Work, Neoliberalism and the "Modern" World*, Maidenhead: Open University Press.

Garrett, P.M. (2013) 'A catastrophic inept, self-serving Church? Re-examining three reports on child abuse in the Republic of Ireland', *Journal of Progressive Human Services*, 24(1): 43–65.

Garrett, P.M (2014) *Children and Families (Critical and Radical Debates in Social Work)*, Bristol: Policy Press.

Garrett, P.M (2018) *Welfare Words. Critical Social Work & Social Policy*, London: Sage.

Garson, B. (1988) *The Electronic Sweatshop: How Computers Are Transforming the Office of the Future into the Factory of the Past*, New York: Simon & Schuster.

Gayle, D. (2016) 'Women's refuges put at risk by benefit changes, says charity', *The Guardian*, 18 May.

Gazzola, N., de Stefano, J., Audet, C. and Thériault, A. (2011) 'Professional identity among counselling psychology doctoral students: a qualitative investigation', *Counselling Psychology Quarterly*, 24(4) (https://doi.org/10.1080/09515070.2011.630572).

Gedalof, I. (2018) *Narratives of Difference in an Age of Austerity*, London: Palgrave Macmillan.

German Retail Blog (2017) 'BRC boss Helen Dickinson talks Brexit', 20 December.

George, M. (2017) 'Angela Rayner outlines 10-point charter for National Education Service', *Times Education Supplement*, 26 September. Available at: https://www.tes.com/news/angela-rayner-outlines-10-point-charter-national-education-service (accessed 7 October 2019).

Gershlick, B., Charlesworth, A., Thorlby, R. and Jones, H. (2017) 'Election briefing: a sustainable workforce – the lifeblood of the NHS and social care', The Health Foundation/King's Fund Centre.

Giddens, A. (1971) *Capitalism and Modern Social Theory: An Analysis of the Writings of Marx, Durkheim and Weber*, Cambridge: Cambridge University Press.

Giddens, A. (1998) *The Third Way: The Renewal of Social Democracy*, Cambridge: Polity.

Gill, R. (2011) *Theory and Practice of Leadership* (2nd edn), London: Sage.

Giridharadas, A. (2019) *Winners Take All: The Elite Charade of Changing the World*, London: Allen Lane.

Glasby, J. and Dickinson, H. (2014) *Partnership Working in Health and Social Care: What is Integrated Care and How Can We Deliver It?* (2nd edn), Bristol: Policy Press.

Glendinning,C., Powell, M. and Rummery, K. (eds) (2002) *Partnerships, New Labour and the Governance of Welfare*, Bristol: Policy Press.

Glyn, A. (2006) *Capitalism Unleashed: Finance, Globalisation and Welfare*, Oxford: Oxford University Press.

Godefroy, S. (2015) *Mental Health & Mental Capacity Law for Social Workers: An Introduction*, London: Sage.

Goffman, E. (1959) *The Presentation of Self in Everyday Life*, Harmondsworth: Penguin Press.

Goffman, E. (1961) *Asylums: Essays on the Social Situation of Mental Patients and Other Inmates*, Harmondsworth: Penguin Press.

Goffman, E. (1963) *Stigma: Notes on the Management of Spoilt Identity*, Harmondsworth: Penguin Press.

Goldin, I. and Kutarna, C. (2016) *Age of Discovery: Navigating the Risks and Rewards of Our New Renaissance*, London: Bloomsbury Publishers.

Goldstein, H. (2000) 'Woodhead abused his position as head of Ofsted', *British Educational Research Journal*, 26: 547–55.

Gomm, R. and Davies, C. (eds) (2000) *Using Evidence in Health and Social Care*, London: Sage.

Goode, W. (1957) 'Community within a Community: The Professions', *American Sociological Review*, 22(2): 194–200.

Goode, W. (1969) 'The theoretical limits of professionalisation', in A. Etzioni (ed.) *The Semi-Professions and Their Organization*, New York: The Free Press, pp. 19–30.

Goodley, D. (2017) *Disability Studies: An Interdisciplinary Introduction* (2nd edn), London: Sage.

Gosport War Memorial Hospital (2018) 'The report of the Gosport Independent Panel', HC 1084, June. Available at: https://www.gosportpanel.independent.gov.uk/.

Gough, I. (1979) *The Political Economy of the Welfare State*, London: Macmillan.

Gough, I. (2017) *Heat, Greed and Human Need: Climate Change, Capitalism and Sustainable Wellbeing*, Cheltenham: Edward Elgar.

Gov.uk (2016) Budget 2016: George Osborne's speech, 16 March. Available at: https://www.gov.uk/government/speeches/budget-2016-george-osbornes-speech (accessed 7 October 2019).

Gov.uk (2018) Consultation outcome. School exclusions review: call for evidence, 16 March. Available at: https://www.gov.uk/government/consultations/school-exclusions-review-call-for-evidence (accessed 7 October 2019).

Gov.uk (2019) Timpson review of school exclusion, May. Available at: https://assets.publishing.service.gov.uk/government/uploads/system/uploads/attachment_data/file/807862/Timpson_review.pdf (accessed 7 October 2019).

Gove, M. (2012) 'Requirements for early education and childcare inspections', letter to Sir Michael Wilshaw, 11 July.

Gramsci, A. (1971) *Selections from the Prison Notebooks*, London: Lawrence and Wishart.

Grant, L. and Kinman, G. (2013) *The Importance of Emotional Resilience for Staff and Students in the Helping Professions*, York: The Higher Education Academy.

Grant, L. and Kinman, G. (2014) *Developing Resilience for Social Work Practice*, London: Palgrave Macmillan.

Gray, A.M. and Birrell, D. (2013) *Transforming Adult Social Care: Contemporary Policy and Practice*, Bristol: Policy Press.

Greener, I. (2018) *Social Policy after the Financial Crisis: A Progressive Response*, Cheltenham: Edward Elgar.

Greenfield, P. (2018) 'Deaths of homeless people up by a quarter in five years', *The Guardian*, 21 December.

Greer, S., Wismar, M. and Figueras, J. (eds) (2016) *Strengthening Health System Governance: Better Policies, Stronger Performance*, Maidenhead: McGraw-Hill.

Griffiths, J. (2018) 'MAYDAY. Happy International Workers' Day!', *The Sun*, 1 May.

Grint, K. (2005) *Leadership: Limits and Possibilities*, Basingstoke: Palgrave Macmillan.

GSCC (General Social Care Council) (2011) 'Professional boundaries evidence for social workers. General Social Care Council'. Available at: www.gscc.org.uk/cmsFiles/Conduct/GSCC Professional Boundaries_evidence_201.Pdf (accessed 7 October 2019).

Gulland, J. (2012) 'Fitting themselves to become wage-earners – conditionality and incapacity for work in the early twentieth century', *Journal of Social Security Law*, 119(2): 51–70.

Hacker, J. and Pierson, P. (2002) 'Business power and social policy: employers and the formation of the American welfare state', *Politics and Society*, 30(2): 277–325.

Ham, C. and Charles, A. (2018) 'Integrated care. Our work on joined-up health and care services', September (www.kingsfund.org.uk/chris-ham).

Hammersley-Fletcher, L., Clarke, M. and McManus, V. (2018) 'Agonistic democracy and passionate professional development in teacher-leaders', *Cambridge Journal of Education*, 48(5): 591–606.

Hanlon, P., Carlisle, S., Hannah, M., Reilly, D. and Lyon, A. (2011) 'Making the case for a "fifth wave" in public health', *Public Health*, 125(1): 30–6.

Hannum, H. (2016) 'Reinvigorating human rights for the twenty-first century', *Human Rights Law Review*, 16(3), September: 409–51 (https://doi.org/10.1093/hrlr/ngw 015).

Harding, E. (2019) 'Number of teachers falls for first time in six years', *Daily Mail*, 5 January.

Hargreaves, A. and O'Connor, M. (2018) 'Leading collaborative professionalism. Centre for Strategic Education (CSE). Seminar Series Paper #27, April, CSE, Victoria.

Hargreaves, F. (2018) 'The Tinder effect? STI testing soars', *Daily Mail*, 1 September.

Harris, J. (2003) *The Social Work Business*, London: Routledge.

Hastings, A., Bailey, N., Bramley, G., Gannon, M. and Watkins, D. (2015) *The Cost of the Cuts: The Impact on Local Government and Poorer Communities*, York: Joseph Rowntree Foundation.

Hastings, A. and Matthews, P. (2014) 'Bourdieu and the big society: empowering the powerful in public service provision', *Policy and Politics*, 43(4): 545–60.

Hay, I. and Beaverstock, J. (2016) *Handbook on Wealth and the Super-Rich*, Cheltenham: Edward Elgar.

Hayek, F. von (1944) *The Road to Serfdom*, London: Routledge.

HCPC (Health and Care Professions Council) (M. Flynn) (2016) 'In search of accountability: a review of the neglect of older people living in care homes investigated as Operation Jasmine (2015) -an update for council'.

Health and Social Act (2013) London: The Stationery Office.

Health Business (2018) 'Rise in sexual assaults on ambulance staff', *Health Business*, 23 April.

Health Foundation/King's Fund (2017) 'One in four social care staff leaving the profession every year', press release, 17 May.

Health Foundation/King's Fund (L. Wenzel, L. Bennett, S. Bottery, R. Murray and B. Sahib) (2018) 'Approaches to social care funding: social care funding options', February.

Healthwatch (2016) 'Are people waiting too long to be assessed for social care support?' *Healthwatch*, 19 July. Available at: https://www.healthwatch.co.uk/news/2016-07-19/are-people-waiting-too-long-be-assessed-social-care-support (accessed 7 October 2019).

Helm, T. (2018) 'McDonnell: Labour will give power to workers through "ownership funds"', *The Observer*, 8 September.

Henrekson, M. and Stenkula, M. (2009) 'Entrepreneurship and public policy', IFN Working Paper No. 804.

Henwood, M. (2018) 'Austerity, outsourcing and councils in crisis', *The Guardian* letters, 14 August.

Heriot Watt University News (2018) 'State of homelessness across Britain revealed – new', 21 December. Available at: https://www.hw.ac.uk/news/articles/2018/state-of-homelessness-across-britain.htm (accessed 7 October 2019).

Heywood, A. (2000) *Key Concepts in Politics*, Basingstoke: Palgrave Macmillan.

Hill, A. (2017) 'The new retirement: how an ageing population is transforming Britain', *The Guardian*, 16 January.

Hill, A. and Bowcott, O. (2018) 'Tory who lost savings in court wants legal aid restored', *The Guardian*, 28 December.

Hill, M. and Hupe, P. (2014) *Implementing Public Policy* (3rd edn), London: Sage.

Hinsliff, G. (2018a) 'Do Brexiters want immigration caps or NHS doctors? They must choose', *The Guardian*, 12 June.

Hinsliff, G. (2018b) 'STI services cut: what is behind Britain's sexual health crisis?', *The Guardian*, 24 July.

HM Inspectorate of Probation (2017) 'Annual report', updated 14 December. Crown Copyright.

Hoel, H. and Cooper, C. (2000) Destructive Conflict and Bullying at Work. Sponsored by the British Occupational Health Research Foundation, School of Management, Manchester: UMIST.

Hogan, L. (2011) 'Clerical and religious child abuse: Ireland and beyond', *Theological Studies*, 72: 170–86.

Holborow, M. (2015) *Language and Neo-Liberalism*, London: Routledge.

Home Office (2016) 'Policy Paper 2010–2015 government policy: legal aid reform'. Available at: https://www.gov/government/policies/making-legal-aid-more-effective (accessed 7 October 2019).

Hood, C. (1995) 'Emerging issues in public administration', *Public Administration*, 73, Spring: 165–83.

House of Commons (2013) 'Foundation years: Sure Start children's centres', House of Commons Education Committee, HC 364-1. Available at: https://publications.parliament.uk/pa/cm201314/cmselect/cmeduc/364/364.pdf (accessed 7 October 2019).

House of Commons (2017) 'Adult social care, ninth report of session 2016–17', HC 1103, Communities and Local Government Committee. Available at: https://publications.parliament.uk/pa/cm201617/cmselect/cmcomloc/1103/1103.pdf (accessed 7 October 2019).

House of Commons (2018) 'Transforming rehabilitation, ninth report of session 2017–19', House of Commons Justice Committee, June. Available at: https://publications.parliament.uk/pa/cm201719/cmselect/cmjust/482/482.pdf (accessed 7 October 2019).

House of Commons Committee of Public Accounts (2018) 'Retaining and developing the teaching workforce'. Seventeenth Report of Session 2017–19. HC 460, 31 January.

Howard, E. (2016) 'Going into legal aid work now is career suicide', *The Guardian*, 6 January.

Howe, D. (1986) *Social Workers and Their Practice in Welfare Bureaucracies*, Aldershot: Gower.

HSCIC (Health and Social Care Information Centre) (2016) 'Personal social services: staff of social services departments, England' (enquiries@nhsdigital.hns.uk).

Hughes, M. and Wearing, M. (2017) *Organisations and Management in Social Work* (3rd edn), London: Sage.

Hugman, R. (1991) *Power in Caring Professions*, Basingstoke: Macmillan.

Humber, L. (2016) 'The impact of neo-liberal market relations of the production of care on the quantity and quality of support for people with learning disabilities', *Critical and Radical Social Work*, 4(2): 149–67.

Hunt, T. (2016) 'Inequality: a problem schools alone can't fix', *The Guardian*, 12 January.

Hunter, P. (2018) 'The local living wage dividend', The Smith Institute. Available at: http://www.smith-institute.org.uk/book/the-local-living-wage-dividend/ (accessed 7 October 2019).

Hupe, P. and Hill, M. (2007) 'Street-level bureaucracy and public accountability', *Public Administration*, 85(2): 279–99.

Hupe, P., Hill, M. and Buffat, A. (eds) (2015) *Understanding Street-Level Bureaucracy*, Bristol: Policy Press.

Hussein, S, Stevens, M. and Manthorpe, J. (2011) 'What drives the recruitment of migrant workers to work in social care in England', *Social Policy and Society*, 10(3): 285–98.

Hutchinson, J. and Crenna-Jennings, W. (2019) 'Unexplained pupil exits from schools: a growing problem?', Working Paper, April, Education Policy Institute. Available at: https://epi.org.uk/publications-and-research/unexplained-pupil-exits/ (accessed 7 October 2019).

Hutton, W. (2018) 'Fanfare for America's heroes of free enterprise. Review of A. Greenspan and A. Wooldridge, *Capitalism in America: A History*', *The Observer*, 18 November.

Huxham, C. and Vangen, S. (2005) 'Enhancing leadership for collaborative advantage: dilemmas of ideology and pragmatism in the activities of partnership managers', *British Journal of Management*, 14: 61–76.

IFS (Institute for Fiscal Studies) (R. Crawford, C. Emmerson and G. Tetlow) (2012) *Public Finance Bulletin* funded by ESRC. Available at: https://www.ifs.org.uk/publications/6400 (accessed 7 October 2019).

IFS (Institute for Fiscal Studies) (Neil Amin Smith and David Phillips) (2019a) *England's Council Funding System is Unsustainable -and Big Choices Loom*, 29 May, London: IFS.

IFS (Institute for Fiscal Studies) (2019b) 'Inequality: the IFS Deaton Review launch', 14 May, The British Academy, London.

Independent Inquiry into Child Sexual Abuse (2017) 'Child sexual abuse within the Catholic and Anglican Churches: a rapid evidence assessment', November, IICSA Research Team.

IPCC (Independent Police Complaints Commission) (2012) 'The abuse of police powers to perpetrate sexual violence', chair Dame Anne Owers, September.

Inman, P. (2016) 'Workers on zero-hours lose £1,000 a year, a study shows', *The Guardian*, 30 December.

Inman, P. (2018) 'Raising minimum wage "could give urban regions a £1bn-plus boost"', *The Guardian*, 3 September.

Inman, P. and Jolly, J. (2018) 'Poor productivity? Just give everyone an extra day off', *The Observer*, 18 November.

Ipsos MORI (2016) 'Enough of Experts? Ipsos MORI Veracity Index. A joint report from Mumsnet and Ipsos MORI using a Veracity Index and online focus groups to explore opinions about trust, information and experts during the EU referendum campaign', Market and Opinion Research International Ltd.

Issimdar, M. (2018) 'Home-schooling in the UK increases 40% over three years', 26 April. Available at: https://www.bbc.co.uk/news/uk-england-42624220 (accessed 7 October 2019).

ITV National News (2016) 'BMA should "stop playing politics" and "put patients first"', 1 September.

ITV National News (2018) 'Gosport GP Jane Barton was "doing her best for patients"', 27 June.

Jay, A. (2014) *Independent Inquiry into Child Sexual Exploitation in Rotherham 1997–2013*, Rotherham: Rotherham Metropolitan Council.

Jay, P. (1979) *Report of the Committee of Enquiry into Mental Handicap Nursing and Care* Vols I and II, Cmnd 7468, London: HMSO.

Jenson, J. (2012) 'Redesigning citizenship regimes: after neo-liberalism: moving towards social investment', in N. Morel, B. Pallier and J. Palme (eds) *Towards a Social Investment Welfare State? Ideas, Policies and Challenges*, Bristol: Policy Press, 61–87.

John Jay College of Criminal Justice (2004) *The Nature and Scope of Sex Abuse of Minors by Catholic Priests and Deacons in the United States 1950–2002*, Washington DC: United States Conference of Catholic Bishops.

Johnson, T. (1982) 'The state and the professions: peculiarities of the British', in A. Giddens and G. MacKenzie (eds) *Social Class and the Division of Labour*, Cambridge: Cambridge University Press, pp. 186–208.

Johnston, C. (2016) 'Bursaries for student nurses will end in 2017, government confirms', *The Guardian*, 21 July.

Jones, K. (1972) *A History of the Mental Health Services*, London: Routledge & Kegan Paul.

Jones, O. (2012) *Chavs: The Demonization of the Working Class* (updated edn), London: Verso.

Jones, O. (2014) 'The Establishment uncovered: how power works in Britain, *The Guardian*, 26 August.

Jones, O. (2018) 'Carillion is no one-off scandal. There are many more to come', *The Guardian*, 17 May.

Jones, R. (2014) *The Story of Baby P: Setting the Record Straight*, Bristol: Policy Press.

Jones, R. (2018) 'If councils lose accountability for children's services then families will lose the help they need', *Community Care Magazine*, 12 December. Available at: https://www.communitycare.co.uk/2018/12/12/ray-jones-councils-lose-accountability-childrens-services-families-will-lose-help-need/ (accessed 7 October 2019).

Jordan, B. (2001) 'Tough love: social work, social exclusion and the Third Way', *British Journal of Social Work*, 31(4): 527–46.

Keenan, M. (2011) *Child Sexual Abuse and the Catholic Church: Gender, Power and Organisational Culture*, New York: Oxford University Press.

Kelly, S (2015) 'The "atomised" council is here to stay, stripped back to the most basic services', *The Guardian*, 2 December.

Kentish, B. (2018) 'Budget 2018: Jeremy Corbyn accuses government of broken promise budget as he dismisses claim austerity is over', *The Independent*, 29 October.

Khele, S, Symons, C. and Wheeler, S. (2008) 'An analysis of complaints to the British Association for Counselling and Psychotherapy 1996–2006', *Counselling and Psychotherapy Research*, 8(2): 124–32 (doi.10:1080/14733140802051408).

Kim, H. and Rehg, M. (2018) 'Faculty performance and morale in higher education: a systems approach', *Systems Research and Behavioral Science*, 35(3): 308–23 (https://doi.org/10.1002/sres.2495).

King's Fund (2018a) 'Nursing student numbers: should we panic yet?' Available at: https://www.kingsfund.org.uk/blog/2018/02/nursing-student-numbers-should-we-panic-yet (accessed 7 October 2019).

King's Fund (2018b) 'The Health Care Workforce in England: Make or Break', 15 November. Available at: https://www.kingsfund.org.uk/publications/health-care-workforce-england (accessed 7 October 2019).

King's Fund Centre (2018a) 'How is the NHS performing?' *Quarterly Monitoring Report*, December.

King's Fund Centre (2018b) 'The NHS budget and how it has changed', 2 July; 'Budget 2018: what it means for health and social care', 9 November.

Kingston, W. (2017) *How Capitalism Destroyed Itself: Technology Displaced by Financial Innovation*, Cheltenham: Edward Elgar.

Kirkpatrick, I., Ackroyd, S. and Walker, R. (2005) *The New Managerialism and Public Service Professions: Change in Health, Social Services and Housing*, New York: Palgrave Macmillan.

Kitzinger, J. (2000) 'Media templates: patterns of association and the (re) construction of meaning over time', *Media, Culture & Society*, 22(1): 61–84.

Klegon, D. (1978) 'The sociology of professions: an emerging perspective', *Work and Occupations*, 5(3), August: 371–410.

Klein, R. (2010) *The New Politics of the NHS – From Creation to Reinvention* (6th edn), Oxford: Radcliffe Publishing.

Knaus, C. (2019) 'Archbishop of Brisbane under investigation over allege response to child abuse information', *The Guardian*, 25 February.

Knoll, J. (2010) 'Teachers' sexual misconduct: grooming patterns and female offenders', *Journal of Child Sexual Abuse*, 19(4): 371–86.

Koch, M. (2012) *Capitalism and Climate Change: Theoretical Discussion, Historical Development and Policy Responses*, Basingstoke: Palgrave Macmillan.

Kramer, R. (ed.) (2006) *Organisational Trust: A Reader*, London: Sage.

Kroger, T. and Yeandle, S. (2013) 'Reconciling work and care: an international analysis', in T. Kröger and S. Yeandle (eds) *Combining Paid Work and Family Care: Policies and Experiences in International Perspective*, Bristol: Policy Press, pp. 3–22.

Kuhlmann, E. and Saks, M (eds) (2008) *Rethinking Professional Governance: International Directions in Health Care*, Bristol: Policy Press.

Kumar, S. (2000) Client empowerment in psychiatry and the professional abuse of clients: where do we stand?, *International Journal of Psychiatry in Medicine*, 30(1): 61–70.

Kushner, B. and Kushner, S. (2013) *Who Needs the Cuts? Myths of the Economic Crisis*, London: Hesperus.

Kynaston, D. (2008) *Austerity Britain 1945–51*, London: Bloomsbury Publishing.

Labour (2018a) 'This policy was yet another example of Theresa May's heartless "hostile environment" – Ashworth', 9 May. Available at: https://labour.org.uk/press/policy-yet-another example-theresa-mays-heartless-hostile-environment-ashworth/ (accessed 7 October 2019).

Labour (2018b) 'Tinkering at the edges will not solve social care crisis – Barbara Keeley interview', 2 October. Available at: https://labour.org.uk/press/tinkering-edges-will-not-solve-social-care-crisis-barbara-keeley/ (accessed 7 October 2019).

Lacey, P. (2001) *Support Partnerships: Collaboration in Action*, London: David Fulton.

Ladkin, D. (2010) *Rethinking Leadership: A New Look at Old Leadership Questions*, Cheltenham: Edward Elgar.

Lambie -Mumford, H. (2015) 'Britain's hunger crisis: where's the social policy?', in Z. Irving, M. Fenger and J. Hudson (eds) *Social Policy Review 27*, Bristol: Policy Press, pp. 13–32.

Larson, M. (1977) *The Rise of Professionalism: A Sociological Analysis*, London: University of California Press.

Larsson, M., Aldegarmann, U. and Aarts, C. (2009) 'Professional role and identity in a changing society: three paradoxes in Swedish midwives' experiences', *Midwifery*, 25(4): 373–81.

Lattuca, L. (2001) *Creating Interdisciplinarity*, Nashville, TN: Vanderbilt University Press.

Lavalette, M. (2011) 'Introduction' in *Radical Social Work Today: Social Work at the Crossroads*, Bristol: Policy Press, pp. 1–7.

Lavalette, M. (2017) 'Austerity, inequality and the context of contemporary social work', *Social Work & Social Sciences Review*, 19(1): 31–9.

Leading Governance (2013) 'The Nolan principles twenty years on', Leading Governance. Available at: https://www.leadinggovernance.com/blog/nolan-principles-20-years (accessed 7 October 2019).

Leathard, A. (ed) (1994) *Going Interprofessional: Working Together for Health and Welfare*, London: Routledge.

Leaton Gray, S. (2006) *Teachers Under Siege*, Stoke on Trent: Trentham Books.

Legal Voice (2017) 'Interview: Sara Ryan talks about justice for Laughing Boy', 1 December. Available at: https://legalvoice.org.uk/interview-sara-ryan-talks-justice-laughing-boy/ (accessed 7 October).

Leonard Cheshire Disability Organisation (2016) 'Care homes, adult day care centres' (www/carehome.co.uk/care_search_results.cfm/searchgroup/36151005LEQA).

Leren, T.H. (2006) 'The importance of student voice', *International Journal of Leadership and Education: Theory and Practice*, 9(4): 363–7.

Lewis, J. and Surender, R. (eds) (2004) *Welfare State Change – Towards a Third Way?*, Oxford: Oxford University Press.

Lewis, J. and West, A. (2017) 'Early childhood education and care in England under austerity: continuity or change in political ideas, policy goals, availability, affordability and quality in a childcare market?', *Journal of Social Policy*, 46(2): 331–48 (doi:10.1017/S0047279416000647).

LGA (Local Government Association) (2017) 'LGA analysis: council tax rises will not fix local government funding crisis', 20 February. Available at: https://www.local.gov.uk/about/news/lga-analysis-council-tax-rises-will-not-fix-local-government-funding-crisis (accessed 7 October 2019).

LGA (Local Government Association) (2018a) 'Children's Services Funding – facts and figures', 11 November. Available at: https://www.local.gov.uk/about/campaigns/bright-futures/bright-futures-childrens-services/childrens-services-funding-facts (accessed 7 October 2019).

LGA (Local Government Association) (2018b) 'Local services face further £1.3 billion government funding cut in 2019/20', 5 October. Available at: www.wired-giv.net/news

Liebenberg, L., Ungar, M. and Ikeda, J. (2015) 'Neo-liberalism and responsibilisation in the discourse of social service workers', *British Journal of Social Work*, 45(3), 1 April: 1006–21.

Lightfoot, L. (2016) 'Nearly half of teachers plan to leave in next five years. Survey shows huge numbers of staff in England at breaking point over their workload', *The Guardian*, www.guardian.com/teacher-network, survey, 22 March.

Lightfoot, L. (2018) 'Let teachers sack heads … and other ideas for a National Education Service', *The Guardian* education forum, 4 September.

Lind, A. (2018) 'Social rights and EU citizenship', in U. Bernitz, M. Mårtensson, L. Oxelheim and T. Persson (eds) *Bridging the Prosperity Gap in the EU: The Social Challenge Ahead*, Cheltenham: Edward Elgar, pp. 22–45.

Lipsey, R. (1979) *An Introduction to Positive Economics* (5th edn), London: Weidenfeld & Nicolson.

Lipsky, M. (1980 and 2010) *Street-Level Bureaucracy: Dilemmas of the Individual in Public Services* (30th anniversary expanded edn), New York: Russell Sage Foundation.

Lister, R. (1997) *Citizenship: Feminist Perspectives*, Basingstoke: Macmillan.

Long, R. and Danechi, S. (2019) 'Off-rolling in English schools', House of Commons Library, Briefing Paper 08444, 10 May.

Longevity Science Panel (2018) *Life Expectancy: Is the Socioeconomic Gap Narrowing? Longevity Science Panel*, London: Department of Health and Social Care.

Lowrey, Y. (2003) 'The entrepreneur and entrepreneurship: a neo-classical approach', Office of Advocacy, US Small Business Administration Economic Research Working Paper, January, SSRN (https://dx.doi.org/10.2139/ssrn.744785).

Lowton, K., Hiley, C. and Higgs, P. (2017) 'Constructing embodied identity in a "new" ageing population: a qualitative study of the pioneer cohort of childhood liver transplant recipients in the UK', *Social Science and Medicine*, 172: 1–9.

Lundgren, K., Needleman, W. and Wohlberg, J. (2005) 'Above all, do no harm: abuse of power by health care professionals', Therapy Exploitation Link Line (TELL).

Lux, J. (2019) 'Understanding the crisis symptoms of representative democracy: the new European governance and France's "political crisis"', *Social Policy and Society*, 18(1): 119–31.

MAC (Migration Advisory Committee) (2018) 'EEA/Migration in the UK. Final report', 18 September. Available at: https://www.gov.uk/government/organisations/migration-advisory-committee (accessed 7 October 2019).

MAC (Migration Advisory Committee) (2019a) 'Corporate report: full review of the shortage occupation list for the UK and Scotland. May 2019'.

MAC (Migration Advisory Committee) (2019b) 'Migration Advisory Committee recommends adding to shortage occupation list', 29 May.

Macdonald, K. and Ritzer, G. (1988) 'The sociology of the professions: dead or alive?', *Work and Occupations*, 15(3): 251–72.

Macdonald, K.M. (1995) *The Sociology of the Professions*, London: Sage.

Machin, A, Machin, T and Pearson, P (2012) 'Maintaining equilibrium in professional role identity: a grounded theory study of health visitors' perceptions of their changing professional practice context', Journal of Advanced Nursing, 68 (7): 1526–37.

MacKian, S. and Simons, J. (eds) (2013) Leading Managing Caring: Understanding Leadership and Management in Health and Social Care, Abingdon: Routledge in association with the Open University.

Macmillan, L., Tyler, C. and Vignoles, A. (2015) 'Who gets the top jobs? The role of family background and networks in recent graduates' access to high-status professions', Journal of Social Policy, 44(3): 487–515.

Madison, B. (2017) 'Professional identity and professionalism', Professional Lawyer, 24(3), November: 1–6.

Maharg, P. (2012) '"Associated life": democratic professionalism and the moral imagination'. Available at: https://openresearch-repository. anu.edu.au/bitstream/1885/11938/4/Maharg%20Associated%20 Life%202013.pdf (accessed 7 October 2019).

Mahmud, T. (2012) 'Debt and discipline', American Quarterly, 64(3): 469–94.

Mahon, R. (2013) 'Social investment according to the OECD/DELSA: a discourse in the making, Global Policy, 4(2): 150–9.

Majaski, C. (2019) 'What is rent-seeking?', Investopedia, 23 April. Available at: https://www.investopedia.com/terms/r/rentseeking. asp (accessed 7 October 2019).

Malerba,F., Mani, S. and Adams, P. (eds) (2017) The Rise to Market Leadership – New Leading Firms from Emerging Countries, Cheltenham: Edward Elgar.

Malin, N. (1997) 'Policy to practise: a discussion of tension, dilemma and paradox in community care', Journal of Learning Disabilities for Nursing, Health and Social Care, 1(3): 131–40.

Malin, N. and Morrow, G. (2007) 'Models of interprofessional working within a Sure Start "Trailblazer" programme', Journal of Interprofessional Care, 21(3): 1–13.

Malin, N. and Morrow, G. (2009) 'Evaluating the role of the Sure Start Plus adviser in providing support for pregnant teenagers and young parents', Health and Social Care in the Community, 17(5): 495–503.

Malin, N., Manthorpe, J., Race, D. and Wilmot, S. (1999) Community Care for Nurses and the Caring Professions, Buckingham: Open University Press.

Maltby, K. (2018) 'Power, and why sexual relations and politics are so problematic', The Guardian, 20 February.

Mambrol, N. (2016) 'The postmodern as "the incredulity towards metanarratives"', *Literary Theory and Criticism*, 3(6), April. Available at: https://literariness.org/2016/04/03/the-postmodern-as-the-incredulity-towards-metanarratives/ (accessed 7 October 2019).

Mance, H. (2016) 'Britain has had enough of experts, says Gove', *Financial Times*, 3 June.

Manthorpe, J. (2002) 'Community care and family policy', in N. Malin, S. Wilmot and J Manthorpe (eds) *Key Concepts and Debates in Health and Social Policy*, Buckingham: Open University Press, pp. 110–22.

Marmot, M. (2015) *The Health Gap: The Challenge of an Unequal World*, London: Bloomsbury Publishing.

Marsh, S. (2017) 'Sharp rise in unexpected deaths of ambulance patients', *The Guardian*, 18 December.

Marsh, S. (2019) 'Mental health patients detained in hospital wards for up to 21 years', *The Guardian*, 23 April.

Marshall, T. (1950 [1987]) *Citizenship and Social Class*, London: Pluto Press.

Marshall, T.H. (1939 [1963]) *The Recent History of Professionalism in Relation to Social Structure and Social Policy*, London: Heinemann.

Marston, G. and McDonald, C. (2012) 'Getting beyond "heroic agency" in conceptualising social workers as policy actors in the twenty-first century', *British Journal of Social Work*, 42(6): 1022–38.

Martin, D. (2018) 'Angela Merkel rejects UK Brexit proposal', Deutsche Welle (DW) news bulletin, 25 September. Available at: https://www.dw.com/en/angela-merkel-rejects-uk-brexit-proposal/a-45627800 (accessed 7 October 2019).

Martinelli, F., Anttonen, A. and Matzke, M. (2017) *Social Services Disrupted – Changes, Challenges and Policy Implications for Europe in Times of Austerity*, Cheltenham: Edward Elgar.

Maslow, A. (1943) 'A theory of human motivation', *Psychological Review*, 50: 370–96.

Maslow, A. (1954) *Motivation and Personality*, New York: Harper & Row.

Mason, R. (2016) 'Ministers to focus on struggling families', *The Guardian*, 19 November.

Matthews-King, A. (2018) 'More than 100,000 NHS posts unfilled, reveal "grim" official figures, *The Independent*, 21 February. Available at: https://www.independent.co.uk/news/health/nhs-posts-staffing-recruitment-official-figures-healthcare-hospitals-a8221961.html (accessed 7 October 2019).

Maybin, J. (2016) *Producing Health Policy: Knowledge and Knowing in Government Policy Work*, London: Palgrave Macmillan.

McCluskey, L. (2016) Speech to TUC annual conference: summary of decisions of the July 2016 Unite policy conference. Available at: https://unitetheunion.org/media/1501/decisions-of-the-policy-conference-2016.pdf (accessed 7 October 2019).

McCulloch, C. (2018) 'Probation Service sacrificed on altar of privatisation', *The Guardian* letters, 27 June.

McIntyre, N. and Weale, S. (2019) 'Academy status forced on 300 primary schools', *The Guardian*, 12 July.

McKenzie, L. (2016) 'Narrative, ethnography and class inequality: taking Bourdieu into a British council estate', in J. Thatcher, N. Ingram, C. Burke and J. Abrahams (eds.) *Bourdieu: The Next Generation*, Oxford: Routledge, pp. 25–36.

McKimm, J. and Phillips, K. (eds) (2009) *Leadership and Management in Integrated Services*, Exeter: Learning Matters.

McKnight, J. (1995) *The Careless Society: Community and Its Counterfeits*, New York: Basic Books.

McLellan Commission (2015) *A Review of the Current Safeguarding Policies, Procedures and Practice within the Catholic Church in Scotland*, Scotland: APS Group. Available at: https://www.bcos.org.uk/Portals/0/McLellan/363924_WEB.pdf (accessed 7 October 2019).

McQueen, C. and Henwood, K. (2002) 'Young men in "crisis": attending to the language of teenage boys' distress', *Social Science and Medicine*, 55(9): 493–509.

McVeigh, T. (2016) '"Reckless" cuts in student nurse funding attacked', *The Times*, 19 June.

Melville-Wiseman, J. (2008) 'Pathologies or apologies: a case study of an incident of professional sexual abuse in the mental health system', unpublished PhD thesis, University of Kent.

Melville-Wiseman, J. (2012) 'Professional sexual abuse in mental health services: capturing practitioner views of a contemporary corruption of care', *Social Work & Social Sciences Review*, 15(3): 26–43 (doi 10.192/09535221x55320).

Mencap (2018) 'Concerns over lack of clinical training causing avoidable learning disability deaths', 15 February. Available at: https://www.mencap.org.uk/press-release/concerns-over-lack-clinical-training-causing-avoidable-learning-disability-deaths (accessed 7 October 2019).

Mendoza, K.-A. (2015) *Austerity: The Demolition of the Welfare State and the Rise of the Zombie Economy*, Oxford: New Internationalist Publications.

Metz, J. (2017) 'The professionalism of professional youth work and the role of values', *Social Work & Society: International Online Journal*, 15(2). Available at: https://www.socwork.net/sws/article/view/528/1029 (accessed 7 October 2019).

Midgley, J., Dahl, E. and Conley Wright, A. (2017) *Social Investment and Social Welfare: International and Critical Perspectives*, Cheltenham: Edward Elgar.

Mikkola, M. (2007) 'Social human rights of migrants under the European Social Charter', *European Journal of Social Security*, 10(1): 25–9.

Milburn, A. (2016) 'Chair of the Social Mobility Commission: state of the nation report on social mobility in Great Britain'. Available at: https://assets.publishing.service.gov.uk/government/uploads/system/uploads/attachment_data/file/569410/Social_Mobility_Commission_2016_REPORT_WEB__1__.pdf (accessed 7 October 2019).

Millar, F. (2016) 'Teacher recruitment "a mess" as every school slugs it out for itself', *The Guardian*, 19 January.

Mind (2017) 'Abuse by health and social care workers'. Available at: https://www.mind.org.uk/information-support/guides-to-support-and-services/abuse/abuse-by-health-and-social-care-workers/#.XZswQDGz-Uk (accessed 7 August 2018).

Mirowski, P. (2013) *Never Let a Serious Crisis Go to Waste: How Neo-Liberalism Survived the Financial Meltdown*, London: Verso.

Missouri Medicine (2017) 'Rural health care: health professions workforce shortage', *Journal of the Missouri State Medical Association*, 114(5): 363–6, September–October.

Mohdin, A. (2018) 'New code for employers on sexual harassment "does not go far enough"', *The Guardian*, 4 September.

Monitor (2018) *Annual Report and Accounts 1 April 2017 to 31 March 2018*, HC 1347, London: NHS Improvement.

Montgomery, D. (1987) *The Fall of the House of Labour: The workplace, the State and American Labour Activism, 1865–1925*, Cambridge: Cambridge University Press.

Moorhead, J. (2016a) School Governors Versus Academy Trustees: What's the Difference? School Governance Teacher Network, 25 May.

Moorhead, J. (2016b) 'Schools are relying on inexperienced staff and supply teachers, survey reveals', *The Guardian*, 22 March.

Moran, M. (2004) *Governing the Health Care State*, Manchester: Manchester University Press.

Morel, N., Palier, B. and Palme, J. (eds) (2012) *Towards a Social Investment Welfare State? Ideas, Policies and Challenges*, Bristol: Policy Press.

Morgan, D. (2019) *Snobbery*, Bristol: Policy Press.

Morris, P. (1969) *Put Away: A Sociological Study of Institutions for the Mentally Retarded*, London: Routledge.

Morris, S. (2018) 'Former teacher says boy imagined "weird" sex on night flight', *The Guardian*, 5 October.

Mulholland, H. (2016) 'Nurse shortages are life-threatening', *The Guardian*, 2 September.

Murphy, J. (2006) 'Building trust in economic space', *Progress in Human Geography*, 30(4): 427–50.

Murphy, S. (2018a) 'Revealed: the bullying culture in Whitehall', *The Guardian*, 13 November.

Murphy, S. (2018b) 'Revealed: the care workers fined £50 for being unwell', *The Guardian*, 24 December.

Murphy, S (2018c) 'Scandal of UK's worst care homes revealed', *The Guardian*, 24 November.

Murphy, S. (2019) 'Agency tried to charge care homes £2,700 a shift for workers', *The Guardian*, 23 February.

Myers, K. (2002) 'Dilemmas of leadership: sexuality and schools', *International Journal of Leadership in Education – Theory and Practice*, 5(4): 285–302.

Mylrea, M., Sen Gupta, T. and Glass, B. (2019) 'Design and evaluation of a professional identity development program for pharmacy students', *American Journal of Pharmaceutical Education*, 83(6): 1320–7.

NAO (National Audit Office) (2014) 'Care Quality Commission: Recruitment and Training of Staff to Build a New Organisational Culture', 22 July. Available at: https://www.nao.org.uk/press-release/capacity-and-capability-to-regulate-the-quality-and-safety-of-health-and-adult-social-care-2/ (accessed 7 October 2019).

NAO (National Audit Office) (2017) 'Retaining and developing the teaching workforce', HC 307, 12 September. Available at: https://www.nao.org.uk/report/supporting-and-improving-the-teaching-workforce/ (accessed 7 October 2019).

NAO (National Audit Office) (2018) 'Sustainability and transformation in the NHS'. Available at: https://www.nao.org.uk/report/sustainability-and-transformation-in-the-nhs/ (accessed 7 October 2019).

Narey, M. (2014) 'Making the education of social workers consistently effective (Report of Sir Martin Narey's independent review of the education of children's social workers)'. Available at: https://assets. publishing.service.gov.uk/government/uploads/system/uploads/ attachment_data/file/287756/Making_the_education_of_social_ workers_consistently_effective.pdf (accessed 7 October 2019).

Narey, M. (2016) 'Residential care in England. Report of Sir Martin Narey's independent review of children's residential care'. Available at: https://www.gov.uk/government/publications/childrens-residential- care-in-england (accessed 7 October 2019).

National Education Union (2018) 'The disgraceful waste of money that is forced academisation', 19 October. Available at: https://www. teachers.org.uk/education-policies/research/discraceful-waste-of- money (accessed 7 October 2019).

National Education Union (2019) Speech by Kevin Courtney, Joint General Secretary, annual conference, Liverpool. Available at: https:// neu.org.uk/annual-conference-2019 (accessed 7 October 2019).

Needham, C. and Glasby, J. (eds) (2014) *Debates in Personalisation*, Bristol: Policy Press.

NESCHA News (2018) 'Sir David Behan CBE interviewed with *The Guardian* on retiring from the CQC', 11 July. Available at: www. guardian.com/society/2018/July/11/cqc-david-behan-care-safer- quality-better (accessed 7 October 2019).

NESTA (2009) 'A review of mentoring literature and best practice'. Available at: https://www.nesta.org.uk/report/a-review-of- mentoring-literature-and-best-practice/ (accessed 7 October 2019).

Newburn, T. (2012) 'Criminal justice', in P. Alcock, M. May and S. Wright (eds) *The Student's Companion to Social Policy*, Chichester: Wiley-Blackwell, pp. 366–74.

Newell, C. and Donelly, L. (2016) 'Junior doctors' strike: leading BMA figure likened Tory policies to Nazi propaganda, *The Telegraph*, 5 January.

Newell, J. (2013) 'Obama: income inequality is "defining challenge of our time" – live', *The Guardian*, 4 December.

Newell, P. and Paterson, M. (2010) *Climate Capitalism: Global Warming and the Transformation of the Global Economy*, Cambridge: Cambridge University Press.

Newman, J. (2005) 'Bending bureaucracy: leadership and multi-level governance', in P. du Gay (ed.) *The Values of Bureaucracy*, Oxford: Oxford University Press, pp. 191–210.

NFER (National Foundation for Educational Research) (J. Worth, S. Lynch, J. Hillary, C. Rennie and J. Andrade) (2018) 'Teacher workforce dynamics in England', 30 October. Available at: https://nfer.ac.uk/teacher-workforce-dynamics-in-england/ (accessed 7 October 2019).

NHS (National Health Service) Employers (2019) Agenda for change NHS pay rates. NHS terms and conditions (AfC) pay scales – annual 1 April, Crown Copyright.

NHS (National Health Service) Employers: Part of the NHS Confederation (2019) NHS terms and conditions (AfC) pay scales. Agenda for change pay rates – annual, 1 April.

NHS (National Health Service) England (2017) 'NHS review of 2016', 1 January. Available at: https://www.england.nhs.uk/2017/01/2016-review/ (accessed 7 October 2019).

NHS (National Health Service) England (2018a) 'NHS launches multi-million pound TV advertising campaign to recruit thousands of nurses in landmark 70th year', 3 July. Available at: https://www.england.nhs.uk/2018/07/nhs-launches-multi-million-pound-tv-advertising-campaign-to-recruit-thousands-of-nurses-in-landmark-70th-year/ (accessed 7 October 2019).

NHS (National Health Service) England (2018b) *Our 2017/18 Annual Report*, HC 1328, Leeds: NHS England.

NHS (National Health Service) Press Association (2014) '"Devastating impact" of NHS blunders revealed in ombudsman's report', *The Guardian*, 29 October.

NHS (National Health Service) Providers (2017) 'Patient safety will be risked this winter without immediate funding and capacity boost for the NHS', 3 September. Available at: https://nhsproviders.org/news-blogs/news/patient-safety-will-be-risked-this-winter-without-immediate-funding-and-capacity-boost-for-the-nhs (accessed 7 October 2019).

NHS (National Health Service) Trust Development Authority (2018) *Annual Report and Accounts 2017/18*, HC 1348, London: NHS Improvement.

Nicholas, E., Qureshi, H. and Bamford, C. (2003) *Outcomes into Practice: Focusing Practice & Information on the Outcomes People Value – A Resource Pack for Managers and Trainers*, York: SPRU, University of York.

NIESR (National Institute of Economic and Social Research) (2016a) (C. Rienzo) 'National evaluation of the troubled families programme: national impact study report', 17 October, Available at: https://www.niesr.ac.uk/publications/national-evaluation-troubled-families-programme-national-impact-study-report (accessed 7 October 2019).

NIESR (National Institute of Economic and Social Research) (2016b) (L. Day, C. Bryson, C. White, S. Purdon, L. Kirchner Sala and J. Portes) 'National evaluation of the Troubled Families Programme: final synthesis report', 17 October. Available at: https://www.niesr.ac.uk/publications/national-evaluation-troubled-families-programme-final-synthesis-report (accessed 2 November 2019).

NIESR (National Institute of Economic and Social Research) (2018) (A. Kara) 'UK economy gathers even more momentum', 10 October. Available at: https://www.niesr.ac.uk/media/press-release-october-gdp-tracker-uk-economy-gathers-even-more-momentum-13504 (accessed 7 October 2019).

NMC (Nursing and Midwifery Council of UK) (2010) *Standards for Medicines Management*, London: NMC.

NMC (Nursing and Midwifery Council of UK) (2015) *The Code: Standards of Conduct, Performance and Ethics for Nurses and Midwives*, London: NMC.

Noel, A. (2006) 'A new global politics of poverty', *Global Social Policy*, 6: 304–33.

Noordegraaf, M (2011) 'Risky business: how professionals and professionals' fields (must) deal with organisational issues', *Organization Studies*, 32(10): 1349–71.

Noordegraaf, M. (2014) 'Fragmented or connective professionalism? Strategies for professionalising the work of strategists and other (organisational) professionals', *Public Administration*, 92: 21–38.

Northouse, P. (2010) *Leadership – Theory and Practice* (5th edn), London: Sage.

NPEU–MBRRACE-UK (2018) *Saving Lives, Improving Mothers' Care – Lessons Learned to Inform Maternity Care from the UK and Ireland, Confidential Enquiries into Maternal Deaths and Morbidity 2014–16*, 1 November. NPEU: Nuffield Department of Population Health, University of Oxford.

Nuffield Trust – Evidence for Better Health Care (2018a) (K. Ridyard and L. Merry) 'Emergency re-admissions to hospital for potentially preventable conditions on the rise, new research shows', 1 June.

Nuffield Trust – Evidence for Better Health Care (2018b) Letter from Nigel Edwards, CEO, to *The Times*, 30 June (a response to a 28 June leading article that argued poorer outcomes are down to the way the NHS is funded).

Nuffield Trust – Evidence for Better Health Care (2019) 'The NHS workforce in numbers: facts on staffing and staff shortages in England', 8 May.

Nutbrown, C. (2012) *Foundations for Quality. The Independent Review of Early Education and Childcare Qualifications. Final Report*, London: DfE.

O'Carroll, L. (2018) 'Javid under fire for plans to slash EU immigration to UK', *The Guardian*, 18 December.

O'Hara, M. (2014) *Austerity Bites: A Journey to the Sharp End of Cuts in the UK*, Bristol: Policy Press.

O'Hara, M. (2018) 'Mental health: "I fell between the cracks in child and adult services"', *The Guardian*, 5 December.

O'Neill, J. (2018) 'I'm an ex-Tory minister: only Labour grasps the public mood', *The Guardian*, 5 October.

O'Sullivan, M. (2018) 'Professional abuse', Available at: http://natcouncilofpsychotherapists.org.uk/Newsletter/Ed001/Professional_Abuse.html (accessed 8 July 2018).

O'Toole, F. (2012) 'Blind search for profits behind care home abuse', *Irish Times*, 14 August.

O'Toole, F. (2018) 'It's too late. Not even the pope can resurrect Catholic Ireland', *The Guardian*, 23 August.

OBR (Office of Budget Responsibility) (2018) *Welfare Trends Report*, Cm 9562, January, London: The Stationery Office.

OECD (Organisation for Economic Co-operation and Development) (2017) *Meeting of the OECD Council at Ministerial Level. Update Report, Inclusive Growth*, 7–8 June, Paris: OECD.

OECD (Organisation for Economic Co-operation and Development) (2018) 'Social mobility in richest countries has stalled since 1990s', 4 July, Paris: OECD.

OECD (Organisation for Economic Co-operation and Development) Data (2018) *Compendium of Productivity Indicators*, Paris: OECD.

Oppenheimer, M. (1975) 'The proletarianization of the professional', *Sociological Review*, Monograph 20, Oxford: Wiley Blackwell.

Orelove, F. and Sobsey, D. (1991) *Educating Children with Multiple Disabilities: A Transdisciplinary Approach*, Baltimore, MD: Paul Brookes.

Osborne, H. (2018) 'Virgin awarded almost £2bn of NHS contracts in past five years', *The Guardian*, 6 August.

Øvretveit, J. (1995) *Purchasing for Health: A Multi-Disciplinary Introduction to the Theory and Practice of Health Purchasing*, Buckingham: Open University Press.

Parker, J. and Bradley, G. (2014) *Social Work Practice* (4th edn), London: Sage/Learning Matters.

Parkin, F. (1979) *Marxism and Class Theory: A Bourgeois Critique*, London: Tavistock Publications.

Parrott, L. and Maguinness, N. (2017) *Social Work in Context: Theory and Concepts*, London: Sage.

Parsons, S. (2019) 'The Matt Ineson IICSA testimony. A crisis of leadership in the Church of England?' Blog, 10 July. Available at: http://survivingchurch.org/2019/07/10/the-matt-ineson-iicsa-testimony-a-crisis-of-leadership-in-the-church-of-england/ (accessed 7 October 2019).

Parsons, T. (1939) 'The professions and the social structure', *Social Forces*, 17: 457–67.

Partington, R. (2018) 'UK autumn budget date falls before crunch Brexit talks', *The Guardian*, 26 September.

Payne, S. (2019) 'Spend £8bn to fix social care "scandal", urge lords', *Financial Times*, 4 July.

Peck, J. (2010) *Construction of Neoliberal Reason*, Oxford: Oxford University Press.

Perraudin, F. (2017) 'More victims of disgraced surgeon "may have been missed"', *The Guardian*, 27 December.

Peters, C. (1982) 'A neo-liberal's manifesto', *The Washington Monthly*, May. Available at: https://www.washingtonpost.com/archive/opinions/1982/09/05/a-neo-liberals-manifesto/21cf41ca-e60e-404e-9a66-124592c9f70d/ (accessed 7 October 2019).

Peterson, C., Park, N. and Sweeney, P. (2008) 'Group well-being: morale from a positive psychology perspective', *Applied Psychology: An International Review*, 57(1), July: 19–36.

Pickard, L. (2019) 'Good value for money? Public investment in "replacement care" for working carers In England', *Social Policy and Society*, 18(3): 365–82.

Pidd, H. (2019) 'Coding project gives prisoners new start – and fills skills gap', *The Guardian*, 23 April.

Pilgrim, D. (1997) 'Some reflections on "quality" and "mental health"', *Journal of Mental Health*, 6(6): 567–76.

Politics Home (2016) 'Theresa May's Conservative conference speech on Brexit: "Britain after Brexit: a vision of a global Britain"', 2 October.

Politics Home (2018) 'Philip Hammond: an uplift in productivity would "put right" many of the challenges facing the country', 3 October.

Pollock, A. (2018) 'Think Carillion is bad? Wait until you see what the government wants to do with the NHS', *New Statesman*, 18 January.

Porter, T.M. (1995) *Trust in Numbers: The Pursuit of Objectivity in Science and Public Life*, Princeton, NJ: Princeton University Press.

Posner, R. (2002) *Anti-Trust Law: An Economic Perspective*, Chicago: University of Chicago Press.

Poulantzas, N. (1975) *Classes in Contemporary Capitalism*, London: New Left Books.

Powell, M. (2019) 'The English National Health Service in a cold climate: a decade of austerity', in E. Heins, C. Needham and J. Rees (eds), *Social Policy Review*, 31, Bristol: Policy Press, pp. 15–32.

Powell, M. and Exworthy, M. (2002) 'Partnerships, quasi-networks and social policy', in C. Glendinning, M. Powell and K. Rummery (eds) *Partnerships, New Labour and the Governance of Welfare*, Bristol: Policy Press, pp. 7–28.

Powell, M. (ed. 1999) *New Labour, New Welfare State*, Bristol: Policy Press.

Power, M. (1999) *The Audit Society: Rituals of Verification*, Oxford: Oxford University Press.

Power, M. (2014) 'Living in an audit society: performance reporting after the global financial crisis', public lecture at the Schools of Social Work and Human Services and Education, the University of Queensland, 9 April.

Powers, J., Mooney, A. and Nunno, M. (1990) 'Institutional abuse – a review of the literature', *Journal of Child and Youth Care* 4(6): 81.

Pre-Learning Alliance/Child Poverty Action Group (CPAG) (Alison Gardham, Chief Executive) (2017) 'Child poverty and local government. The story so far', 29 March.

Prescott, T. and Caleb-Solly, P. (2017) 'Robotics in social care: a connected care ecosystem for independent living', *UK-RAS White Papers*, UK-RAS NETWORK. Available at: www.ukras.org.

Press Association (2019) 'UK wages worth up to a third less than in 2008, study shows', 31 January.

Pridham, G. (2008) 'Status quo bias or institutionalisation for reversibility? The EU's political conditionality, post-accession tendencies and democratic consideration in Slovakia', *Journal of Europe-Asia Studies*, 60(3): 423-54.

Provost, C. (2016) 'The privatisation of UK aid', Global Justice Now. aidWATCH, April. Available at: https://www.globaljustice.org.uk/sites/default/files/files/resources/the_privatisation_of_uk_aid.pdf (accessed 7 October 2019).

Public Health Agency (2019) *Business Plan 2018–2019*, Belfast: HSC Public Health Agency.

PULSE (2016) 'Junior doctors are angry because of BMA "misrepresentation", claims Hunt', 8 February. Available at: http://www.pulsetoday.co.uk/news/hot-topics/junior-doctor-contract/junior-doctors-are-angry-because-of-bma-misrepresentation-claims-hunt/20031075.article (accessed 7 October 2019).

Putnam, R. (2015) *Our Kids: The American Dream in Crisis*, New York: Simon & Schuster.

PwC (PricewaterhouseCoopers) (2005) *Academies Evaluation: Second Annual Report*, London: DfES.

Quaglia, R. and Corso, M. (2014) 'Student voice: pump it up', *Principal Leadership Journal*, Corwin University, Australia, September: 29–32.

Quinn, B. (2016) 'Surgeons operated on wrong parts of patients, CQC finds: culture of bullying at Brighton and Sussex Trust', *The Guardian*, 17 August.

Quinn, B. and Campbell, D. (2016) 'NHS vows to transform mental health services with extra £1bn a Year', *The Guardian*, 15 February.

Quinn, S. and Owen, S. (2016) 'Digging deeper: understanding the power of "student voice"', *Australian Journal of Education*, 60(1), February: 60–72.

Race, D. (1999) 'Values, assumptions and ideologies', in N. Malin, J. Manthorpe, D. Race and S. Wilmot, *Community Care for Nurses and the Caring Professions*, Buckingham: Open University Press, pp. 57–79.

Race, D. (2007) *Intellectual Disability: Social Approaches*, Maidenhead: Open University Press/McGraw-Hill Education.

Ramlogan, R. and Rigby, J. (2012) 'The impact and effectiveness of entrepreneurship policy: Compendium of evidence on the effectiveness of innovation policy intervention', Manchester Institute of Innovation Research, Manchester Business School, University of Manchester. Available at: http://research.mbs.ac.uk/innovation/ (accessed 7 October 2019).

Ray, B. (2017) 'A review of research on home-schooling and what might educators learn?', *Pro-Posicoes. Scielo*, 28(2):85–103.

RCM (Royal College of Midwives) (2017) 'Agency, bank and overtime spending in UK maternity units in 2016'. Available at: https://www.rcm.org.uk/media/2371/rcm-report-spending-on-agency-midwives-in-england.pdf (accessed 7 October 2019).

RCN (Royal College of Nursing) (2016a) BMA Letter to PM David Cameron Regarding Bursaries. Nursing Grants-rcnfoundation.org.uk, www.rcn-foundation.org.uk. Removing Nurse Bursaries -Latest Policy Updates – nuffieldtrust.org.uk, www.nuffieldtrust.org.uk.

RCN (Royal College of Nursing) (2016b) *Annual Report*. Available at https://www.rcn.org.uk/professional-development/publications/pub-005871 (accessed 2 November 2019).

RCN Magazines (2018) '"We must stop this": RCN chief executive announces launch of major safe staffing campaign', 13 May.

Reay, D. (2018) 'Miseducation: inequality, education and the working classes', *International Studies in Sociology of Education*, 27(4): 453–6.

Reclaiming Education (2018) *A New Education Programme for Labour*, Conference Proceedings, 22 May, House of Commons Committee Room 9.

Reinert, H. and Reinert, E. (2006) 'Creative destruction in economics: Nietzsche, Sombart, Schumpeter' in J. Backhaus and W. Drechsler (eds) Friedrich Nietzsche 1844–2000, New York: Springer, pp. 55–85.

Report of the Committee on Local Authority and Allied Personal Social Services (Seebohm Committee) (1968) (Seebohm Report) Cmnd 3703, July.

Repper, J. and Perkins, R. (2009) *Social Inclusion and Recovery* (2nd edn), London: Balliere Tindall.

Reyes, R. (2018) 'The Church stands with the poor. Corrupt leaders, beware', *Church Times*, 16 March.

Ribbens McCarthy, J. and Edwards, R. (2011) *Key Concepts in Family Studies*, London: Sage.

Rickards, T. (2015) *Dilemma of Leadership* (3rd edn), London: Routledge.

Roaf, C. (2002) *Coordinating Services for Included Children*, Buckingham: Open University Press.

Roberts, N. (2016) 'Junior doctors could strike next week as talks deadline looms', *GP News*, 4 January.

Roberts, N. (2016a) 'Junior doctor strike key to future of general practice', *GP News*, 9 February.

Robinson, M. and Cottrell, D. (2005) 'Health professionals in multidisciplinary and multi- agency teams: changing professional practice', *Journal of Interprofessional Care*, 19(6), December: 547–60.

Rogers, A. and Pilgrim, D. (2014) *A Sociology of Mental Health and Illness* (5th edn), Maidenhead: Open University Press.

Rogers, J., Bright, L. and Davies, H. (2015) *Social Work with Adults*, London: Sage.

Rogers, T. (2016) 'It's not academisation that worries me the most, it's "academicisation": focusing on academic over vocational', *Times Education Supplement*, 15 April.

Rogowski, S. (2011) 'Managers, managerialism and social work with children and families. The deformation of a profession?', *Practice*, 23(3): 157–67.

Rogowski, S. (2016) *Social Work with Children and Families: Reflections of a Critical Practitioner*, Abingdon: Routledge.

Rolfe, S. (2018) 'Governance and governmentality in community participation: the shifting sands of power, responsibility and risk', *Social Policy and Society*, 17(4): 579–98.

Romero, M. and Pérez, N (2016) 'Conceptualising the foundation of inequalities in care work', *American Behavioural Scientist*, 60(2): 172–88.

Rose, M. (1971) *The English Poor Law 1870–1930 Documents*, London: Barnes & Noble.

Rourke, J. (2008) 'Increasing the number of rural physicians', *Canadian Medical Association Journal*, 178(3): 322–5.

Royal Commission into Institutional Responses to Child Sexual Abuse (2017) *Analysis of Claims of Child Sexual Abuse Made with Respect to Catholic Church Institutions in Australia*, Sydney: Royal Commission into Institutional Responses to Child Sexual Abuse.

Runciman, D. (2016) *How Democracy Ends*, London: Profile Publications.

Rushton, P. (2018) 'Austerity – a critical history of the present', in P. Rushton and C. Donovan (eds) *Austerity Policies: Bad Ideas in Practice*, Basingstoke: Palgrave Macmillan, pp. 21–44.

Rustin, S. (2016) 'It's your school. It's personal: meet the parents who are fighting back', *The Guardian*, 12 July.

Ryan, F. (2018) 'Now disabled people face a kind of internment', *The Guardian*, 10 May.

Ryan, S. (2018) *Justice for Laughing Boy: Connor Sparrowhawk – A Death by Indifference*, London: Jessica Kingsley.

Sabbagh, D. (2018) 'Gordon Brown speaks out on "fundamental" issue of anti-Semitism', *The Guardian*, 2 September.

Sainsbury, E. (1977) *The Personal Social Services*, London: Pitman.

Sako, M. (1992) *Price, Quality and Trust*, Cambridge: Cambridge University Press.

Saks, M. (1994) 'The alternatives to medicine', in J. Gabe, D. Kelleher and G. Williams (eds) *Challenging Medicine*, London: Routledge, pp. 84–103.

Saks, M. (1995) *Professions and the Public Interest – Medical Power, Altruism and Alternative Medicine*, London: Routledge.

Salmon, G. and Rapport, F. (2005) 'Multi-agency Voices: a thematic analysis of multi-agency working practices within the setting of a child and adolescent mental health service', *Journal of Interprofessional Care*, 19(5): 429–43.

Sanderson, M., Allen, P. and Osipovic, D. (2017) 'The regulation of competition in the National Health Service (NHS): what difference has the Health and Social Care Act 2012 made?', *Health Economics, Policy and Law*, 12(1): 1–19.

Sanghara, K. and Wilson, C. (2006) 'Stereotypes and attitudes about child sex abusers: a comparison of experience and inexperienced professionals in sex offender treatment', *Legal and Criminal Psychology – The British Psychology Journal*, September (doi: 10 1348/135532505x68818).

Satel, S. (2007) 'In praise of stigma', in J.E. Henningfield, P.B. Santora and W. Bickel (eds) *Addiction Treatment: Science and Policy for the Twenty-First Century*, Baltimore, MD: Johns Hopkins University Press, pp. 147–51.

Saul, J. (1992) *Voltaire's Bastards: The Dictatorship of Reason in the West*, London: Sinclair Stevenson.

Saunders, P. (1983) *Urban Politics: A Sociological Interpretation*, London: Hutchinson.

Savage, M. and Wright, M. (2016) 'Cameron wasted £1bn on troubled families', *The Times*, 18 October.

Savedoff, W. and Smith, P. (2016) 'Measuring Governance: Accountability, Management and Research', in S. Greer, M. Wismar and J. Figueras (eds) *Strengthening Health System Governance: Better Policies, Stronger Performance*, Maidenhead: Open University Press, pp. 85–104.

Sayer, D. (2014) 'Five reasons why the REF is not fit for purpose', *The Guardian*, 15 December.

Schedlitzki, D. and Edwards, G. (2014) *Studying Leadership: Traditional and Critical Approaches*, London: Sage.

Schaible, L. (2018) 'The impact of the police professional identity on burnout', *Policing: An International Journal*, 41(1): 129–43 (https://doi.org/10.1108/PIJPSM-03-2016-0047).

Schoener, G. (1995) 'Assessment of professionals who have engaged in boundary violations', *Psychiatric Annals* (25(2): 95–9.

Scholte, J. (2005) *Globalization: A Critical Introduction* (2nd edn), London: Macmillan.

Schumpeter, J. (1928) 'Unternehmer', in E. Ludwig, A. Weber and F. Wieser (eds) *Handworterbuch der Staatswissenschaften*, Vol. 8 (4th edn) Jena: Gustav Fischer, pp. 476–87.

Schumpeter, J. (1934) *The Theory of Economic Development*, London: Harper.

Schumpeter, J. (1942) *Capitalism, Socialism and Democracy*, 2nd edn, Floyd, VA: Impact Books.

Scott, P. (2018) 'This toxic Brexit hurts universities, linking us to Trump and the rest', *The Guardian*, 6 November.

Scourfield, P. (2012) 'Caretelization revisited and the lesson of Southern Cross', *Critical Social Policy*, 32(1): 137–49.

Scourfield, P. (2013) 'Even further beyond street-level bureaucracy', *British Journal of Social Work*, 45: 914–31.

Scull, A. (1979) *Museums of Madness*, Harmondsworth: Penguin.

Seabrook, J. (2013) *Pauperland: Poverty and the Poor in Britain*, London: Hurst & Company.

Secretary of State for Health (2002) *Learning from Bristol: The Department of Health's Response to the Report of the Public Inquiry into Children's Heart Surgery at the Bristol Royal Infirmary*, Cm 5363, London: The Stationery Office.

Sennett, R. (1998) *The Corrosion of Character*, New York and London: W.W. Norton & Company.

Seymour, R. (2014) *Against Austerity: How We Can Fix the Crisis They Made*, London: Pluto Press.

Shaw, C. (2015) 'Education has never mattered more, so why won't the UK invest in it properly?', *The Guardian*, 26 March.

Shaxson, N. (2018) *The Finance Curse: How Global Finance Is Making Us All Poorer*, London: Bodley Head.

Shelter (2019) *Building for Our Future: A Vision for Social Housing. The Final Report of Our Commission on the Future of Social Housing*, London: Shelter.

Shepherd, S. (2017) 'There's a gulf between academics and university management – and it's growing' *The Guardian*, 27 July.

Shermer, E.T. (2014) 'Review', *Journal of Modern History*, 86(4), December: 884–90.

Sherwood, H. (2019) 'Archbishop of Canterbury calls for mandatory reporting of sexual abuse', *The Guardian*, 11 July.

Shore, C. (2008) 'Audit culture and illiberal governance: universities and the politics of accountability', *Anthropological Theory*, 8(3): 278–98.

Shore, C. and Wright, S. (1999) 'Audit culture and anthropology: neo-liberalism in British higher education', *The Journal of the Royal Anthropological Institute*, 5(4): 557–75.

Siddique, H. (2015) 'Hospitals told to shed staff as NHS funding crisis deepens', *The Guardian*, 15 November.

Siddique, H. (2018) 'One third of dementia patients not getting right care – Age UK', *The Guardian*, 13 February.

Siddique, H. (2019) 'Skilled workers – call to put more jobs on visa list', *The Guardian*, 30 May.

Sikes, P. (2006) 'Scandalous stories and dangerous liaisons: when female pupils and male teachers fall in love', *Journal: Sex Education*, 6(3): 265–80.

Skidelsky, R. and Fraccaroli, N. (eds) (2017) *Austerity vs Stimulus: The Political Future of Economic Recovery*, London: Palgrave Macmillan.

Slater, D. and Tonkiss, F. (2001) *Market Society*, Cambridge: Polity Press.

Slaughter, A (2017) 'Three responsibilities every government has towards its citizens', 13 February, World Economic Forum/New America.

Slaughter, S. and Leslie, L. (1997) *Academic Capitalism: Politics, Policies and the Entrepreneurial University*, Boston, MD: Johns Hopkins University Press.

Smith, D. (2001) 'The changing idea of a university', in D. Smith and K. Langlow (eds) *The Idea of a University*, London: Jessica Kingsley, pp. 148–74.

Smith, D. (2004 ed.) *Social Work and Evidence-Based Practice*, London: Jessica Kingsley.

Snyder, T. (2018) *The Road to Unfreedom*. New York: Crown Publishing Group.

Social Mobility Commission (2016) 'State of the nation 2016: social mobility in Great Britain', 16 November. Available at: https://www.gov.uk/government/publications/state-of-the-nation-2016 (accessed 7 October 2019).

Southwell, A. (2017) 'De-professionalisation of the academy', *Quillette*, 17 April. Available at: https://quillette.com/2017/04/13/de-professionalization-academy/ (accessed 7 October 2019).

Sparrow, A. (2016) 'Junior doctors risk being struck off GMC', *The Guardian*, 5 September.

Springer, S., Birch, K. and MacLeavy, J. (2016) *The Handbook of Neoliberalism*, London: Routledge.

Standing, G. (2014) *The Precariat: The New Dangerous Class*, London: Bloomsbury Academic.

Steinmetz, G. (1993) *Regulating the Social: The Welfare State and Local Politics in Imperial Germany*, Princeton, NJ: Princeton University Press.

Stewart, H. (2017) 'Theresa May adopts contrite tone after Tory MPs vent anger over election', *The Guardian*, 10 June.

Stiglitz, J. (2013) *The Price of Inequality*, London: Penguin.

Stone, J. (2016) 'Junior doctors' strikes: BMA announces three 48-hour walkouts over contract', *The Independent*, 7 March.

Swallow, T. (2018) 'Windrush and other failures in British immigration policy', 4 October. Available at: https://www.theguardian.com/uk-news/2018/oct/04/windrush-and-other-failures-in-british-immigration-policy (accessed 7 October 2019).

Swedberg, R. (1998) *Max Weber and the Idea of Economic Sociology*, Princeton, NJ: Princeton University Press.

Swerling, G. (2019) 'The Archbishop of Canterbury banned abuse victim from cathedral grounds', *Daily Telegraph*, 11 July.

Szmukler, G. and Rose, N. (2013) 'Risk assessment in mental health care: values and costs', *Behavioural Science and the Law*, 31(1): 125–40.

Taylor, D. (2014) 'Councils using online auctions to find carers for elderly people', *The Guardian*, 28 August.

Taylor, F. (2003) *Scientific Management*, London Routledge.

Taylor, M. (2016) 'Failing children's services to be taken over by rival councils under proposed changes', *The Guardian*, 15 April.

Taylor-Gooby, P. (2008) 'The new welfare state settlement in Europe', *European Societies*, 10(1): 3–24.

Taylor-Gooby, P. and Stoker, G. (2011) 'The coalition programme: a new vision for Britain or politics as usual?', *The Political Quarterly*, 82(1): 4–15.

The Russell Group of Universities (2018) 'Policy: evidence and impact exchange', 3 July. Available at: https://russellgroup.ac.uk/policy/policy-documents/evidence-and-impact-exchange/ (accessed 7 October 2019).

The Telegraph (2019) 'Bursaries for student nurses and midwives to be scrapped by government', 21 July. Available at: https://www.telegraph.co.uk/news/2016/07/21/bursaries-for-student-nurses-and-midwives-to-be-scrapped-by-gove/ (accessed 2 November 2019).

Think Ahead: 'Fast-track mental health work'. Available at: https://thinkahead.org/?gclid=EAIaIQobChMIt7i3hLOK5QIVBUTTCh0VPQbNEAAYASAAEgLy9PD_BwE (accessed 7 October 2019).

Thomas, C. (2007) *Sociologies of Disability and Illness: Contested Ideas in Disability Studies and Medical Sociology*, London: Palgrave Macmillan.

Thompson, M. (2016) *Enough Said: What's Gone Wrong with the Language of Politics*, London: Bodley Head.

Thompson, N. (2016) *The Authentic Leader*, London: Palgrave Macmillan.

Tickle, L. (2017) 'Mother courage: trading pregnancy for help', *The Guardian*, 25 January.

Toren, N. (1972) *Social Work: The Case of a Semi-Profession*, London: Sage.

Townsend, P. (1962) *The Last Refuge: A Survey of Residential Institutions and Homes for the Aged in England and Wales*, London: Routledge & Kegan Paul.

Toynbee, A. (1948) *Civilization on Trial*, New York: Oxford University Press.

Toynbee, P. (2015) 'Hunt's hit squad is a danger to our national health', *The Guardian*, 22 September.

Toynbee, P. (2016) 'Our nurses are being cast into a perfect Brexit storm', *The Guardian*, 14 October.

Toynbee, P. (2017) 'The social care crisis drags on, thanks to May's cowardice', *The Guardian*, 22 May.

Travis, A. (2018) 'Fears for NHS staff shortages after visa ceiling reached again', *The Guardian*, 18 August.

Treanor, J. (2016) 'Chancellor insists foreign worker plan not aimed at banks', *The Guardian*, 7 October.

Treanor, J. and Watt, N. (2016) 'Mark Carney fears Brexit would leave UK relying on "kindness of strangers"', *The Guardian*, 26 January.

Trinder, L. and Reynolds, S. (2008) *Evidence-Based Practice: A Critical Appraisal*, Oxford: Blackwell Science.

Triseliotis, J. (1995) 'Adoption: evolution or revolution, in British Agencies for Adoption and Fostering', *Selected BAAF Seminar Papers 1994/1995*, London: BAAF.

Triseliotis, J. (1997) 'Foster care and adoption', in M. Davies (ed.) *The Blackwell Companion to Social Work*, Oxford: Blackwell, pp. 331–6.

Truth, Justice and Healing Council (2014) 'Activity report', December.

TUC (Trades Union Congress) (2018) 'Wage growth is stuck in the slow lane, says TUC', 12 June. Available at: https://www.tuc.org.uk/news/wage-growth-stuck-slow-lane-says-tuc (accessed 7 October 2019).

Tunstill, J. (2016) 'In defence of progressive social work', *Social Work & Social Sciences Review*, 18(2): 3–6.

Tunstill, J. and Blewett, J. (2019) 'Pruned, policed and privatised: the social work knowledge base for children's services in a period of austerity', unpublished paper.

Turner, C. and Hodge, M. (1970) 'Occupations and professions', in J.A. Jackson (ed.) *Professions and Professionalisation. Sociological Studies, 3*, London: Cambridge University Press, pp. 19–50.

Tyler, I. (2013) *Revolting Subjects: Social Abjection and Resistance in Neoliberal Britain*, London: Zed Books.

UEA (University of East Anglia) (2018) 'Critical Reinventions: 12 May. Programme for 2nd symposium on de-professionalisation held by UEA Centre for the Creative and the Critical'.

UKHCA (United Kingdom Home Care Association) (2015) *The Home Care Deficit. A Report on the Funding of Older People's Home Care across the United Kingdom, Version 1, March 2015*, Wallington: UKHCA.

UN Convention on the Rights of the Child (2014) 'Concluding observations on the Second Periodic Report of the Holy See', CRC/C/VAT/CO/2, 25 February.

UNESCO/OECD (2014) 'Investing in education. Analysis of the 1999 World Education Indicators', UNESCO/OECD World Education Indicators Programme.

UNISON (2012) 'UNISON challenges councils to embrace ethical care charter'. Available at: www.unison. org.uk/news/article/2012/11/unison-challenges-councils-to-embrace-ethical-care-charter/ (accessed 7 October 2019).

UNISON (2013) UNISON'S Ethical Care Charter, London: UNISON.

UNISON (2018a) 'UNISON calls for a new set of principles for public service contracts', 8 February. Available at: https://www.unison.org.uk/news/press-release/2018/02/unison-calls-new-set-principles-public-service-contracts/ (accessed 7 October 2019).

UNISON (2018b) 'Stress and the Staffing Crisis' Conference. London: UNISON Centre.

United Lincolnshire Hospitals Trust (2018) 'Overview: departments and services'. Available at: https://www.nhs.uk/Services/Trusts/Overview/DefaultView.aspx?id=1990 (accessed 7 October 2019).

Usborne, S. (2018) 'Effectively we've been made into border guards', The Guardian, 1 August.

UUK (Universities UK) (2018) Minding Our Future: Starting a Conversation about the Support of Student Mental Health, 11 May, London: Universities UK.

Vallas, S. (1990) 'The concept of skill: a critical review', Work and Occupations, 17(4): 379–98.

Van der Aa, P. and van Berkel, R. (2015) 'Fulfilling the promise of professionalism in street-level practice', in P Hupe, M. Hill and A. Buffat (eds) Understanding Street-Level Bureaucracy, Bristol: Policy Press, pp. 263–78.

Van Oorschot, W., Roosma, F., Meuleman, B. and Reeskens, T. (2017) The Social Legitimacy of Targeted Welfare: Attitudes to Welfare Deservingness, Cheltenham: Edward Elgar.

Vaughan, R. (2017) 'Tories to make the Ebacc compulsory', TES Connect (accessed 30 August 2017).

Venugopal, R. (2015) 'Neoliberalism as concept', Economy and Society, 44(2): 165–87.

Verita (2015) 'Independent investigation into governance arrangements' (report for Cambridge University Hospitals NHS Foundation Trust), October. Available at: https://www.verita.net/wp-content/uploads/2016/04/Independent-investigation-into-governance-arrangements-in-the-paediatric-haematology-and-oncology-service-at-Cambridge-University-Hospitals-NHS-Foundation-Trust-following-the-Myles-Bradbury-case.pdf (accessed 7 October 2019).

Wardhaugh, J. and Wilding, P. (1993) 'Towards an explanation of the corruption of care', *Critical Social Policy*, 13(37): 4–31.

Weale, S. (2015a) 'Schools hit by record £1.3bn supply staff bill, says Labour', *The Guardian*, 14 December.

Weale, S. (2015b) 'Without Kids Company I'd be dead or in prison – its closure was a big shock to me', *The Guardian*, 22 September.

Weale, S. (2016a) 'Parents see fees go up after big fall in number of childminder places', *The Guardian*, 8 February.

Weale, S. (2016b) 'Third of new teachers quit within five years: unions blame workload and constant changes', *The Guardian*, 5 August.

Weale, S. (2018a) 'Call for urgent action to improve mental health services for students', *The Guardian*, 11 May.

Weale, S. (2018b) 'New scheme aims to aid mental health of university students', *The Guardian*, 15 July.

Weale, S. (2019a) 'More than 49,000 pupils "disappeared" from English schools – study', *The Guardian*, 18 April.

Weale, S. (2019b) 'Parents face obligation to register children being educated at home', *The Guardian*, 2 April.

Weale, S. and McIntyre, N. (2018) 'Crisis looms for special needs education', *The Guardian*, 23 October.

Weaver, M. (2016) 'What you need to know about the junior doctors' strike', *The Guardian*, 1 September.

Webb, S. (ed. 2017) *Professional Identity and Social Work*, Abingdon: Routledge.

Weber, M. (1947) *The Theory of Social and Economic Organisation* (trans. T. Parsons), New York: Hodge Press.

Weber, M. (1949) *The Methodology of the Social Sciences* (trans. and ed. E. Shils and H. Finch), New York: Free Press.

Weber, M. (1966) *The Theory of Social and Economic Organisation* (trans. A.M. Henderson and T. Parsons), New York: New York Philosophical Library.

Weber, M. (1976 [1930]) *The Protestant Ethic and The Spirit of Capitalism*, London: Allen & Unwin.

Weber, M. (1978) *Economy and Society*, Berkeley: University of California Press.

Weber, S. (1987) 'The limits of professionalism', in S. Weber (ed.) *Institution and Interpretation: Theory and History of Literature*, Vol. 31, Minneapolis: University of Minnesota Press, pp. 19–32.

Webster, R. (2017) 'Probation court work back on track', blog, 23 June.

Welter, F. (2012) 'All you need is trust. A critical review of the trust and entrepreneurship literature', *International Small Business Journal: Researching Entrepreneurship*, 30(3): 193–212.

West, A. (2016) *Nursery Education and Reducing Social Inequalities: An International Comparison of Early Childhood Education and Care*, Paris: Cnesco.

White, S. (2001) 'The ambiguities of the Third Way', in S. White (ed.) *New Labour: The Progressive Future?*, London: Palgrave Macmillan, pp. 3–17.

Whitty, G. (2008) 'Changing modes of teacher professionalism: traditional, managerial, collaborative and democratic', in B. Cunningham (ed.) *Exploring Professionalism*, Bedford Way Papers, London: Institute of Education, University of London, pp. 28–49.

Wilby, P. (2016) 'Parents out, chief executives in: our schools will be anything by free', *The Guardian*, 21 March.

Wilkinson, R. and Pickett, K. (2010) *The Spirit Level: Why Equality Is Better for Everyone*, London: Penguin.

Williams, M. (2016) *Key Concepts in the Philosophy of Social Research*, London: Sage.

Williams, P. (2012) 'The role of leadership in learning and knowledge for integration: managing community care', *Journal of Integrated Care*, 20(3): 164–74.

Williams, R. (2018) 'Recruitment: the care provider rewriting the rules', *The Guardian*, 28 November.

Wilmot, S. (2003) *Ethics, Power and Policy – The Future of Nursing in the NHS*, Basingstoke: Palgrave Macmillan.

Wingrave, M. and McMahon, M. (2016) 'Professionalisation through academicisation: valuing and developing the early years sector in Scotland', *Professional Development in Education*, 42(5), 13 October: 710–31.

Wintour, P. (2015) '"Anti-austerity unpopular with voters" finds inquiry into Labour's election loss', *The Guardian*, 4 August.

Wolfensberger, W., Nirje, B., Olshansky, S., Perske, R. and Roos, P. (1972) *The Principle of Normalisation in Human Services*, Toronto: NIMR.

Wolfensberger, W. (1998) *Social Role Valorisation* (3rd edn), Syracuse, New York: Syracuse University, Training Institute on Human Service Planning, Leadership and Change Agency.

Woll, C. (2014) *The Power of Inaction: Bank Bailouts in Comparison.* Cornell Studies in Political Economy, Ithaca, NY: Cornell University Press.

Wood, J., Westwood, S. and Thompson, G. (2015) *Youth Work: Preparation for Practice*, London: Routledge.

Wood, S. (ed.) (1982) *The Degradation of Work? Skill, Deskilling and the Labour Process*, London: Hutchinson.

World Economic Forum (2019) 'These are the OECD's most productive economies', 15 February.

Wright, S. (2016) 'Conceptualising the active welfare subject: welfare reform in discourse, policy and lived experience', *Policy and Politics*, 44(2): 235–52 (doi: 10.1332/030557314x13904856745154).

Index